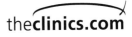
theclinics.com

SURGICAL CLINICS
OF NORTH AMERICA

Breast Cancer

GUEST EDITOR
Lisa A. Newman, MD, MPH

CONSULTING EDITOR
Ronald F. Martin, MD

April 2007 • Volume 87 • Number 2

SAUNDERS

An Imprint of Elsevier, Inc.
PHILADELPHIA   LONDON   TORONTO   MONTREAL   SYDNEY   TOKYO

W.B. SAUNDERS COMPANY
A Division of Elsevier Inc.

1600 John F. Kennedy Blvd., Suite 1800, Philadelphia, PA 19103-2899

http://www.theclinics.com

SURGICAL CLINICS OF NORTH AMERICA
April 2007
Editor: Catherine Bewick

Volume 87, Number 2
ISSN 0039–6109
ISBN-13: 978-1-4160-4370-6
ISBN-10: 1-4160-4370-5

Reprints. For copies of 100 or more of articles in this publication, please contact the commercial Reprints Department Elsevier Inc., 360 Park Avenue South, New York, New York 10010-1710. Tel. (212) 633-3813, Fax: (212) 462-1935, email: reprints@elsevier.com

The ideas and opinions expressed in *The Surgical Clinics of North America* do not necessarily reflect those of the Publisher. The Publisher does not assume any responsibility for any injury and/or damage to persons or property arising out of or related to any use of the material contained in this periodical. The reader is advised to check the appropriate medical literature and the product information currently provided by the manufacturer of each drug to be administered to verify the dosage, the method and duration of administration, or contraindications. It is the responsibility of the treating physician or other health care professional, relying on independent experience and knowledge of the patient, to determine drug dosages and the best treatment for the patient. Mention of any product in this issue should not be construed as endorsement by the contributors, editors, or the Publisher of the product or manufacturers' claims.

Surgical Clinics of North America (ISSN 0039–6109) is published bimonthly by Elsevier Inc., 360 Park Avenue South, New York, NY 10010-1710. Months of publication are February, April, June, August, October, and December. Business and Editorial Offices: 1600 John F. Kennedy Blvd., Suite 1800, Philadelphia, PA 19103-2899. Customer Service Office: 6277 Sea Harbor Drive, Orlando, FL 32887-4800. Periodicals postage paid at New York, NY and additional mailing offices. Subscription prices are $220.00 per year for US individuals, $347.00 per year for US institutions, $110.00 per year for US students and residents, $270.00 per year for Canadian individuals, $424.00 per year for Canadian institutions, $286.00 for international individuals, $424.00 per year for international institutions and $143.00 per year for Canadian and foreign students/residents. To receive student/resident rate, orders must be accompanied by name of affiliated institution, date of term, and the *signature* of program/residency coordinator on institution letterhead. Orders will be billed at individual rate until proof of status is received. Foreign air speed delivery is included in all *Clinics* subscription prices. All prices are subject to change without notice. POSTMASTER: Send address changes to *Surgical Clinics*, Elsevier Periodicals Customer Service, 6277 Sea Harbor Drive, Orlando, FL 32887-4800. **Customer Service: 1-800-654-2452 (US). From outside of the US, call 1-407-345-1000.**

The Surgical Clinics of North America is also published in Spanish by McGraw-Hill Interamericana Editores S.A., P.O. Box 5-237 06500 Mexico D.F. Mexico; and in Portuguese by Interlivros Edicoes Ltda., Rua Comandante Coelho 1085, CEP 21250, Rio de Janeiro, Brazil; and in Greek by Paschalidis Medical Publications, Athens Greece.

The Surgical Clinics of North America is covered in *Index Medicus, EMBASE/Excerpta Medica, Current Contents/Clinical Medicine, Current Contents/Life Sciences, Science Citation Index*, and *ISI/BIOMED.*

Printed in the United States of America.

CONSULTING EDITOR

RONALD F. MARTIN, MD, Staff Surgeon, Marshfield Clinic, Marshfield, Wisconsin; Lieutenant Colonel, Medical Corps, United States Army Reserve

GUEST EDITOR

LISA A. NEWMAN, MD, MPH, FACS, Associate Professor of Surgery and Director, Breast Care Center, University of Michigan Comprehensive Cancer Center; and Department of Surgery, University of Michigan, Ann Arbor, Michigan

CONTRIBUTORS

AMY K. ALDERMAN, MD, MPH, VA Center for Practice Management and Outcomes Research, Ann Arbor VA Health Care System, Ann Arbor, Michigan

GILDY V. BABIERA, MD, Department of Surgical Oncology, The University of Texas M. D. Anderson Cancer Center, Houston, Texas

DAWN M. BARNES, MD, House Officer, Department of Surgery, University of Michigan Health System, Ann Arbor, Michigan

KEIVA L. BLAND, MD, Division of Breast Surgical Oncology, Department of Surgery, University of Arkansas for Medical Sciences, Little Rock, Arkansas

AMY C. DEGNIM, MD, Assistant Professor of Surgery, Department of Surgery, Mayo Clinic and Mayo Foundation, Mayo Clinic College of Medicine, Rochester, Minnesota

REGINA M. FEARMONTI, MD, Fellow, Breast Surgical Oncology, Department of Surgical Oncology, The University of Texas M. D. Anderson Cancer Center, Houston, Texas

JENNIFER GASS, MD, Departments of General Surgery and Oncology, Women's & Infants Breast Health Center, Providence, Rhode Island

NORA HANSEN, MD, Director, Lynn Sage Comprehensive Breast Center/Northwestern University, Chicago, Illinois

AWORI J. HAYANGA, MD, House Officer, Department of Surgery, University of Michigan, Ann Arbor, Michigan

EMILY HU, MD, Section of Plastic Surgery, Department of Surgery, University of Michigan Medical Center, Ann Arbor, Michigan

RESHMA JAGSI, MD, DPhil, Assistant Professor, Department of Radiation Oncology, University of Michigan Hospitals, Ann Arbor, Michigan

V. SUZANNE KLIMBERG, MD, Division of Breast Surgical Oncology, Department of Surgery, University of Arkansas for Medical Sciences; and Department of Pathology, University of Arkansas for Medical Sciences, Little Rock, Arkansas

HENRY M. KUERER, MD, PhD, Director of Breast Surgical Oncology Training Program and Associate Professor of Surgery, Department of Surgical Oncology, The University of Texas M. D. Anderson Cancer Center, Houston, Texas

JULIE E. LANG, MD, Department of Surgical Oncology, The University of Texas M. D. Anderson Cancer Center, Houston, Texas

MARIE CATHERINE LEE, MD, Multidisciplinary Breast Fellow, Department of Surgery, University of Michigan Hospitals, Ann Arbor, Michigan

ELEFTHERIOS P. MAMOUNAS, MD, MPH, FACS, Chairman, NSABP Breast Committee, Associate Professor of Surgery, Director, Aultman Health Foundation Cancer Center, Canton, Ohio

MONICA MORROW, MD, G Willing Pepper Chair in Surgery, Department of Surgical Oncology, Fox Chase Cancer Center, Philadelphia, Pennsylvania

ERIKA A. NEWMAN, MD, House Officer, Department of Surgery, University of Michigan, Ann Arbor, Michigan

LISA A. NEWMAN, MD, MPH, FACS, Associate Professor of Surgery and Director, Breast Care Center, University of Michigan Comprehensive Cancer Center; and Department of Surgery, University of Michigan, Ann Arbor, Michigan

MARTIN J. O'SULLIVAN, MD, Breast Fellow, Department of Surgical Oncology, Fox Chase Cancer Center, Philadelphia, Pennsylvania

TIMOTHY M. PAWLIK, MD, Assistant Professor of Surgery, Department of Surgery, Johns Hopkins School of Medicine, Johns Hopkins Hospital, Baltimore, Maryland

AEISHA RIVERS, MD, Surgical Breast Fellow, Lynn Sage Comprehensive Breast Center/Northwestern University, Chicago, Illinois

S. EVA SINGLETARY, MD, Professor, Department of Surgical Oncology, The University of Texas M.D. Anderson Cancer Center, Houston, Texas

MARGARET THOMPSON, MD, Division of Breast Surgical Oncology, Department of Surgery, University of Arkansas for Medical Sciences, Little Rock, Arizona

FRANK A. VICINI, MD, Chief of Oncology and Clinical Professor, Beaumont Cancer Institute, William Beaumont Hospital, Royal Oak, Michigan

ANGELIQUE F. VITUG, MD, Breast Cancer Center, University of Michigan, Ann Arbor, Michigan

VICTOR G. VOGEL, MD, MHS, FACP, Director, Magee/UPCI Breast Cancer Prevention Program; Professor of Medicine and Epidemiology, University of Pittsburgh School of Medicine, Magee-Womens Hospital, Pittsburgh, Pennsylvania

JENNIFER F. WALJEE, MD, MPH, General Surgery House Officer, Department of Surgery, Breast Care Center, University of Michigan, Ann Arbor, Michigan

SHAHEEN ZAKARIA, MD, Department of Surgery, Mayo Clinic and Mayo Foundation, Mayo Clinic College of Medicine, Rochester, Minnesota

CONTENTS

The National Surgical Adjuvant Breast Project (NSABP) is a clinical trials cooperative group funded by the National Cancer Institute that has been responsible for the majority of prospective, randomized studies that have defined standards of breast cancer care in the United States during the past 4 decades. This article summarizes the design of and findings from a selection of their landmark studies. Results from their many successfully completed trials have been reported as subset analyses, pooled analyses, and retrospective studies. This article focuses on presenting the study designs, aims, and primary endpoint results of these studies.

Until recently, the primary message of breast health awareness programs was that early detection is a woman's best protection against breast cancer, because there was no way to prevent it. Currently, however, tamoxifen is approved for chemoprevention of breast cancer in high-risk women, and studies are underway evaluating other medications that may decrease breast cancer risk. Data have also become available regarding the efficacy of surgical strategies to reduce breast cancer risk. Any prevention method, however, will have associated risk of complications or adverse effects, and determining the net risk/benefit ratio depends on the ability to accurately quantify a woman's baseline likelihood of developing breast cancer. This article reviews available methods for assessing and reducing breast cancer risk.

With availability of genetic testing and development of statistical models for risk stratification, more women are being identified as having increased risk for breast cancer. A number of risk-reducing treatment options with varying efficacy exist for them, including frequent surveillance, chemoprevention, prophylactic salpingo-oophorectomy (PSO), and prophylactic mastectomy (PM). Those most likely to benefit from PM are BRCA gene carriers and those who have a strong family history of breast cancer. Prevetive PM remains controversial, however. There are no randomized controlled trials to substantiate the potential benefit or harms of PM. This article describes the high-risk women in whom PM may be considered, and summarizes data on the efficacy of PM as a treatment for the prevention of breast cancer.

This article summarizes the modern evidence-based management of ductal carcinoma in situ. The data addressing the surgical issues, including indications for mastectomy and the use of sentinel node biopsy, are presented. The randomized trials examining the role of radiation therapy after breast-conserving surgery and the use of tamoxifen in ductal carcinoma in situ are discussed. Factors to consider in developing a management strategy for the individual patient are elucidated in the final section.

The axillary nodal status is accepted universally as the most powerful prognostic tool available for early stage breast cancer. The removal of level I and level II lymph nodes at axillary node dissection (ALND) is the most accurate method to assess nodal status, and it is the universal standard; however, it is associated with several adverse long-term sequelae. Lymphatic mapping with sentinel lymph node biopsy has emerged as an effective and safe alternative to the ALND for detecting axillary metastases. This article discusses some lymphatic mapping methodology.

(BCT) is an area of intensive clinical investigation. This article describes evolving methods of APBI in comparison to WBI and in the setting of ongoing clinical trials.

The benefits of adjuvant systemic therapy in reducing risk of distant relapse from breast cancer have been recognized for several decades. The intent of adjuvant therapy is to eliminate the occult micrometastatic breast cancer burden before it progresses into clinically apparent disease. Successful delivery of effective adjuvant systemic therapy as a complement to surgical management of breast cancer has contributed to the steady declines in breast cancer mortality observed internationally over the past 2 decades. Ongoing clinical and translational research in breast cancer seeks to improve the efficacy of systemic agents for use in the conventional postoperative (adjuvant) setting.

The indications and benefits of postmastectomy radiation therapy (PMRT) continue to evolve. Advances in systemic adjuvant therapy and targeted therapy for breast cancer are likely to play an increasingly important role in control of locoregional as well as distant disease. Ongoing scrutiny of patterns of chest wall failure will be required to define the net benefit derived from PMRT. This article discusses the 2001 American Society of Clinical Oncology guidelines for PMRT and current practices using PMRT in selected groups of patients who have breast cancer.

The intact primary in patients diagnosed with Stage IV breast cancer is generally reserved for palliative indications. Haagensen and Stout's 1943 criteria of inoperability for carcinoma of the breast, including tumor fixation to the chest wall, ulceration, and peau d'orange, hold true. Surgery alone is unlikely to prolong life in such patients. Improvements in breast cancer screening and awareness mean fewer patients having inoperable breast cancer. The current problem is that imagining studies reveal some patients to have oligometastatic disease with an intact primary. This article considers surgical treatment as part of multimodal Stage IV breast cancer treatment for such patients. Several challenges to previous dogma to never operate on Stage IV breast cancer patients except with palliative intent have arisen.

FORTHCOMING ISSUES

RECENT ISSUES

The Clinics are now available online!

www.theclinics.com

ELSEVIER
SAUNDERS

SURGICAL
CLINICS OF
NORTH AMERICA

Surg Clin N Am 87 (2007) xv–xvii

Foreword

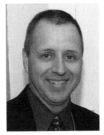

Ronald F. Martin, MD
Consulting Editor

When it was first agreed that I would serve as Consulting Editor to the *Surgical Clinics of North America* it was with the agreement between the publishers and me that we would try to explore topics that had true relevance to the general surgeon. Although at the time that seemed like a straightforward objective, it has proved to me to be a more elusive concept than I might have originally thought. The topic of breast care is particularly illustrative of how difficult it can be to characterize what it is that a general surgeon should know and what a general surgeon should do.

One of the first difficulties to address is; what is the difference between limiting one's practice and developing a specialty practice. I would think that most surgeons know of surgeons who limit their practice to certain problems and then claim to be specialists. One might argue that a surgeon who limits her or his scope of practice is able to maintain a focus of development that would allow for development of extraordinary knowledge in that area. Others may argue that additionally focused formal fellowship specialty training is mandatory to be considered a specialist. We as a discipline have not addressed this dilemma well and perhaps we cannot. The American Board of Surgery is clear and specific about its inclusion of the diagnostic and operative management of patients who have breast problems being within the scope of a fully trained general surgeon. There are also fellowship-trained breast surgeons, either by specific additional training in breast surgery or as part of a surgical oncology fellowship, who feel that the training provided by standard residency training is inadequate to be considered fully qualified in the management of patients who have breast disorders.

doi:10.1016/j.suc.2007.03.015
surgical.theclinics.com

Technically both may be right or wrong. It is unclear to me who would be the final arbiter of such a disagreement.

Another point of contention that was made very clear to me at a recent systemwide meeting in the large multispecialty clinic in which I work was the concept of "Captain of the Ship." It was proposed at that meeting that we discuss limitations on the process of performing and choosing biopsy options and timing. One of the arguments that was put forth was that a general surgeon should be consulted before every biopsy, no matter how performed. This would effectively eliminate the ability for a physician to directly request a biopsy performed by someone other than a surgeon. This rings as a battle cry to some of you reading this and some will squirm as they imagine their clinic space filled with patients requiring urgent consultation before stereotactic biopsy of benign disease.

Like many of the readers of this series I was trained to believe that general surgeons can do just about everything better, faster, cheaper, and with fewer problems than any other specialty. Although my ego would like me to believe that is true, I am not sure that my intellect will allow me to accept it as a blanket statement anymore (not that it ever should have). Although we as surgeons may envision ourselves as Captains of Ships, I don't believe it is written anywhere that we actually are. Also, our ability to force anyone else to believe that is pretty limited. If we are to convince anyone of our value to the patient who has breast problems we shall have to do so by providing superior service to our patients and referring physicians and providers.

The comprehensive care of the patient who has complex breast problems is for the most part multidisciplinary at this time. It is the extremely rare surgeon who solely prescribes chemotherapy or delivers radiation therapy. It would seem to me that given the complexities of skill sets, from diagnostic imaging to extirpation and adjuvant therapy, most general surgeons involved in this kind of care are more likely to become valuable team members in a service line than sole providers. And because that is the case the expectation that we will *always* be the Captain of the Ship is probably unlikely to be a philosophy shared by our other valued team members. Perhaps we should rethink our positions in some situations to optimally care for the patient.

A last point refers to breast care related to other disorders. Breast care, and specifically breast cancer, is an extraordinarily well-funded health care concern. It is most likely funded disproportionately to other similarly devastating health care problems. There certainly many reasons for this—public awareness through the media, celebrity backing of funding events, and public perception relative to actual data, to name a few. In a national or international strategy (or lack thereof) to address health care research and funding, the process of open competition for what seems to be limited global funding may either be brilliant market pressure strategy or complete abdication of establishing priority by central powers; most likely the answer lies in between.

As in many situations, the answers to the questions posed above are certainly not absolute. Any considered response to these challenges requires a sound understanding of the underlying subject matter. Dr. Newman and her colleagues have assembled an excellent collection of articles so that the considered reader can be well versed in the issues as they present from the surgeon's viewpoint. At the minimum a thorough understanding of these topics will make one a better team member; perhaps it will better qualify one for a leadership position.

Ronald F. Martin, MD
Department of Surgery
Marshfield Clinic
1000 North Oak Avenue
Marshfield, WI 54449, USA

E-mail address: martin.ronald@marshfieldclinic.org

ELSEVIER
SAUNDERS

Surg Clin N Am 87 (2007) xix–xx

SURGICAL
CLINICS OF
NORTH AMERICA

Preface

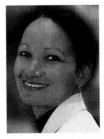

Lisa A. Newman, MD, MPH, FACS
Guest Editor

This issue of the *Surgical Clinics of North America* is dedicated to surgical trainees at the level of house officers and fellows. The evaluation and management of both benign and malignant diseases of the breast are likely to demand a substantial fraction of a general surgeon's practice, yet general surgery residents frequently receive their breast pathology education in a fragmented fashion. Exposure to outpatient clinics and office-based management (where much of the decision-making processes in breast cancer take place) is limited, and surgical breast procedures are often assigned to junior trainees, who do not necessarily understand the subtle judgment that is required in planning incisions, skin flaps, and extent of breast resections. The surgical chief resident must finish his/her training program with the requisite number of breast procedures documented in their case log, but the majority of them may have been performed during the first half of the residency, and there may have been very little exposure to considerations regarding neoadjuvant therapy versus postoperative adjuvant therapy, postmastectomy radiation, and breast cancer risk reduction. Our goal was to develop a collection of articles that cover essential areas of surgical as well as nonsurgical breast cancer management.

We have therefore compiled 18 articles that focus on several important aspects of breast disease management; most of the articles have been coauthored by surgery trainees so that resident-level perspectives are provided. These articles can be categorized in general as having an emphasis on one of the following areas: (1) contemporary surgical treatment strategies (eg, lymphatic mapping and breast reconstruction); (2) new systemic therapy

doi:10.1016/j.suc.2007.03.008 *surgical.theclinics.com*

strategies (adjuvant and neoadjuvant); (3) breast cancer risk reduction (surgical and medical); and (4) novel research directions that trainees should consider (eg, disparity-related research and breast tumor ablation techniques).

We are deeply indebted to the many experts that contributed to this issue and are confident that their efforts will prove quite useful to surgical trainees as they prepare for their board examinations and, more importantly, a future involving care of breast cancer patients. Furthermore, we are extremely grateful to Catherine Bewick and her editorial staff for their patience and guidance throughout the publication process.

Lisa A. Newman, MD, MPH, FACS
Department of Surgery, Breast Care Center
University of Michigan
1500 East Medical Center Drive, 3308 CGC
Ann Arbor, MI 48109, USA

E-mail address: lanewman@med.umich.edu

ELSEVIER
SAUNDERS

SURGICAL
CLINICS OF
NORTH AMERICA

Surg Clin N Am 87 (2007) 279–305

Review of Breast Cancer Clinical Trials Conducted by the National Surgical Adjuvant Breast Project

Lisa A. Newman, MD, MPH, FACS[a],*,
Eleftherios P. Mamounas, MD, MPH, FACS[b]

[a]Breast Care Center, University of Michigan, 1500 East Medical Center Drive, 3308 CGC, Ann Arbor, MI 48109-0932, USA
[b]Department of Surgery, Aultman Health Foundation Cancer Center, 2600 Sixth Street, SW, Canton, OH 44710, USA

The National Surgical Adjuvant Breast Project (NSABP) is a National Cancer Institute (NCI)-funded clinical trials cooperative group that for the past 48 years has conducted multiple randomized clinical trials on the loco-regional and adjuvant systemic therapy of early-stage breast cancer, as well as on breast cancer chemoprevention. Results from many of these trials have undoubtedly been responsible for defining new standards of breast cancer care in the United States and worldwide. This article summarizes the design, primary aims, and main results from selected NSABP trials evaluating loco-regional and adjuvant systemic therapy questions.

National Surgical Adjuvant Breast Project protocols of loco-regional management of invasive breast cancer

National Surgical Adjuvant Breast Project B-04

The B-04 trial is arguably one of the most important of the NSABP trials, but to understand its value some historical perspective is necessary [1–7]. Before the twentieth century breast cancer was viewed as a uniformly fatal disease, generally without any available or attempted treatment options. The advent of the Halstedian radical mastectomy at the turn of the twentieth century represented a major advance for breast cancer patients. This

---

* Corresponding author.
E-mail address: lanewman@umich.edu (L.A. Newman).

0039-6109/07/$ - see front matter © 2007 Published by Elsevier Inc.
doi:10.1016/j.suc.2007.02.005   *surgical.theclinics.com*

operation called for the en bloc radical resection of the breast, overlying skin, pectoralis muscles, and axillary lymph nodes. Although radical mastectomy (RM) was certainly associated with substantial morbidity, it served a valuable purpose at a time when most women presented with locally advanced disease that warranted an aggressive surgical approach. The benefits of successful extirpation of these bulky tumors relative to achieving loco-regional control of the disease as well as occasional long-term survival were readily appreciated, and Halsted thereby ushered in an era in which breast cancer was perceived as a disease that progressed in an anatomically stepwise fashion, with likelihood of cure being dependent on the surgeon's ability to resect beyond the last site of breast or nodal involvement. In deference to this theory, subsequent attempts to surgically conquer breast cancer included the extended RM (RM plus resection of the internal mammary nodes) and the RM coupled with resection of supraclavicular nodes. Unfortunately, these procedures succeeded only in increasing treatment morbidity, without any appreciable improvement in survival.

The NSABP therefore set out to design a large prospective randomized clinical trial to examine whether reducing the extent of surgery for breast cancer might not compromise outcome. The corollary message of this study was that improvement in breast cancer survival was dependent upon achieving control of distant organ micrometastases, either by early detection (when the risk of such involvement is reduced), or by developing nonsurgical, systemic treatment strategies. In the 1970 to 1974 accrual time frame, however, there were no effective systemic therapies available for breast cancer, and so the B-04 trial was designed as a "pure" comparison of different loco-regional approaches for the management of resectable breast cancer.

The NSABP B-04 trial was set up as two companion trials conducted in parallel: one trial for patients who had clinically node-negative breast cancer, and the other for patients who had clinically node-positive disease. Because the RM was the standard-of-care management at that time, this operation was included as the control arm for both trials. One thousand seventy-nine patients who had clinically node-negative disease were randomized to one of three different treatment arms: RM (362 patients); total mastectomy (TM)—complete removal of the breast, but sparing the pectoralis musculature and axillary nodes), plus loco-regional/axillary irradiation (352 patients); or TM alone, with no targeted axillary treatment (365 patients). For patients presenting with clinically-suspicious disease in the axilla, it would be unethical to leave gross disease untreated, and thus 586 patients were randomized to one of only two treatment arms: RM (292 patients) or TM plus radiation (294 patients).

Survival analyses from the B-04 trial have been reported on multiple occasions, and the results have been consistent. As hypothesized by the study design, there were no significant differences in overall survival among the three arms in the clinically node-negative patients, even with 25 years of follow-up: 25% for the RM arm; 19% for the TM/radiation arm; and 26% for the TM-alone arm. Similarly, there were no overall survival differences between the two arms in the clinically node-positive patients (overall survival: 14% for each arm).

Several other important observations emerged from the B-04 trial. First, the inadequacy of clinical axillary evaluation was demonstrated; among patients thought to have clinically node-negative disease, pathologic evaluation of the axillary specimen in the RM arm revealed that 40% of cases were actually node-positive. Because of randomization, one would assume that 40% of the patients randomized to TM followed by radiation or randomized to TM alone were also node-positive at presentation and had disease that was either radiated or not treated at all. The axillary failure rate in the TM-alone arm was only 19%, however, indicating that microscopic, occult disease in the axilla is not necessarily destined to progress into clinically overt disease. Furthermore, the similar overall survival among the three arms suggests that an axillary lymph node dissection (ALND) for the clinically negative axilla is largely prophylactic, and that outcome is not likely to be significantly compromised by deferring ALND until there is clinical evidence of disease in the axilla. Going one step further, because the axillary failure rate in the TM plus radiation arm was only 3%, it could also be argued that a TM plus axillary radiation is an alternative effective approach.

The B-04 trial results continue to be used as the basis for arguments against routine ALND, even in the current era of lymphatic mapping, when the nodal status can be readily documented by a lower-morbidity sentinel lymph node biopsy (SLNB). It must be kept in mind, however, that the B-04 trial was not powered statistically to detect a small survival difference between the three arms, and thus a modest outcome contribution from the axillary dissection could not be ruled out by this trial. Also, nearly one-quarter of the TM cases included some axillary nodal tissue, and the extent of this "inadvertent" nodal resection was inversely associated with risk of axillary failure. Furthermore, among the patients who had clinically node-positive disease, axillary radiation proved to be inferior to ALND with regard to axillary recurrence, justifying the concept that surgical resection provides optimal control of grossly-apparent disease. Lastly, by the latter part of the 1970s, adjuvant tamoxifen and chemotherapy entered the breast cancer treatment arena, and because their use was reserved at the time for node-positive patients, ALND remained an essential component of primary breast cancer treatment.

National Surgical Adjuvant Breast Project B-06

The results of the B-04 trial had a significant influence in challenging the need for radicality in breast cancer surgery, and helped pave the way for the conduct of the NSABP B-06 trial evaluating even less radical surgical procedures for the treatment of early-stage breast cancer [8–10]. Furthermore, in the decade that followed completion of the B-04 trial, increase in breast cancer awareness and expansion of mammographic screening programs resulted in more patients presenting with smaller primary cancers. This favorable trend provided motivation for efforts to evaluate the safety and efficacy of breast-sparing surgery for early-stage breast cancer. The B-06 trial was therefore designed for women who had operable primary breast cancer no larger than 4 cm in greatest diameter. Between 1976 and 1984, 2163 patients were randomized to one of three different treatment arms: (1) modified radical mastectomy (MRM)—the standard of care referent group; (2) lumpectomy, ALND, and breast radiation; or (3) lumpectomy and ALND. After 20 years of follow-up [10], there continue to be no significant differences in overall survival, disease-free survival, or distant disease-free survival between the group of patients who underwent MRM and the groups treated with lumpectomy with or without breast radiation. The hazard ratios for death comparing the lumpectomy-alone and lumpectomy-plus-radiation arms to the mastectomy arm were 1.05 (95% CI, 0.90–1.23) and 0.97 (95% CI, 0.83–1.14), respectively.

Despite lack of significant differences in overall survival, significant differences in local control of the disease were observed among the three arms of the B-06 trial. In-breast recurrence occurred in 39.2% of the patients randomized to lumpectomy alone, compared with 14.3% in those randomized to lumpectomy plus breast irradiation. Chest wall recurrence was observed in 10.2% of the patients in the mastectomy arm. Nearly three quarters of the local recurrences in the lumpectomy-alone arm occurred within the first 5 years after surgery, compared with the lumpectomy and irradiation arm, in which 40% of recurrences occurred within the first 5 years. Thus the NSABP B-06 trial established the safety of breast-conserving surgery for early-stage invasive breast cancer, and demonstrated the importance of adjuvant breast radiation to minimize risk of in-breast recurrence. Furthermore, along with other randomized trials—including those conducted by the Milan group evaluating quadrantectomy [11,12]—the B-06 trial was instrumental in establishing breast-conserving surgery plus radiotherapy as the preferred method of local treatment for patients who have operable breast cancer.

National Surgical Adjuvant Breast Project B-21

One of the unresolved questions following disclosure of the results from the B-06 trial, as well as those from the Milan trial, was whether all patients who had invasive breast cancer undergoing lumpectomy needed postoperative radiotherapy [13]. It was hypothesized that patients who had small tumors (≤1 cm) could potentially be spared from radiotherapy because they have lower rates of local recurrence. It was further argued at that time (1990 Consensus Development Conference), that patients who have negative nodes and tumors 1 cm or smaller might not even need adjuvant systemic therapy because of their good prognosis. Because the B-06 trial (as well as the B-14 trial, described below) did not include a sufficient number of patients who had tumors 1 cm or smaller to adequately address the radiotherapy and the tamoxifen questions respectively, NSABP Protocol B-21 was designed to address these questions. Women who had node-negative invasive breast cancer 1 cm or less in diameter treated with lumpectomy and axillary dissection were randomized tamoxifen alone for 5 years, breast radiation plus tamoxifen for 5 years, or breast radiation plus placebo for 5 years. A total of 1009 patients were randomized (tamoxifen: n = 336, radiation and placebo: n = 336, radiation and tamoxifen: n = 337). Recently published results [13] demonstrated that radiation and placebo resulted in a 49% lower hazard rate of in-breast recurrence than did tamoxifen alone; radiation and tamoxifen resulted in a 63% lower rate of in-breast recurrence than did radiation and placebo. When compared with tamoxifen alone, radiation and tamoxifen resulted in an 81% reduction in hazard rate of in-breast recurrence. Cumulative incidence of in-breast recurrence through 8 years was 16.5% with tamoxifen alone, 9.3% with radiation and placebo, and 2.8% with radiation and tamoxifen. Radiation reduced in-breast recurrence below the level achieved with tamoxifen alone, regardless of estrogen receptor status. Survival in the three groups was 93%, 94%, and 93%, respectively ($P = .93$). Thus, this trial demonstrated that in the group of node-negative patients who had small invasive tumors treated by lumpectomy, tamoxifen was not as effective as breast radiation in controlling the disease in the breast. It further demonstrated that the combination of tamoxifen and breast radiation results in better local control of the disease in the breast than either modality alone.

National Surgical Adjuvant Breast Project B-32

In the 1990s, SLNB was developed as an alternative method for evaluating the axilla in early-stage breast cancer patients (Fig. 1) [14,15]. In 1993, Krag and colleagues [16] reported on isotope lymphatic mapping, and in 1994, Giuliano and colleagues [17] reported on blue-dye lymphatic mapping. Both investigators showed the feasibility of identifying a sentinel node in breast cancer patients. Subsequent studies were largely performed with dual-agent mapping and with a concomitant ALND, so that accuracy rates could be defined. These studies confirmed the presence of a learning curve with this technique, but generally demonstrated reasonably low false-negative rates (averaging 8% in one meta-analysis) coupled with very high (more than 90%) identification rates [18]. As a result, sentinel node biopsy was enthusiastically adopted by many surgeons, and has been endorsed by several authoritative groups. Nonetheless, rigorous evaluation of its short- and long-term outcomes in the setting of a prospective, randomized clinical trial was necessary.

The NSABP B-32 Protocol was therefore established to compare SLNB alone with sentinel node biopsy followed by an axillary dissection in

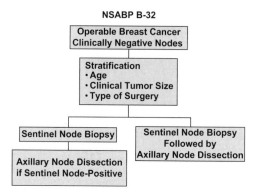

Fig. 1. Randomization schema for NSABP Protocol 32.

clinically node-negative patients who had operable breast cancer. Patients were randomized to undergo SLNB and mandatory concomitant ALND (group 1) or SLNB followed by ALND only if the sentinel node revealed metastatic disease (group 2). Patients in the sentinel node biopsy alone group who were found to have a positive sentinel node were required to also undergo full axillary dissection. In addition to its main objective, which was to compare the two procedures in terms of outcome, the study addressed a number of important biologic questions, such as the prognostic significance of immunohistochemically detected tumor cells in lymph nodes when a routine haematoxylin and eosin (H & E) stain, is negative. Between 1999 and 2004, 5611 patients were randomized. Although the trial is not mature for survival analysis yet, technical reports on the performance of the procedure have shown an identification rate of 97% and a false-negative rate of 9.7%. The proportion of patients who had metastatic sentinel nodes was 26% for both arms of the study. In nearly two thirds of the cases the sentinel nodes were the only sites of metastatic adenopathy [14].

National Surgical Adjuvant Breast Project B-39

Whole-breast irradiation (delivered in 5-day per week fractions over a 5 or 6 week period) represents the standard approach of breast irradiation in patients who have early-stage breast cancer treated with lumpectomy [19]; however, most true in-breast recurrences occur near the lumpectomy cavity, and in-breast events that occur in separate quadrants are frequently new primary breast tumors that develop after more prolonged follow-up. The incidence of these second primaries is not necessarily affected by the delivery of post-lumpectomy radiation therapy.

These patterns of local failure following lumpectomy have motivated a renewed interest in accelerated partial breast irradiation (APBI) techniques. The advantages of APBI include the feasibility of completing adjuvant breast irradiation within a week, and the potential for repeating breast-sparing surgery when another in-breast event occurs outside of the irradiated lumpectomy bed. In addition, given the short duration of the regimen, breast irradiation can precede the administration of adjuvant chemotherapy in patients who require treatment with both modalities. Before APBI can be considered in place of whole breast irradiation, however, large-scale randomized clinical trials must compare the clinical safety and efficacy of these two approaches. One such trial, currently conducted in North America by the NSABP and the Radiation Therapy Oncology Group (RTOG) is NSABP B-39/RTOG 0413. This trial will randomize 3000 women to receive either conventional whole-breast irradiation or APBI. Participating institutions have the option of delivering APBI via high-dose multicatheter brachytherapy, high-dose single-catheter balloon brachytherapy, or three-dimensional conformal external beam radiation therapy. The primary endpoint of the trial is in-breast tumor recurrence. The trial opened in March 2005 and is expected to complete its accrual in 2007.

National Surgical Adjuvant Breast Project B-37

Despite the consistent finding that the development of in-breast recurrence or other loco-regional recurrence is associated with considerable increase in the risk of subsequent distant failure, there is very little evidence on the value of additional systemic therapy at the time of in-breast recurrence or other loco-regional recurrence [14]. To date there have been no reported randomized trials on the worth of administering additional "adjuvant" chemotherapy at the time of loco-regional recurrence. One of the reasons for this is that until the development of taxanes, there were no candidate non–cross-resistant regimens with promising activity that could be tested in this setting; however, the demonstration of significant antitumor activity with taxanes in patients resistant to anthracyclines provided the opportunity to revisit the above question in a randomized clinical trial. Such a currently ongoing trial is the International Breast Cancer Study Group (IBCSG) 27-02/NSABP B-37, which randomizes patients who have resected in-breast recurrence or other loco-regional recurrence to chemotherapy or observation (in addition to hormonal therapy for hormone-receptor–positive tumors) [14]. A total of 977 patients will be recruited to this trial, which is currently open for accrual.

National Surgical Adjuvant Breast Project protocols for the management of ductal carcinoma in situ

The introduction and widespread use of mammography has contributed to a dramatic increase in the incidence of small, localized, nonpalpable ductal carcinoma in situ (DCIS), an entity with excellent prognosis after local therapy alone. Currently, Surveillance Epidemiology and End Results (SEER) data reveal that DCIS accounts for approximately 20% of all breast cancers diagnosed in the United States, with age-adjusted incidence rates of 30 cases per 100,000 women, and approximately 47,000 cases detected each year [20]. The steadily increasing number of screen-detected DCIS cases has led to a greater appreciation for the biologic heterogeneity of this pre-invasive lesion, generating questions regarding alternative treatment needs.

National Surgical Adjuvant Breast Project B-17

As randomized trials demonstrated the value of breast-conserving surgery in patients who have invasive breast cancer, an obvious question arose relative to the value of this procedure in patients who have noninvasive disease (Fig. 2) [21–24]. Based on the results of the B-06 and other trials described above, in the early 1980s there was a paradox in the surgical treatment of early-stage breast cancer, with invasive disease being treated progressively more with lumpectomy, whereas mastectomy remained the recommended surgical treatment for noninvasive disease. Thus, it became imperative at the time to test the value of breast conservation in patients who have DCIS. The NSABP was the first group to conduct such a prospective randomized trial. The NSABP B-17 trial compared lumpectomy alone with lumpectomy plus breast radiation in 818 patients who had localized ductal carcinoma in-situ. A mastectomy control group was not included, given the acceptance of lumpectomy based on the results of the B-06 trial, as well as the excellent prognosis of patients who had localized DCIS. Recently updated results from the B-17 trial after 12 years of follow-up [24] continue to indicate—as previously reported [21,22]—that radiotherapy significantly decreases the rate of invasive and noninvasive ipsilateral breast tumor recurrence. The cumulative incidence of noninvasive ipsilateral breast cancer recurrence as a first event was significantly reduced with breast radiation from 14.6% to 8.0% ($P = .001$). More importantly, the cumulative

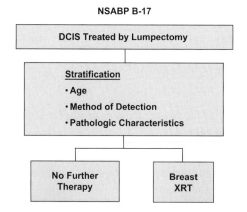

Fig. 2. Randomization schema for NSABP Protocol 17.

incidence of invasive ipsilateral recurrence was also significantly reduced from, 16.8% to 7.7% ($P = .00001$). No difference in overall survival has been observed between the two groups (86% versus 87%, $P = .80$), and over two thirds of the deaths occurring in this trial were not breast-cancer related. In a subset of 623 out of 814 evaluable patients from this trial, pathologic features were analyzed relative to their prognostic significance for ipsilateral breast cancer recurrence [23]. Only the presence of moderate/ marked comedo necrosis was a statistically significant independent predictor of risk for ipsilateral breast cancer recurrence in both treatment groups, and breast radiation markedly reduced the annual hazard rates for ipsilateral breast cancer recurrence in all subgroups of patients.

National Surgical Adjuvant Breast Project B-24

Most cases of DCIS will demonstrate elevated expression of the estrogen receptor, and use of a selective estrogen receptor modulator such as tamoxifen is therefore a reasonable consideration for decreasing risk of recurrence in patients who have DCIS and are treated with lumpectomy (Fig. 3) [24,25]. The NSABP therefore built upon the B-17 experience, which established lumpectomy and breast irradiation as the standard of care for resected, localized DCIS, and designed the B-24 trial to evaluate adjuvant tamoxifen therapy in addition to lumpectomy and breast irradiation. This protocol randomized 1800 DCIS patients to lumpectomy and breast irradiation, followed by 5 years of tamoxifen versus placebo. Updated results after 7 years of follow-up continue to demonstrate, as previously reported [25], that the addition of tamoxifen significantly improved disease-free survival from 77.1% to 83.0% ($P = .002$). This improvement was mainly the result of a reduction in the incidence of invasive and noninvasive breast cancer events in the ipsilateral as well as in the contralateral breast. The cumulative incidence of all ipsilateral and contralateral breast cancer events was reduced by 39%; from 16.0% in the placebo group to 10.0% in the tamoxifen group

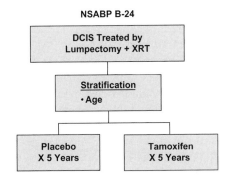

Fig. 3. Randomization schema for NSABP Protocol 24.

$(P = .0003)$ [24]. When the rate of all invasive breast cancer events was evaluated, tamoxifen resulted in a 45% reduction $(P = .0009)$. When the rate of non-invasive breast cancer events was evaluated, the addition of ta- moxifen resulted in a 27%, nonsignificant reduction $(P = .11)$. When the effect of tamoxifen was examined according to the location of the first event, the cumulative incidence of ipsilateral breast cancers was reduced by 31% (11.1% with tamoxifen versus 7.7% with placebo, $P = .02$), and the cumu- lative incidence of contralateral breast cancers was reduced by 47% (4.9% versus 2.3%, $P = .01$).

In 2002, Allred and colleagues [26] presented data from the NSABP B-24 trial assessing the tamoxifen benefit according to the estrogen receptor sta- tus of the primary DCIS tumor. Out of the 1804 patients participating in the trial, information on the status of estrogen receptor was available for 628 patients (327 placebo, 301 tamoxifen). Seventy-seven percent of the patients had estrogen receptor (ER)-positive tumors, and in those patients the effec- tiveness of tamoxifen was clear (RR for all breast cancer events: 0.41, $P = .0002$). Significant reductions in breast cancer events were seen in both the ipsilateral and the contralateral breast. In patients who had ER-negative tumors, little benefit was observed (RR for all breast cancer events: 0.80, $P = .51$), but the total number of events in this cohort was too small to rule out a small, clinically meaningful benefit. When these results are taken together with those evaluating the effect of tamoxifen in patients who had invasive breast cancer and negative estrogen receptors, however, they are consistent with the observation that tamoxifen has no appreciable benefit in reducing rates of recurrence or rates of contralateral breast cancer in patients with ER-negative tumors. Furthermore, these results suggest that routine assess- ment of estrogen receptor status should now be performed also in patients who have DCIS to determine their candidacy for tamoxifen therapy.

National Surgical Adjuvant Breast Project B-35

In the 1990s, significant enthusiasm developed with the demonstration of considerable activity and favorable toxicity profile with third-generation ar- omatase inhibitors in patients who have hormone-responsive, advanced breast cancer. As a result, several clinical trials have evaluated aromatase in- hibitors as adjuvant therapy in patients who had early-stage breast cancer. The first one to report results was the Arimidex or Tamoxifen Alone or in Combination (ATAC) trial that randomized more than 9000 early-stage breast cancer patients to receive anastrozole, tamoxifen, or the combination of anastrozole and tamoxifen, as adjuvant hormonal therapy. Besides yield- ing provocative results regarding the activity of anastrozole in the adjuvant treatment of ER-positive postmenopausal breast cancer, this trial was the first to demonstrate that the risk of contralateral new primary breast cancers was significantly reduced with anastrozole when compared with tamoxifen (odds ratio 0.42; $P = .007$) [27]. These results were eventually confirmed in other similar trials evaluating aromatase inhibitors in the adjuvant setting, and provided a rationale for the evaluation of aromatase inhibitors in patients who have DCIS and for those at high risk for developing invasive breast cancer. These findings prompted the design and implementation of NSABP B-35, a Phase III trial that randomized postmenopausal DCIS patients treated with breast conservation therapy and breast irradiation to tamoxifen versus anastrozole for 5 years. The primary aim of the study is to evaluate the effectiveness of anastrozole compared with tamoxifen in preventing the subsequent occurrence of breast cancer (local, regional, and distant recurrences, and contralateral breast cancer). In addition, the trial will ascertain the effects of anastrozole on patient symptoms and quality of life as compared with tamoxifen. This protocol has completed is accrual goal after accruing over 3100 patients, and is currently awaiting maturation of follow-up.

National Surgical Adjuvant Breast Project trials of adjuvant systemic therapy in patients who have negative axillary nodes

During the last 20 years the NSABP has played a significant role in the establishment of adjuvant chemotherapy and adjuvant hormonal therapy for the treatment of breast cancer patients who have negative nodes. Beginning in the early 1980s, several important trials were conducted evaluating the worth of combination chemotherapy and the worth of tamoxifen in such patients.

Studies in patients who have estrogen-receptor negative tumors: National Surgical Adjuvant Breast Project B-13, B-19, and B-23

The first trial (NSABP B-13) (Fig. 4) randomized patients who had negative nodes and negative estrogen receptors to surgery alone or surgery followed by 12 months of adjuvant chemotherapy with methotrexate and sequentially administered 5-FU (M-F) followed by leucovorin. Findings through 14 years of follow-up [28] demonstrate that the improvements in disease-free and overall survival from M-F, previously reported after 5 [29] and 8 [30] years, have persisted ($P < .0001$ in the former and $P = .02$ in the latter). A statistically significant benefit in disease-free survival was evident both for women 50 years of age or older ($P = .005$) as well as in those 50 years old or younger ($P = .001$). A statistically significant benefit in terms of survival was evident only in women 50 years of age or older ($P = .02$); however, there was no statistically significant evidence of an interaction between treatment group and age relative to overall survival ($P = .34$).

A subsequent trial in the same patient population (NSABP B-19) (Fig. 5) attempted to determine whether the alkylating agent cyclophosphamide contributed additional benefit when administered with methotrexate and 5-FU (CMF regimen, as developed by the Milan Group). A total of

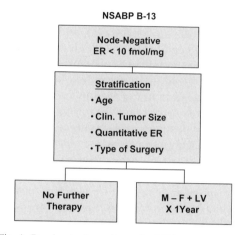

Fig. 4. Randomization schema for NSABP Protocol 13.

1095 patients were randomized to receive either six courses of M-F or six courses of CMF. Through 8 years of follow-up [28], just as first reported after 5 years [30], the results continue to demonstrate a statistically significant disease-free and overall survival advantage with CMF over M-F ($P = .003$ an $P = .03$, respectively). Those advantages were most evident in women aged 50 or younger ($P = .0004$ and $P = .007$, respectively). As was also observed in the B-13 study, there was no evidence of a statistically significant interaction between treatment and age group relative to disease-free survival ($P = .22$) and overall survival ($P = .08$).

Following completion of the B-19 trial, Protocol B-23 attempted to address whether tamoxifen has a role in patients who have ER-negative tumors. Patients who had negative nodes and ER-negative tumors were randomized to four cycles of adjuvant doxorubicin/cyclophosphamide

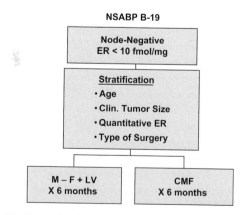

Fig. 5. Randomization schema for NSABP Protocol 19.

(AC) or six cycles of adjuvant CMF with or without tamoxifen. The rationale for evaluating tamoxifen in patients who have ER-negative tumors came both from preclinical and clinical observations [31–33]. More recently, however, an increasing body of evidence has demonstrated that tamoxifen confers no significant advantage in patients who have ER-negative tumors. The results of the B-23 trial confirmed these latter observations and demonstrated no significant prolongation in disease-free survival or overall survival with the addition of tamoxifen to chemotherapy [34]. The results of the B-23 trial also confirmed (in the node-negative setting) the previous observation from the NSABP B-15 trial (in node-positive patients) that four cycles of AC were equivalent to six cycles of CMF in terms of disease-free and overall survival prolongation. One interesting observation in this trial was that tamoxifen did not confer a significant reduction in the incidence of contralateral breast cancer, as has been shown in patients who had ER-positive tumors and negative nodes [28,35]. Explanation for this discrepancy was recently provided by a retrospective review of several NSABP trials, which found that there was significant concordance between the ER-status of the primary breast cancer and that of contralateral breast cancer [36]. Thus in about 80% of patients who initially present with an ER-negative primary and who develop contralateral breast cancer, the contralateral breast tumor is also ER-negative, making the potential chemopreventative effect of tamoxifen negligible in this population of patients.

Studies in patients who have estrogen-receptor positive tumors: National Surgical Adjuvant Breast Project B-14 and B-20

In parallel to the studies evaluating chemotherapy and tamoxifen in patients who had node-negative, ER-negative breast cancer, the NSABP launched a series of trials evaluating tamoxifen and the combination of tamoxifen plus chemotherapy in patients who had node-negative, ER-positive disease.

The NSABP B-14 trial randomized patients after surgery to 5 years of tamoxifen or 5 years of placebo. Published results from this trial through 10 years of follow-up [37] continue to demonstrate a statistically significant disease-free survival benefit from tamoxifen (69% versus 57%, $P < .0001$). In addition, a significant survival advantage was demonstrated in this update (80% versus 76%; $P = .02$). Tamoxifen therapy continued to demonstrate a significant reduction in the rate of contralateral breast cancer (4.0% versus 5.8%, $P = .007$). The significant advantage for disease-free and overall survival with tamoxifen has now persisted through 15 years of follow-up [38].

One of the most common questions asked while the NSABP B-14 trial was being conducted related to the optimal duration of tamoxifen administration. To answer the question of optimal tamoxifen duration beyond 5 years, patients randomized to tamoxifen who were alive and recurrence-free following 5 years of treatment were asked to be re-randomized to 5 additional years of tamoxifen or 5 years of placebo [37]. Originally reported results, through 4 years from re-randomization, demonstrated a significant disadvantage in disease-free survival (86% versus 92%, $P = .003$) and distant disease-free survival (90% versus 96%, $P = .01$) for patients who continued tamoxifen for more than 5 years versus those who discontinued the drug at 5 years. Overall survival was 96% for those who discontinued tamoxifen compared with 94% for those who continued ($P = .08$). Updated results, through 7 years from the time of re-randomization, continue to demonstrate no additional benefit from the prolonged tamoxifen administration [39]. In fact, a slight advantage continues to exist for patients who discontinued tamoxifen after 5 years relative to those who continued to receive it (disease-free survival: 82% versus 78%, $P = .03$; relapse-free survival: 94% versus 92%, $P = .13$; overall survival: 94% versus 91%, $P = .07$, respectively). The lack of benefit from additional tamoxifen therapy was independent of age or other characteristics.

An important observation from the B-14 trial was that through 10 years of follow-up of tamoxifen-treated patients who had ER-positive, node-negative breast cancer, the disease-free survival (69%) and survival (80%) were not as good as originally thought for this group of patients, generally considered to have favorable prognosis [37]. These numbers further decreased after 14 years of follow-up [28], with disease-free survival being around 60% and overall survival around 75%. These results underscore the need for further improvement in this group of patients. Subsequent to the B-14 trial, the NSABP conducted Protocol B-20, which evaluated the worth of adding chemotherapy to tamoxifen in patients who had negative nodes and positive estrogen receptors. Between 1988 and 1993, 2363 patients were randomized to receive either tamoxifen for 5 years, or tamoxifen plus six cycles of sequential methotrexate and 5-fluorouracil followed by leucovorin (MFT) or tamoxifen plus six cycles of cyclophosphamide, methotrexate and 5-fluorouracil (CMFT). Through 5 years of follow-up, the combination of chemotherapy plus tamoxifen resulted in significantly better disease-free survival than tamoxifen alone (90% for MFT versus 85% for tamoxifen, $P = .01$; 89% for CMFT versus 85% for tamoxifen, $P = .001$). A similar benefit was observed in overall survival (97% for MFT versus 94% for tamoxifen, $P = .05$; 96% for CMFT versus 94% for tamoxifen, $P = .03$) [40]. The reduction in recurrence and mortality was greatest in patients aged 49 years or less. No subgroup of patients evaluated in this study failed to benefit from chemotherapy. The results from the B-20 study were recently updated with 12 years of follow-up, and continue to demonstrate a significant improvement in disease-free survival and a borderline significant improvement in overall survival with the addition of chemotherapy to tamoxifen when compared with tamoxifen alone [38].

An important remaining question following the disclosure of the NSABP B-14 and NSABP B-20 trials is whether we can identify subgroups of these

node-negative, ER-positive patients at low risk for recurrence when treated with tamoxifen alone, who can be spared chemotherapy administration. In the past few years, genomic profiling of the primary breast tumor has shown considerable promise toward that goal. Using archival paraffin block material from the NSABP B-14 and NSABP B-20 trials, Genomic Health (Redwood City, California), in collaboration with the NSABP, developed and validated a reverse transcriptase polymerase chain reaction (RT-PCR)-based 21-gene assay (also known as 21-gene recurrence score) that predicts outcome and benefit from hormonal therapy and chemotherapy in these patients [41,42]. This assay (OncoType DX) is currently commercially-available for use in ER-positive, node-negative patients. According to the results of this assay, ER-positive, node-negative breast cancer patients who have a low recurrence score have low risk of recurrence and receive little benefit from the addition of adjuvant chemotherapy to hormonal therapy, although those who have a high recurrence score receive significant benefit from the addition of adjuvant chemotherapy to hormonal therapy and should be offered both. A prospective randomized clinical trial, Trial Assigning IndividuaLized Options for Treatment (Rx) (TAILORx), is currently being conducted to evaluate whether the addition of adjuvant chemotherapy to hormonal therapy is necessary for patients who have an intermediate recurrence score.

National Surgical Adjuvant Breast Project trials evaluating aromatase inhibitors in patients who have hormone-receptor positive, invasive breast cancer

National Surgical Adjuvant Breast Project B-33

The results from the NSABP B-14 trial demonstrating no additional benefit from continuing tamoxifen therapy for longer than 5 years [39], as well as the appreciation of continued risk for recurrence in patients who had hormone-receptor positive breast cancer after 5 years of tamoxifen [43] lead several investigators to consider additional adjuvant hormonal therapy interventions following completion of tamoxifen therapy [44,45]. During the past several years, abundant information became available demonstrating substantial antitumor activity with the use of aromatase inhibitors in patients who had advanced breast cancer and who suffered a recurrence during or after tamoxifen therapy. Thus, attempting to further reduce the risk of subsequent recurrence in patients who remain disease free after completion of adjuvant tamoxifen by administering aromatase inhibitors became an important clinical research question. Based on the above rationale, the NSABP developed Protocol B-33, a randomized trial comparing exemestane (a steroidal, third-generation aromatase inhibitor) with placebo in postmenopausal patients who complete 5 years of tamoxifen and are recurrence-free.

The primary aim of the B-33 trial was to determine whether exemestane will prolong disease-free survival, and secondary aims were to determine whether exemestane will prolong overall survival, and to evaluate the effect of exemestane and that of tamoxifen withdrawal on fracture rate, bone mineral density, markers of bone turnover, levels of lipids and lipoproteins, and quality of life. Between May 2001 and October 2003, a total of 1598 patients were randomized out of the 3000 required to complete the study. In October 2003, however, accrual to this study was terminated early per recommendation of the NSABP Data Monitoring Committee when results from a similar adjuvant trial (NCIC MA.17) became available demonstrating significant improvement with letrozole after 5 years of tamoxifen [46]. As a result of these findings, all patients in the NSABP B-33 trial were unblinded and 5 years of exemestane was offered to both groups at no cost. Despite the premature closure of the trial (50% of the target accrual) and the ensuing crossover to exemestane (about 50% of patients), original assignment to exemestane versus placebo resulted in borderline improvement in disease-free survival and in a significant improvement in relapse-free survival of a similar magnitude to that seen in the NCIC MA.17 trial with letrozole [44].

National Surgical Adjuvant Breast Project B-42

Aromatase inhibitors have demonstrated significant activity in the adjuvant setting either as up-front therapy, as sequential therapy after 2 to 3 years of adjuvant tamoxifen, or as extended adjuvant therapy after 5 years of tamoxifen. Based on the above results, aromatase inhibitors are increasingly used as adjuvant therapy in these three clinical situations. No data currently exist on the optimal duration of aromatase inhibitor therapy. The durations of therapy employed in the previously conducted trials were arbitrarily chosen based on previous experience with tamoxifen or for purposes of study design (ie, to match the duration of tamoxifen). Based on the experience with tamoxifen (as described previously), it is by no means intuitive that prolonging the use of adjuvant aromatase inhibitors would necessarily result in increased benefit when compared with shorter duration. Thus, there is a need to definitively address the question of aromatase inhibitor duration in a prospective randomized trial. NSABP B-42 is a Phase III, randomized, placebo-controlled, double-blind clinical trial that aims to determine whether prolonged adjuvant hormonal therapy with letrozole will improve disease-free survival in postmenopausal women who have ER-positive or progesterone receptor (PgR)-positive breast cancer, and who have completed 5 years of hormonal therapy with either 5 years of an aromatase inhibitor or up to 3 years of tamoxifen followed by an aromatase inhibitor. The study will also determine whether prolonged letrozole therapy will improve survival, breast cancer-free survival, and time to distant recurrence. It will also examine whether prolonged letrozole therapy will increase the incidence of osteoporotic-related fractures and arterial thrombotic events.

Women eligible for the study must have had Stage I, II, or IIIA breast cancer at the time of their original diagnosis, and must be disease-free after completing 5 years of hormonal therapy consisting of an aromatase inhibitor or tamoxifen followed by an aromatase inhibitor. The sample size for the study is 3840 patients, who will be accrued over a period of 5.25 years. The study opened to accrual in August 2006. To have a predominantly letrozole-treated population for the B-42 trial, patients who have taken a minimum of 2 years of hormonal therapy with tamoxifen or an aromatase inhibitor may be offered letrozole at no cost until they complete 5 years of initial adjuvant hormonal therapy, through the B-42 Registration Program. Participation in the Registration Program is not required for enrollment in the B-42 randomized trial, and patients who have received letrozole through the Registration Program are not required to enroll in B-42.

Recent National Surgical Adjuvant Breast Project trials of adjuvant systemic therapy in patients who have positive axillary nodes

National Surgical Adjuvant Breast Project B-28

In the 1990s, the demonstration of significant antitumor activity with taxanes in patients who had advanced breast cancer provided the rationale for evaluating these agents in the adjuvant setting [47,48]. Thus, in 1995 the NSABP initiated a randomized trial (NSABP B-28) to evaluate the worth of paclitaxel following standard-dose Adriamycin and cyclophosphamide (AC) chemotherapy in breast cancer patients who had positive axillary nodes. Eligible patients were randomly assigned to receive four cycles of AC chemotherapy or four cycles of AC followed by four cycles of paclitaxel at 225 mg/m^2 given as a 3-hour infusion. A total of 3060 patients were randomized. With a median follow-up of 64.6 months, a significant improvement in disease-free survival (DFS) was observed in favor of the paclitaxel-containing arm (5-year DFS: 76% versus 72%, RR: 0.83, $P = .006$). Improvement in overall survival (OS) was small and not statistically significant (five-year OS: 85% for both groups, RR: 0.93, $P = .46$) [47]. The results of the B-28 trial were similar to those previously reported by Cancer and Leukemia Group B (CALGB) from a trial of similar design (CALGB 9344) [48], and supported the sequential addition of a taxane after AC chemotherapy in patients who have positive nodes.

National Surgical Adjuvant Breast Project B-30

The next logical step in the clinical development of taxanes as adjuvant treatment for breast cancer was to compare regimens of sequential AC followed by a taxane (as administered in the first-generation adjuvant studies with taxanes) with combination regimens of taxanes plus other active existing agents. Thus far, doxorubicin and docetaxel are among the most active agents against breast cancer. Combinations of doxorubicin with paclitaxel have demonstrated excellent response rates in Phase II studies in patients who have advanced breast cancer, but have also been associated with a significant increase in cardiotoxicity [49,50]. Similar cardiotoxicity was not seen in Phase I and II studies when docetaxel was used in combination with doxorubicin, although the increased efficacy was maintained [51–54]. Based on the above studies, as well as Phase III trials in patients who had advanced breast cancer demonstrating increased efficacy with doxorubicin-docetaxel (AT) over AC [55] and with doxorubicin-docetaxel-cyclophosphamide (TAC) over 5-fluorouracil-doxorubicin-cyclophosphamide (FAC) [56], the NSABP B-30 study was designed to directly compare the sequential regimen of AC followed by docetaxel with the combination of doxorubicin plus docetaxel and with the triple combination of doxorubicin plus docetaxel plus cyclophosphamide. This trial was initiated in 1999 and has completed accrual in 2004 after accruing 5351 patients. Results from this trial are not yet available.

National Surgical Adjuvant Breast Project B-31

During the 1990s, a substantial amount of information accumulated in support of a significant role for the HER-2/neu oncogene in breast cancer as a therapeutic target for antibody development [57,58]. In the advanced disease setting, trastuzumab has activity as a single agent [59], and significantly increases the efficacy of chemotherapy in terms of response rates, time to progression, and overall survival [60]; however, this improvement was associated with a substantial increase in cardiac toxicity, particularly when an anthracycline-containing regimen was combined with trastuzumab. The NSABP B-31 trial was designed to evaluate the role of trastuzumab in the adjuvant setting. Results from the B-31 trial on the benefit of adjuvant trastuzumab in node-positive patients who had HER-2/neu-positive breast cancer represent one of the most exciting advances in the contemporary era of adjuvant clinical trials. The B-31 trial compared doxorubicin and cyclophosphamide followed by paclitaxel every 3 weeks with this same chemotherapy regimen plus 1 year of trastuzumab given concurrently with paclitaxel in node-positive, HER-2/neu positive patients. The North Central Cancer Treatment Group Trial N9831 conducted a similar trial that compared AC followed by weekly paclitaxel versus the same chemotherapy plus trastuzumab either concurrently with paclitaxel or sequentially for 1 year. The N9831 trial also randomized 191 high-risk/node-negative patients. Based on the similarities between the two trials, a decision was made to perform a joint analysis by combining the control arms and the concurrent trastuzumab arms from both trials. Interim analysis of the joined dataset lead to early disclosure of the results because of the magnitude of outcome difference in favor of adjuvant trastuzumab. The joined analysis revealed that with a median follow-up of 2 years, adjuvant trastuzumab reduced the risk of treatment failure by 52% (hazard ratio 0.48; $P < .0001$), and the risk of death by 33% ($P = .015$) [57]. In the B-31 study, cardiac-related events occurred in 4.1% of the patients in the trastuzumab arm compared with 0.8% of the patients in the control arm. Cases of congestive heart failure were more common among older patients, and among patients who had a decrease in ejection fraction following doxorubicin/paclitaxel chemotherapy [58].

National Surgical Adjuvant Breast Project trials of neoadjuvant chemotherapy

The establishment of lumpectomy as the surgical treatment of choice for the majority of patients who have operable breast cancer, and the demonstration of significant improvements in disease-free survival and overall survival with adjuvant systemic chemotherapy in patients who have positive as well as in those who have negative axillary nodes, have offered clinical justification for considering the use of systemic chemotherapy before surgical resection (preoperative or neoadjuvant chemotherapy). In addition, several preclinical and clinical observations have provided a biological rationale as to why such an intervention may have an advantage over the administration of chemotherapy in the conventional postoperative fashion [61–64]. Although several single-institution, nonrandomized clinical series evaluated preoperative chemotherapy in patients who had operable breast cancer, before such treatment could become standard clinical practice it had to be evaluated in prospective randomized clinical trials.

National Surgical Adjuvant Breast Project B-18

In 1988, the NSABP initiated Protocol B-18, a randomized trial in patients who had operable breast cancer that compared preoperative versus postoperative administration of adjuvant chemotherapy (four cycles of doxorubicin/cyclophosphamide) (Fig. 6) [65–68]. The primary aim of the study was to determine whether preoperative chemotherapy will more effectively prolong disease-free survival and overall survival than the same chemotherapy given postoperatively. Secondary aims of the study included the evaluation of clinical and pathologic response of primary breast cancer to preoperative chemotherapy, the determination of the down-staging effect of preoperative chemotherapy in the axillary nodes, and the determination of whether preoperative chemotherapy increases the rate of breast-conserving surgery. In addition, the study attempted to determine whether primary breast cancer response to preoperative chemotherapy correlates with disease-free survival and overall survival. Between October 1988 and April 1993, 1523 patients were accrued in to the trial. Results on the effect of preoperative chemotherapy on tumor response [65,66] indicate that following administration of preoperative chemotherapy, 36% of patients obtained

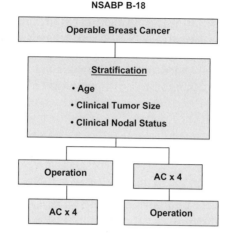

Fig. 6. Randomization schema for NSABP Protocol 18.

a clinical complete response and 43% of patients obtained a clinical partial response, for an overall response rate of 79%. More importantly, 13% of the patients achieved a pathologic complete response (absence of invasive tumor in the breast specimen following neoadjuvant chemotherapy). Administration of preoperative chemotherapy resulted in significant pathologic axillary lymph node down-staging in 37% of the patients presumed to be node-positive at the time of administration of preoperative chemotherapy. Patients receiving preoperative chemotherapy were significantly more likely to receive a lumpectomy than were patients receiving postoperative chemotherapy (67% versus 60%, $P = .002$). When the two treatment groups were compared in terms of outcome [67], there were no differences in disease-free survival, distant disease-free survival, or overall survival between the two groups. There was evidence of significant correlation between pathologic response of primary breast tumors to preoperative chemotherapy and disease-free and overall survival. Patients achieving a pathologic complete response (pCR) had a statistical significant improvement in disease-free survival and overall survival compared with those who had a clinical complete response but residual invasive carcinoma in the breast specimen (pINV) or those who had a clinical partial response (cPR) or a clinical nonresponse (cNR). When the prognostic effect of pCR was examined after adjusting for other known clinical prognostic factors such as clinical nodal status, clinical tumor size, and age, pCR remained a significant independent predictor for disease-free survival and a borderline significant predictor for overall survival. Recently updated outcome results from the B-18 study continue demonstrate that the equivalence between preoperative and postoperative chemotherapy and the significant correlation between pCR and outcome has persisted through 9 years of follow-up [68].

The B-18 Protocol also provided an opportunity to study patterns of loco-regional failure as a function of preoperative versus postoperative systemic therapy. At 9 years, the rate of ipsilateral breast tumor recurrence (IBTR) was slightly higher in the preoperative group (10.7% versus 7.6%), although this difference was not statistically significant [68]. Risk of local recurrence was somewhat higher in the subset of lumpectomy patients that were down-staged to become breast-conserving therapy (BCT)-eligible in comparison with the BCT patients who were BCT candidates at presentation [67]. This subset of down-staged BCT cases was predominantly comprised of T_3 tumors, however, and because local recurrence is an indication of underlying tumor biology, it would be expected that the more advanced stage lesions might have increased local recurrence rates, regardless of surgery type and treatment sequence. Also, radiation boost doses were not consistently used in the lumpectomy patients, and tamoxifen therapy was only used in patients over 50 years of age. Both of these interventions, if implemented uniformly, might have influenced local recurrence rates in down-staged tumors.

National Surgical Adjuvant Breast Project B-27

The results from the B-18 trial strengthened the biologic and clinical rationale for continuing to evaluate the role of preoperative chemotherapy in patients who have operable breast cancer (Fig. 7) [69–73]. The demonstration of significant antitumor activity with taxanes in patients who had advanced breast cancer provided the opportunity to take the results from the NSABP B-18 trial a step further. In 1995 the NSABP implemented Protocol B-27, a randomized trial that evaluated the worth of docetaxel when administered in the preoperative or the postoperative setting following four cycles of preoperative AC chemotherapy [70]. The main objective of the study was to determine whether the addition of four cycles of preoperative or postoperative docetaxel, following four cycles of preoperative AC, could more effectively prolong disease-free survival and overall survival in

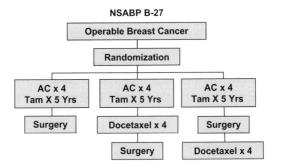

Fig. 7. Randomization schema for NSABP Protocol 27.

patients who had operable breast cancer than four cycles of preoperative AC alone. Secondary objectives were to determine whether the addition of preoperative docetaxel following preoperative AC could increase the rate of loco-regional response, pathologic complete response, pathologic axillary nodal down-staging, and breast-conserving surgery. Additional secondary objectives were to determine whether any benefit from the addition of postoperative docetaxel after preoperative AC might be limited to specific subgroups of patients; for example, those who have residual positive nodes after preoperative AC. The trial opened in December 1995 and closed in December 2000 after accruing 2411 patients.

Although the addition of preoperative docetaxel to preoperative AC significantly increased the rates of pCR in the breast (26.1% versus 13.7%; $P < .001$) and significantly decreased the rates of pathologically positive nodes, it did not significantly increase further the rate of breast conservation [71]. Furthermore, disease-free survival and overall survival were not significantly prolonged with the addition of preoperative or postoperative docetaxel [72]; however, achievement of pCR remained a significant independent predictor of improved outcome, thus validating the use of this endpoint as a surrogate marker for the effectiveness of systemic therapy agents.

Incidentally, the B-27 Protocol also provided a valuable opportunity to study the accuracy of lymphatic mapping and SLNB in women treated with neoadjuvant chemotherapy [73]. Although there was no specific protocol for lymphatic mapping as part of the study, 428 patients underwent SLNB followed by completion axillary lymph node dissection. The study authors reported that 89% of patients had successful mapping of the sentinel nodes (90% with radiocolloid alone, 77% with blue dye alone, and 88% with the combination of both tracers). The false-negative rate was 11%, and this is comparable to the false-negative rate observed in multicenter studies of sentinel node biopsy before systemic therapy.

Summary

This article has summarized the results from several of the pivotal NSABP breast cancer clinical trials, which in a step-wise fashion evaluated various loco-regional and systemic therapy questions in the management of patients who had operable breast cancer. Results from these trials have contributed to the reduction in the extent of surgery for invasive and non-invasive breast cancer, to the establishment of breast radiation as an effective method of controlling in-breast recurrence following lumpectomy, and more importantly, to significant improvements in overall survival with adjuvant systemic therapy. Recently conducted trials aimed to further reduce the extent of surgical resection in the breast and axilla by evaluating neoadjuvant chemotherapy and sentinel node biopsy, to optimize adjuvant chemotherapy and adjuvant hormonal therapy by evaluating taxanes, aromatase inhibitors, and molecular targeted therapies such as trastuzumab.

References

[1] Fisher B, Montague E, Redmond C, et al. Comparison of radical mastectomy with alternative treatments for primary breast cancer. A first report of results from a prospective randomized clinical trial. Cancer 1977;39(6 Suppl):2827–39.

[2] Fisher ER, Palekar A, Rockette H, et al. Pathologic findings from the National Surgical Adjuvant Breast Project (Protocol No. 4). V. Significance of axillary nodal micro- and macro-metastases. Cancer 1978;42(4):2032–8.

[3] Fisher ER, Palekar AS, Gregorio RM, et al. Pathological findings from the national surgical adjuvant breast project (Protocol No. 4). IV. Significance of tumor necrosis. Hum Pathol 1978;9(5):523–30.

[4] Fisher ER, Redmond C, Fisher B. Pathologic findings from the National Surgical Adjuvant Breast Project (Protocol No. 4). VI. Discriminants for five-year treatment failure. Cancer 1980;46(4 Suppl):908–18.

[5] Fisher B, Montague E, Redmond C, et al. Findings from NSABP Protocol No. B-04—comparison of radical mastectomy with alternative treatments for primary breast cancer. I. Radiation compliance and its relation to treatment outcome. Cancer 1980;46(1):1–13.

[6] Fisher B, Wolmark N, Redmond C, et al. Findings from NSABP Protocol No. B-04: comparison of radical mastectomy with alternative treatments. II. The clinical and biologic significance of medial-central breast cancers. Cancer 1981;48(8):1863–72.

[7] Fisher B, Redmond C, Fisher ER, et al. Ten-year results of a randomized clinical trial comparing radical mastectomy and total mastectomy with or without radiation. N Engl J Med 1985;312(11):674–81.

[8] Fisher B, Bauer M, Margolese R, et al. Five-year results of a randomized clinical trial comparing total mastectomy and segmental mastectomy with or without radiation in the treatment of breast cancer. N Engl J Med 1985;312(11):665–73.

[9] Fisher ER, Sass R, Fisher B, et al. Pathologic findings from the National Surgical Adjuvant Breast Project (Protocol 6). II. Relation of local breast recurrence to multicentricity. Cancer 1986;57(9):1717–24.

[10] Fisher B, Anderson S, Bryant J, et al. Twenty-year follow-up of a randomized trial comparing total mastectomy, lumpectomy, and lumpectomy plus irradiation for the treatment of invasive breast cancer. N Engl J Med 2002;347(16):1233–41.

[11] Veronesi U, Saccozzi R, Del Vecchio M, et al. Comparing radical mastectomy with quadrantectomy, axillary dissection, and radiotherapy in patients with small cancers of the breast. N Engl J Med 1981;305(1):6–11.

[12] Veronesi U, Cascinelli N, Mariani L, et al. Twenty-year follow-up of a randomized study comparing breast-conserving surgery with radical mastectomy for early breast cancer. N Engl J Med 2002;347(16):1227–32.

[13] Fisher B, Bryant J, Dignam JJ, et al. Tamoxifen, radiation therapy, or both for prevention of ipsilateral breast tumor recurrence after lumpectomy in women with invasive breast cancers of one centimeter or less. J Clin Oncol 2002;20(20):4141–9.

[14] Wickerham DL, Costantino JP, Mamounas EP, et al. The landmark surgical trials of the National Surgical Adjuvant Breast and Bowel Project. World J Surg 2006;30(7):1138–46.

[15] Julian T, Krag D, Brown A. Preliminary technical results of NSABP B-32, a randomized Phase III clinical trial to compare sentinel node resection to conventional axillary dissection in clinically-node-negative breast cancer patients. Abstract No. 14. Presented at the San Antonio breast cancer Symposium. San Antonio (TX); December 2004.

[16] Krag DN, Weaver DL, Alex JC, et al. Surgical resection and radiolocalization of the sentinel lymph node in breast cancer using a gamma probe. Surg Oncol 1993;2(6):335–9 [discussion: 340].

[17] Giuliano AE, Kirgan DM, Guenther JM, et al. Lymphatic mapping and sentinel lymphadenectomy for breast cancer. Ann Surg 1994;220(3):391–8 [discussion: 398–401].

[18] Kim T, Giuliano AE, Lyman GH. Lymphatic mapping and sentinel lymph node biopsy in early-stage breast carcinoma: a metaanalysis. Cancer 2006;106(1):4–16.

[19] Julian TB, Mamounas EP. Partial breast irradiation: continuing the retreat from Halstedian breast cancer management. Oncology Issues 2006;21(1):16–8.

[20] Ries L, Eisner M, Kosary CL, et al. SEER cancer statistics review, 1973–1999. Available at: http://seer.cancer.gov/csr/1973_1999/. Accessed March 1, 2007.

[21] Fisher B, Costantino J, Redmond C, et al. Lumpectomy compared with lumpectomy and radiation therapy for the treatment of intraductal breast cancer. N Engl J Med 1993;328(22):1581–6.

[22] Fisher B, Dignam J, Wolmark N, et al. Lumpectomy and radiation therapy for the treatment of intraductal breast cancer: findings from National Surgical Adjuvant Breast and Bowel Project B-17. J Clin Oncol 1998;16(2):441–52.

[23] Fisher ER, Dignam J, Tan-Chiu E, et al. Pathologic findings from the National Surgical Adjuvant Breast Project (NSABP) eight-year update of Protocol B-17: intraductal carcinoma. Cancer 1999;86(3):429–38.

[24] Fisher B, Land S, Mamounas E, et al. Prevention of invasive breast cancer in women with ductal carcinoma in situ: an update of the national surgical adjuvant breast and bowel project experience. Semin Oncol 2001;28(4):400–18.

[25] Fisher B, Dignam J, Wolmark N, et al. Tamoxifen in treatment of intraductal breast cancer: National Surgical Adjuvant Breast and Bowel Project B-24 randomised controlled trial. Lancet 1999;353(9169):1993–2000.

[26] Allred C, Bryant J, Land S, et al. Estrogen receptor expression as a predictive marker of the effectiveness of tamoxifen in the treatment of DCIS: findings from NSABP Protocol B-24 [abstract 30]. Breast Cancer Res Treat 2002;76:S36.

[27] Julian T, Land S, Wolmark N. NSABP B-35: a clinical trial to compare anastrazole and tamoxifen for postmenopausal patients with ductal carcinoma in situ undergoing lumpectomy with radiation therapy. Breast Diseases: A Yearbook Quarterly 2003;14,(2):121–2.

[28] Fisher B, Jeong JH, Dignam J, et al. Findings from recent National Surgical Adjuvant Breast and Bowel Project adjuvant studies in Stage I breast cancer. J Natl Cancer Inst Monogr 2001; 30:62–6.

[29] Fisher B, Redmond C, Dimitrov NV, et al. A randomized clinical trial evaluating sequential methotrexate and fluorouracil in the treatment of patients with node-negative breast cancer who have estrogen-receptor-negative tumors. N Engl J Med 1989;320(8):473–8.

[30] Fisher B, Dignam J, Mamounas EP, et al. Sequential methotrexate and fluorouracil for the treatment of node-negative breast cancer patients with estrogen receptor-negative tumors: eight-year results from National Surgical Adjuvant Breast and Bowel Project (NSABP) B-13 and first report of findings from NSABP B-19 comparing methotrexate and fluorouracil with conventional cyclophosphamide, methotrexate, and fluorouracil. J Clin Oncol 1996; 14(7):1982–92.

[31] Controlled trial of tamoxifen as single adjuvant agent in management of early breast cancer. Analysis at six years by Nolvadex Adjuvant Trial Organisation. Lancet 1985;1(8433): 836–40.

[32] Breast Cancer Trials Committee. Adjuvant tamoxifen in the management of operable breast cancer: the Scottish Trial. Report from the Breast Cancer Trials Committee, Scottish Cancer Trials Office (MRC), Edinburgh. Lancet 1987;2(8552):171–5.

[33] Baum M, Brinkley DM, Dossett JA, et al. Improved survival among patients treated with adjuvant tamoxifen after mastectomy for early breast cancer. Lancet 1983;2(8347):450.

[34] Fisher B, Anderson S, Tan-Chiu E, et al. Tamoxifen and chemotherapy for axillary node-negative, estrogen receptor-negative breast cancer: findings from National Surgical Adjuvant Breast and Bowel Project B-23. J Clin Oncol 2001;19(4):931–42.

[35] Fisher B, Costantino J, Redmond C, et al. A randomized clinical trial evaluating tamoxifen in the treatment of patients with node-negative breast cancer who have estrogen-receptor-positive tumors. N Engl J Med 1989;320(8):479–84.

[36] Swain S, Wilson J, Mamounas E, et al. Estrogen receptor (ER) status of primary breast cancaer is predictive of ER status of contralateral breast cancer (CBC) [abstract 150]. Proceedings of the American Society of Clinical Oncology 2002;21:38a.

[37] Fisher B, Dignam J, Bryant J, et al. Five versus more than five years of tamoxifen therapy for breast cancer patients with negative lymph nodes and estrogen receptor-positive tumors. J Natl Cancer Inst 1996;88(21):1529–42.

[38] Fisher B, Jeong JH, Bryant J, et al. Treatment of lymph-node-negative, oestrogen-receptor-positive breast cancer: long-term findings from National Surgical Adjuvant Breast and Bowel Project randomised clinical trials. Lancet 2004;364(9437):858–68.

[39] Fisher B, Dignam J, Bryant J, et al. Five versus more than five years of tamoxifen for lymph node-negative breast cancer: updated findings from the National Surgical Adjuvant Breast and Bowel Project B-14 randomized trial. J Natl Cancer Inst 2001;93(9):684–90.

[40] Fisher B, Dignam J, Wolmark N, et al. Tamoxifen and chemotherapy for lymph node-negative, estrogen receptor-positive breast cancer. J Natl Cancer Inst 1997;89(22):1673–82.

[41] Paik S, Shak S, Tang G, et al. A multigene assay to predict recurrence of tamoxifen-treated, node-negative breast cancer. N Engl J Med 2004;351(27):2817–26.

[42] Paik S, Shak S, Tang G, et al. Expression of the 21 genes in the Recurrence Score assay and tamoxifen clinical benefit in the NSABP study B-14 of node negative, estrogen receptor positive breast cancer [abstract 510]. J Clin Oncol 2005;23(16s):6s.

[43] Saphner T, Tormey DC, Gray R. Annual hazard rates of recurrence for breast cancer after primary therapy. J Clin Oncol 1996;14(10):2738–46.

[44] Mamounas E, Jeong JH, Wickerham L, et al. Benefit from exemestane (EXE) as extended adjuvant therapy after 5 years of tamoxifen (TAM): intent-to-treat analysis of NSABP B-33 [abstract 49]. Breast Cancer Res Treat 2006;100(Suppl 1):S22.

[45] Mamounas EP. Adjuvant exemestane therapy after 5 years of tamoxifen: rationale for the NSABP B-33 trial. Oncology (Williston Park) 2001;15(5 Suppl 7):35–9.

[46] Goss PE, Ingle JN, Martino S, et al. A randomized trial of letrozole in postmenopausal women after five years of tamoxifen therapy for early-stage breast cancer. N Engl J Med 2003;349(19):1793–802.

[47] Mamounas EP, Bryant J, Lembersky B, et al. Paclitaxel after doxorubicin plus cyclophosphamide as adjuvant chemotherapy for node-positive breast cancer: results from NSABP B-28. J Clin Oncol 2005;23(16):3686–96.

[48] Henderson IC, Berry DA, Demetri GD, et al. Improved outcomes from adding sequential paclitaxel but not from escalating doxorubicin dose in an adjuvant chemotherapy regimen for patients with node-positive primary breast cancer. J Clin Oncol 2003;21(6):976–83.

[49] Gianni L, Munzone E, Capri G, et al. Paclitaxel by 3-hour infusion in combination with bolus doxorubicin in women with untreated metastatic breast cancer: high antitumor efficacy and cardiac effects in a dose-finding and sequence-finding study. J Clin Oncol 1995;13(11):2688–99.

[50] Gehl J, Boesgaard M, Paaske T, et al. Combined doxorubicin and paclitaxel in advanced breast cancer: effective and cardiotoxic. Ann Oncol 1996;7(7):687–93.

[51] Dieras V. Docetaxel in combination with doxorubicin: a Phase I dose-finding study. Oncology (Williston Park) 1997;11(6 Suppl 6):17–20.

[52] Misset JL, Dieras V, Gruia G, et al. Dose-finding study of docetaxel and doxorubicin in first-line treatment of patients with metastatic breast cancer. Ann Oncol 1999;10,(5):553–60.

[53] Nabholtz JM, Mackey JR, Smylie M, et al. Phase II study of docetaxel, doxorubicin, and cyclophosphamide as first-line chemotherapy for metastatic breast cancer. J Clin Oncol 2001;19(2):314–21.

[54] Sparano JA, O'Neill A, Schaefer PL, et al. Phase II trial of doxorubicin and docetaxel plus granulocyte colony-stimulating factor in metastatic breast cancer: Eastern Cooperative Oncology Group Study E1196. J Clin Oncol 2000;18(12):2369–77.

[55] Nabholtz JM, Falkson CI, Campos D. Doxorubicin and docetaxel (AT) is superior to standard doxorubicin and cyclophosphamide (AC) as 1st line CT for MBC: randomized Phase III trial [abstract 485]. Breast Cancer Res Treat 1999;57:84.

[56] Mackey JR, Paterson A, Dirix LY, et al. Final results of the Phase III randomized trial comparing doxetaxel (T), doxorubicin (A) and cyclophosphamide (C) to FAC as first line chemotherapy (CT) for patients (pts) with metastatic breast cancer (MBC) [abstract 137]. Proceedings of the American Society of Clinical Oncology 2002;21:35a.

[57] Romond EH, Perez EA, Bryant J, et al. Trastuzumab plus adjuvant chemotherapy for operable HER2-positive breast cancer. N Engl J Med 2005;353(16):1673–84.

[58] Tan-Chiu E, Yothers G, Romond E, et al. Assessment of cardiac dysfunction in a randomized trial comparing doxorubicin and cyclophosphamide followed by paclitaxel, with or without trastuzumab as adjuvant therapy in node-positive, human epidermal growth factor receptor 2-overexpressing breast cancer: NSABP B-31. J Clin Oncol 2005; 23(31):7811–9.

[59] Cobleigh MA, Vogel CL, Tripathy D, et al. Efficacy and safety of Herceptin (humanized anti-Her2 antibody) as a single agent in 222 women with Her2 overexpression who relapsed following chemotherapy for metastatic breast cancer [abstract]. Proceedings of the American Society of Clinical Oncology 1998;17:97a.

[60] Slamon DJ, Leyland-Jones B, Shak S, et al. Use of chemotherapy plus a monoclonal antibody against HER2 for metastatic breast cancer that overexpresses HER2. N Engl J Med 2001;344(11):783–92.

[61] Skipper HE. Kinetics of mammary tumor cell growth and implications for therapy. Cancer 1971;28(6):1479–99.

[62] Goldie JH, Coldman AJ. A mathematic model for relating the drug sensitivity of tumors to their spontaneous mutation rate. Cancer Treat Rep 1979;63(11–12):1727–33.

[63] Gunduz N, Fisher B, Saffer EA. Effect of surgical removal on the growth and kinetics of residual tumor. Cancer Res 1979;39(10):3861–5.

[64] Fisher B, Gunduz N, Saffer EA. Influence of the interval between primary tumor removal and chemotherapy on kinetics and growth of metastases. Cancer Res 1983;43(4):1488–92.

[65] Fisher B, Rockette H, Robidoux A, et al. Effect of preoperative therapy for breast cancer (BC) on local-regional disease: first report of NSABP B-18 [abstract 57]. Proceedings of the American Society of Clinical Oncology 1994;13:64.

[66] Fisher B, Brown A, Mamounas E, et al. Effect of preoperative chemotherapy on local-regional disease in women with operable breast cancer: findings from National Surgical Adjuvant Breast and Bowel Project B-18. J Clin Oncol 1997;15(7):2483–93.

[67] Fisher B, Bryant J, Wolmark N, et al. Effect of preoperative chemotherapy on the outcome of women with operable breast cancer. J Clin Oncol 1998;16(8):2672–85.

[68] Wolmark N, Wang J, Mamounas E, et al. Preoperative chemotherapy in patients with operable breast cancer: nine-year results from National Surgical Adjuvant Breast and Bowel Project B-18. J Natl Cancer Inst Monogr 2001;30:96–102.

[69] Fisher B, Mamounas EP. Preoperative chemotherapy: a model for studying the biology and therapy of primary breast cancer. J Clin Oncol 1995;13(3):537–40.

[70] Mamounas EP. NSABP Protocol B-27. Preoperative doxorubicin plus cyclophosphamide followed by preoperative or postoperative docetaxel. Oncology (Williston Park) 1997;11(6 Suppl 6):37–40.

[71] Bear HD, Anderson S, Brown A, et al. The effect on tumor response of adding sequential preoperative docetaxel to preoperative doxorubicin and cyclophosphamide: preliminary results from National Surgical Adjuvant Breast and Bowel Project Protocol B-27. J Clin Oncol 2003;21(22):4165–74.

[72] Bear HD, Anderson S, Smith RE, et al. Sequential preoperative or postoperative docetaxel added to preoperative doxorubicin plus cyclophosphamide for operable breast cancer: National Surgical Adjuvant Breast and Bowel Project Protocol B-27. J Clin Oncol 2006;24(13): 2019–27.

[73] Mamounas EP, Brown A, Anderson S, et al. sentinel node biopsy after neoadjuvant chemotherapy in breast cancer: results from National Surgical Adjuvant Breast and Bowel Project Protocol B-27. J Clin Oncol 2005;23(12):2694–702.

ELSEVIER
SAUNDERS

SURGICAL
CLINICS OF
NORTH AMERICA

Surg Clin N Am 87 (2007) 307–316

Breast Cancer Risk Assessment and Risk Reduction

Lisa A. Newman, MD, MPH, FACS[a,*], Victor G. Vogel, MD, MHS, FACP[b]

[a]Breast Care Center, 1500 East Medical Center Drive, 3308 CGC, University
of Michigan, Ann Arbor, MI 48109, USA
[b]University of Pittsburgh Cancer Institute, Breast Cancer Prevention Program,
University of Pittsburgh School of Medicine, Magee-Womens Hospital, 300 Halket Street,
Room 3524 Pittsburgh, PA 15213-3180, USA

Until recently, the primary message of breast health awareness programs has been that early detection is a woman's best protection against breast cancer, because there was no way to prevent the disease. Currently, however, tamoxifen is approved by the Food and Drug Administration (FDA) for chemoprevention of breast cancer in high-risk women, and studies are underway to evaluate other medications that may decrease the risk of breast cancer. Data have also become available regarding the efficacy of surgical strategies to reduce breast cancer risk. Any prevention method, however, will have associated risk of complications or adverse effects, and determining the net risk/benefit ratio depends on the ability to quantify accurately a woman's baseline likelihood of developing breast cancer. This article reviews available methods for assessing and reducing risk breast cancer.

Breast cancer risk assessment

The most common means of estimating an individual woman's risk of developing breast cancer is by application of a statistical tool known as the Gail model. The Gail model was derived from data from an American Cancer Society study regarding feasibility of mammographic screening of the American female population, the Breast Cancer Detection and Demonstration Project (BCDDP). Breast cancer risk factors generated from a case control subset of BCDDP participants are combined with estimates of baseline risk

---

* Corresponding author.
E-mail address: lanewman@umich.edu (L.A. Newman).

0039-6109/07/$ - see front matter © 2007 Elsevier Inc. All rights reserved.
doi:10.1016/j.suc.2007.01.010   *surgical.theclinics.com*

generated from the Surveillance, Epidemiology, and End Results (SEER) program incidence data to compute individualized, absolute estimates of breast cancer risk [1]. Risk factor components of the Gail model include age at time of counseling, age at menarche, age at first live birth, history of prior breast biopsies, and first-degree relatives who have breast cancer.

The Gail model was modified for determination of eligibility to participate in the National Surgical Adjuvant Breast Project (NSABP) chemoprevention trials, and the modified version was made available as a Web-based program (http://www.nci.nih.gov/bcrisktool/). These modifications allowed for prediction of invasive breast cancer only; they accounted for risk related to history of atypical hyperplasia; and they included adjustments to predict risk in African American women [2]. Women aged 35 years and older were deemed eligible to participate in the first chemoprevention trial if they had a 5-year risk of at least 1.7%.

Model accuracy for predicting number of breast cancers detected in independent cohorts of white American women has been validated in studies of screened Texas women [3], the Nurses' Health Study [4,5], and the placebo arm of the NSABP's first Breast Cancer Prevention Trial (BCPT) [2]. Limitations of the Gail model (and its modifications) include the facts that it does not account for paternal cancer history or the extended family cancer history, and its uncertain validity for assessing risk in non-white American women. Although the model is well-suited for identifying cohorts of women who are appropriate to participate in a chemoprevention trial, its discriminatory accuracy at the individual level has been assessed as modest [5].

Alternative strategies for estimating breast cancer risk have therefore been explored, such as random periareolar fine-needle aspiration biopsy (RPFNA) [6,7], ductal lavage [8], mammographic density [9,10], and endogenous hormone levels [11–13]. RPFNAs have limited applicability because of the invasive nature, ductal lavage enjoyed limited popularity because of the specialized training and equipment required, and measurement of circulating hormones is associated with substantial interlaboratory variability in technology. Mammographic density, however, has recently generated substantial enthusiasm as a powerful feature that can be incorporated into accurate breast cancer statistical models, with improved discriminatory accuracy compared with the standard Gail model [14,15]. Unfortunately, however, mammographic density is not a standardized component of routine mammographic reporting [16].

Medical risk reduction with chemoprevention

The ability to manipulate hormonally breast tissue and thereby reduce proliferative changes that would otherwise evolve into cancer has been recognized over the past several decades. Women using tamoxifen for a unilateral breast cancer were seen to have a 47% lower risk of second primary/ contralateral breast cancer compared with breast cancer patients not treated with tamoxifen. These data motivated implementation of the first large-scale chemoprevention trial conducted in the United States, the NSABP P-1 study [17]. This was a prospective, placebo-controlled, randomized study of tamoxifen in 13,880 high-risk women. Eligibility criteria to participate in the P-1 study included aged least 60 years; a 5-year Gail model breast cancer risk estimate of more than 1.66%; and history of lobular carcinoma in situ (LCIS). After 54 months median follow-up, the trial was unblinded early because of the magnitude of difference in breast cancer incidence between the treated and control arms of the study, revealing that tamoxifen lowered breast cancer risk by 49%. It is therefore now considered standard of care to evaluate breast cancer risk factor information in women and to counsel high-risk women about the options of chemoprevention.

Unfortunately, however, making a commitment to 5 years of tamoxifen is not easy, because several potentially severe adverse reactions can be associated with this therapy. Tamoxifen's effects on estrogen receptors in the uterus, vascular system, and central nervous system increase risks of uterine cancer, thromboembolic phenomena (deep vein thrombosis and pulmonary emboli), and vasomotor symptoms (eg, hot flashes, night sweats), respectively. Partially offsetting these risks are tamoxifen's estrogen agonist effects on the skeletal system and lipid profile, resulting in a reduced incidence of osteoporosis and lower serum cholesterol levels. NSABP P-1 study participants in the premenopausal age range were relatively protected from adverse tamoxifen effects [17]; however, the safety of tamoxifen during fetal development has not been established, and chemoprevention with this agent is therefore contraindicated in women who are contemplating pregnancy. Otherwise, tamoxifen has a favorable risk-benefit ratio in high-risk premenopausal women.

Complicating the chemoprevention decision process further is the fact that tamoxifen will only reduce the incidence of estrogen receptor-positive tumors. Tamoxifen has no impact on the occurrence of estrogen receptor-negative disease, a potentially significant issue in counseling women who harbor mutations in one of the breast cancer susceptibility genes. Subset analysis of genetically-tested NSABP P-1 participants demonstrated that tamoxifen does not reduce breast cancer risk in BRCA1 gene mutation carriers; however, it does appear to offer some chemoprevention benefit in BRCA2 mutation carriers [18]. This is consistent with prior studies revealing that BRCA2 mutation-associated tumors are similar in histopathology to sporadic breast cancer, whereas BRCA1 cancers are more likely to be estrogen receptor-negative and aneuploid.

The ideal selective estrogen receptor modulator (SERM) would retain antiproliferative activity in the breast, but without subjecting the patient to the negative risks. Raloxifene is a SERM that is approved by the FDA for management of postmenopausal osteoporosis, and preliminary evidence from its use in this setting suggested that it would have similar activity as tamoxifen in breast cancer prevention, but with fewer adverse effects. The NSABP's second chemoprevention trial, the Study of Tamoxifen and Raloxifene (STAR), randomized more than 19,000 high-risk postmenopausal

Table 1
Phase III trials of breast cancer providing data on chemoprevention

Study	Primary chemoprevention study?	N	Eligibility criteria	Age range	Randomization	Intended treatment duration (years)	Median follow-up	Breast cancer hazard (95% confidence interval)
Royal Marsden [24,25]	Yes	2471	High risk, family history	30–70	Tam versus placebo	5–8	70 months	1.06 (0.7–1.7) tam versus placebo
NSABP P-01 [17,24]	Yes	13,388	≥1.67% 5-year risk LCIS Age >60 years	35–	Tam versus placebo	5	54.6 months	0.51 (0.39–0.66)
Italian Tamoxifen Study Group [24,26–28]	Yes	5408	S/p hysterectomy	35–70	Tam versus placebo	5	81.2 months	All: 0.75 (0.48–1.18) No HRT: 0.99 (0.59–1.68) HRT: 0.36 (0.14–0.91)
IBIS [24,29]	Yes	7139	RR >2	35–70	Tam versus placebo	5	50 months	0.68 (0.50–0.92)
Tamoxifen Chemoprevention Overview Analysis [24]	Yes, collective review	28,406	NA	NA	Tam versus placebo	NA	70.6×10^3 women years	0.62 (0.54–0.72)
MORE [24,30]	No	7705	Postmenopausal osteoporosis	Median 66.5	Raloxifene versus placebo	4	36 months	0.28 (0.17–0.46)
CORE [33]	Yes	5213	Postmenopausal osteoporosis	Mean 65.8	Raloxifene versus placebo	8	95 months	0.34 (0.18–0.66)
STAR [19,20,34]	Yes	19,747	Postmenopausal; ≥1.67% 5-year risk LCIS	Mean 58.5	Tam versus raloxifene	5	47 months	1.02 (0.82–1.28) Tam versus raloxifene; invasive breast cancer hazard

Study	Risk reduction	n	Population	Age	Comparison	Years	Follow-up	Hazard Ratio
Fenritimide/ 4-HPR [31]	Yes	1574	Early-stage unilateral breast cancer	28–67	4HPR versus placebo	7	97 months	Premenopausal: 0.66 (0.41–1.07) Postmenopausal: 1.32 (0.82–2.15)
Tamoxifen Adjuvant Therapy Overview Analysis [24,35]	No	14,170	Operable breast cancer	NA	Tam versus no adjuvant therapy	≥5 (average, 5 years)	60 months	0.54 (0.43–0.69)
ATAC [23]	No	9366	Postmenopausal, early-stage breast cancer	Mean 64 years	Anastrozole versus Tam versus Tam + anastrozole	5	33.3 months	0.42 (0.22–0.79)

The reader should note that the Royal Marsden Trial was designed statistically to develop pilot data for the IBIS trial. The Hazard Ratio for risk reduction in the ATAC Trial refers to reduction in risk of new contralateral primary breast cancer.

Abbreviations: ATAC, Anastrozole Alone or in Combination with Tamoxifen versus Tamoxifen Alone; CORE, Continuing Outcomes Relevant to Evista; HRT, hormone replacement therapy; IBIS, International Breast Cancer Intervention Study; MORE, Multiple Outcomes of Raloxifene Evaluation; Tam, tamoxifen; s/p, status post.

women to receive one of these two SERMs for 5 years. Premenopausal women were ineligible for STAR participation because of the absence of data on raloxifene's effects in young, ovulating women.

Results of the STAR trial were released recently [19,20], demonstrating comparable effectiveness for tamoxifen and raloxifene in preventing invasive breast cancer (incidence 4.3 per 1000 versus 4.4 per 1000; relative risk (RR) 1.02; 95% confidence interval [CI], 0.82–1.28). Surprisingly, women randomized to receive raloxifene had a slightly higher (but not statistically significant) incidence of ductal carcinoma in situ compared with the tamoxifen arm (2.11 per 1000 versus 1.51 per 1000; RR 1.40; 95% CI 0.98–2.00). The two study arms were similar in risk for ischemic heart disease, osteoporotic fractures, and stroke. Raloxifene was associated with less morbidity from thromboembolic phenomena and cataracts, and a trend for fewer uterine cancers was also observed in the raloxifene arm. A quality-of-life analysis revealed low symptom severity in both study arms, but slight increases in vasomotor symptoms, leg cramps, and bladder problems were reported in the tamoxifen arm [21].

One theory of breast carcinogenesis proposes that risk of malignant transformation is related to lifetime exposure of breast tissue to cyclic extremes in the levels of circulating hormones. Accordingly, it is postulated that stabilization of estrogen levels will decrease the incidence of mammary neoplasia. Studies of gonadotropin-releasing hormone agonists in conjunction with low-dose hormone replacement therapy are therefore underway as a means of testing this hypothesis, and preliminary results have shown that this approach can successfully decrease mammographic density [22]; however, longer follow-up is needed to evaluate actual chemoprevention efficacy.

Recent data on the efficacy of aromatase inhibitors for adjuvant therapy in breast cancer have revealed that these agents also possess significant chemoprevention activity [23]. Table 1 [17,23–35] summarizes reported data on the risk-reducing strength of various medical therapies.

Surgical risk reduction with prophylactic oophorectomy or prophylactic mastectomy

Premenopausal prophylactic oophorectomy and prophylactic mastectomy are additional options as surgical strategies for breast cancer risk reduction. Surgical menopause before age 35 years is an established protective factor against breast cancer risk. Availability of BRCA testing has resulted in the identification of women from hereditary breast-ovarian cancer families, and these women are especially motivated to consider prophylactic removal of the ovaries. Published case-control data (Level II evidence) by Rebbeck and colleagues [36] and Kauff and colleagues [37] have confirmed that prophylactic oophorectomy in this setting can decrease breast cancer incidence by approximately 50%. Premature menopause, however, is associated with an increased risk of osteoporosis and atherosclerotic cardiovascular disease. Interestingly, the breast cancer protection afforded by prophylactic oophorectomy was not diminished by hormone replacement therapy in the Rebbeck and colleagues [36] study.

Prophylactic mastectomy is a dramatic and extreme maneuver to decrease breast cancer risk, yet only recently has its efficacy in high-risk women been documented. Early reports of prophylactic mastectomy in humans [38,39] demonstrated a 1% to 2% failure rate, but these studies were flawed by limited follow-up, and by the inclusion of many women who were probably at low-risk for developing breast cancer. Women at risk for hereditary breast cancer would potentially be most susceptible to a failed prophylactic mastectomy, as in these cases any microscopic amount of residual breast tissue would harbor the germ line predisposition for malignant transformation.

Hartmann and colleagues [40], have made valuable contributions to our understanding of the efficacy of prophylactic mastectomy through their meticulous scrutiny of the Mayo Clinic database. This analysis yielded 639 prophylactic mastectomy patients who had documented increased risk on the basis of family history of breast or ovarian cancer. These high-risk patients were further stratified into very high-risk (214 patients) and moderately high-risk (425 patients) subsets based on extent of family history. Outcome regarding number of subsequent breast cancers occurring among the very-high-risk subset was compared with the number of breast cancers developing among the female siblings of these patients. For the moderate-risk patients, efficacy of the prophylactic surgery was evaluated by calculating the number of expected cancers based on summing of the individual Gail model risk estimates for the entire group. Survival analyses were performed by projecting anticipated longevity based on population-based data. With a median follow-up of approximately 14 years, seven breast cancers were detected in the prophylactic mastectomy patients (three in the very-high risk subset and four in the moderate-risk subset) consistent with a 90% reduction in breast cancer risk and mortality in both categories of high-risk patients.

Subsequent study of the Hartmann database [41] reported results of prophylactic mastectomy in women who were also found to be BRCA mutation carriers, and confirmed an equivalent magnitude of breast cancer risk reduction. Similarly, Meijers-Heijboer and colleagues [42] reported outcome for 76 BRCA-mutation carriers followed prospectively after having undergone prophylactic mastectomy, and found no tumors developing with an average follow-up of nearly 3 years. Hence, reliable evidence does indicate that prophylactic mastectomy will effectively and substantially reduce the incidence of breast cancer in high-risk women, although the protection conferred is not complete.

Summary

Options for breast cancer risk assessment continue to evolve, and risk reduction strategies are expanding as well. Breast cancer screening and diagnostic work-up for abnormalities should always be prioritized, but healthy women also deserve to receive appropriate counseling regarding their level of risk for breast cancer. Referral to genetic counseling services or to a breast specialist with expertise in chemoprevention should be provided as necessary.

References

[1] Gail MH, Brinton LA, Byar DP, et al. Projecting individualized probabilities of developing breast cancer for white females who are being examined annually. J Natl Cancer Inst 1989; 81(24):1879–86.

[2] Costantino JP, Gail MH, Pee D, et al. Validation studies for models projecting the risk of invasive and total breast cancer incidence. J Natl Cancer Inst 1999;91(18):1541–8.

[3] Bondy ML, Lustbader ED, Halabi S, et al. Validation of a breast cancer risk assessment model in women with a positive family history. J Natl Cancer Inst 1994;86(8):620–5.

[4] Spiegelman D, Colditz GA, Hunter D, et al. Validation of the Gail et al. model for predicting individual breast cancer risk. J Natl Cancer Inst 1994;86(8):600–7.

[5] Rockhill B, Spiegelman D, Byrne C, et al. Validation of the Gail et al. model of breast cancer risk prediction and implications for chemoprevention. J Natl Cancer Inst 2001;93(5): 358–66.

[6] Fabian CJ, Kimler BF, Zalles CM, et al. Short-term breast cancer prediction by random peri-areolar fine-needle aspiration cytology and the Gail risk model. J Natl Cancer Inst 2000; 92(15):1217–27.

[7] Fabian C. Benign breast tissue sampling for prevention studies. Breast J 2000;6(4):215–9.

[8] Dooley WC, Ljung BM, Veronesi U, et al. Ductal lavage for detection of cellular atypia in women at high risk for breast cancer. J Natl Cancer Inst 2001;93(21):1624–32.

[9] Boyd NF, Lockwood GA, Martin LJ, et al. Mammographic densities and risk of breast cancer among subjects with a family history of this disease. J Natl Cancer Inst 1999;91(16): 1404–8.

[10] Boyd NF, Rommens JM, Vogt K, et al. Mammographic breast density as an intermediate phenotype for breast cancer. Lancet Oncol 2005;6(10):798–808.

[11] Key T, Appleby P, Barnes I, et al. Endogenous sex hormones and breast cancer in post-menopausal women: reanalysis of nine prospective studies. J Natl Cancer Inst 2002;94(8): 606–16.

[12] Cauley JA, Lucas FL, Kuller LH, et al. Elevated serum estradiol and testosterone concentrations are associated with a high risk for breast cancer. Study of Osteoporotic Fractures Research Group. Ann Intern Med 1999;130(4 Pt 1):270–7.

[13] Cummings SR, Lee JS, Lui LY, et al. Sex hormones, risk factors, and risk of estrogen receptor-positive breast cancer in older women: a long-term prospective study. Cancer Epidemiol Biomarkers Prev 2005;14(5):1047–51.

[14] Chen J, Pee D, Ayyagari R, et al. Projecting absolute invasive breast cancer risk in white women with a model that includes mammographic density. J Natl Cancer Inst 2006; 98(17):1215–26.

[15] Barlow WE, White E, Ballard-Barbash R, et al. Prospective breast cancer risk prediction model for women undergoing screening mammography. J Natl Cancer Inst 2006;98(17): 1204–14.

[16] Bondy ML, Newman LA. Assessing breast cancer risk: evolution of the Gail model. J Natl Cancer Inst 2006;98(17):1172–3.

[17] Fisher B, Costantino JP, Wickerham DL, et al. Tamoxifen for prevention of breast cancer: report of the National Surgical Adjuvant Breast and Bowel Project P-1 Study. J Natl Cancer Inst 1998;90(18):1371–88.

[18] King MC, Wieand S, Hale K, et al. Tamoxifen and breast cancer incidence among women with inherited mutations in BRCA1 and BRCA2: National Surgical Adjuvant Breast and Bowel Project (NSABP-P1) Breast Cancer Prevention Trial. JAMA 2001;286(18):2251–6.

[19] Vogel VG, Costantino JP, Wickerham DL, et al. Effects of tamoxifen vs raloxifene on the risk of developing invasive breast cancer and other disease outcomes: the NSABP Study of Tamoxifen and Raloxifene (STAR) P-2 trial. JAMA 2006;295(23):2727–41.

[20] Land SR, Wickerham DL, Costantino JP, et al. Patient-reported symptoms and quality of life during treatment with tamoxifen or raloxifene for breast cancer prevention: the NSABP Study of Tamoxifen and Raloxifene (STAR) P-2 trial. JAMA 2006;295(23):2742–51.

[21] Land S. Quality-of-life valuations of advanced breast cancer by New Zealand women. Pharmacoeconomics 2006;24(4):415–6 [author reply: 416–7].

[22] Gram IT, Ursin G, Spicer DV, et al. Reversal of gonadotropin-releasing hormone agonist induced reductions in mammographic densities on stopping treatment. Cancer Epidemiol Biomarkers Prev 2001;10(11):1117–20.

[23] Baum M, Budzar AU, Cuzick J, et al. Anastrozole alone or in combination with tamoxifen versus tamoxifen alone for adjuvant treatment of postmenopausal women with early breast cancer: first results of the ATAC randomised trial. Lancet 2002;359(9324):2131–9.

[24] Cuzick J, Powles T, Veronesi U, et al. Overview of the main outcomes in breast-cancer prevention trials. Lancet 2003;361(9354):296–300.

[25] Powles T, Eeles R, Ashley S, et al. Interim analysis of the incidence of breast cancer in the Royal Marsden Hospital tamoxifen randomised chemoprevention trial. Lancet 1998; 352(9122):98–101.

[26] Veronesi U, Maisonneuve P, Rotmensz N, et al. Italian randomized trial among women with hysterectomy: tamoxifen and hormone-dependent breast cancer in high-risk women. J Natl Cancer Inst 2003;95(2):160–5.

[27] Veronesi U, Maisonneuve P, Sacchini V, et al. Tamoxifen for breast cancer among hysterectomised women. Lancet 2002;359(9312):1122–4.

[28] Veronesi U, Maisonneuve P, Costa A, et al. Prevention of breast cancer with tamoxifen: preliminary findings from the Italian randomised trial among hysterectomised women. Italian Tamoxifen Prevention Study. Lancet 1998;352(9122):93–7.

[29] First results from the International Breast Cancer Intervention Study (IBIS-I): a randomised prevention trial. Lancet 2002;360(9336):817–24.

[30] Cauley JA, Norton L, Lippman ME, et al. Continued breast cancer risk reduction in postmenopausal women treated with raloxifene: 4-year results from the MORE trial. Multiple Outcomes of Raloxifene Evaluation. Breast Cancer Res Treat 2001;65(2):125–34.

[31] Veronesi U, De Palo G, Marubini E, et al. Randomized trial of fenretinide to prevent second breast malignancy in women with early breast cancer. J Natl Cancer Inst 1999;91(21): 1847–56.

[32] Nagata C, Takatsuka N, Inaba S, et al. Effect of soymilk consumption on serum estrogen concentrations in premenopausal Japanese women. J Natl Cancer Inst 1998;90(23): 1830–5.

[33] Martino S, Cauley JA, Barrett-Connor E, et al. Continuing outcomes relevant to Evista: breast cancer incidence in postmenopausal osteoporotic women in a randomized trial of raloxifene. J Natl Cancer Inst 2004;96(23):1751–61.

[34] Vogel VG, Costantino JP, Wickerham DL, et al. The study of tamoxifen and raloxifene: preliminary enrollment data from a randomized breast cancer risk reduction trial. Clin Breast Cancer 2002;3(2):153–9.

[35] Tamoxifen for early breast cancer: an overview of the randomised trials. Early Breast Cancer Trialists' Collaborative Group. Lancet 1998;351(9114):1451–67.

[36] Rebbeck TR, Levin AM, Eisen A, et al. Breast cancer risk after bilateral prophylactic oophorectomy in BRCA1 mutation carriers. J Natl Cancer Inst 1999;91(17):1475–9.

[37] Kauff ND, Satagopan JM, Robson ME, et al. Risk-reducing salpingo-oophorectomy in women with a BRCA1 or BRCA2 mutation. N Engl J Med 2002;346(21):1609–15.

[38] Pennisi VR, Capozzi A. Subcutaneous mastectomy data: a final statistical analysis of 1500 patients. Aesthetic Plast Surg 1989;13(1):15–21.

[39] Woods JE, Meland NB. Conservative management in full-thickness nipple-areolar necrosis after subcutaneous mastectomy. Plast Reconstr Surg 1989;84(2):258–64 [discussion: 265–6].

[40] Hartmann LC, Schaid DJ, Woods JE, et al. Efficacy of bilateral prophylactic mastectomy in women with a family history of breast cancer. N Engl J Med 1999;340(2):77–84.

[41] Hartmann LC, Sellers TA, Schaid DJ, et al. Efficacy of bilateral prophylactic mastectomy in BRCA1 and BRCA2 gene mutation carriers. J Natl Cancer Inst 2001;93(21):1633–7.

[42] Meijers-Heijboer H, van Geel B, van Putten WL, et al. Breast cancer after prophylactic bilateral mastectomy in women with a BRCA1 or BRCA2 mutation. N Engl J Med 2001; 345(3):159–64.

ELSEVIER
SAUNDERS

SURGICAL
CLINICS OF
NORTH AMERICA

Surg Clin N Am 87 (2007) 317–331

Prophylactic Mastectomy

Shaheen Zakaria, MD, Amy C. Degnim, MD*

*Department of Surgery, Mayo Clinic and Mayo Foundation, Mayo Clinic College
of Medicine, 200 First Street SW, Rochester, MN 55905, USA*

With availability of genetic testing and development of statistical models for risk stratification, more women are being identified as having an increased risk for breast cancer. A number of risk-reducing treatment options with varying efficacy exist for such women. These include frequent surveillance with clinical examination and imaging, chemoprevention, prophylactic salpingo-oophorectomy (PSO), and prophylactic mastectomy (PM). The individuals most likely to benefit from PM are BRCA gene carriers and those who have a strong family history of breast cancer. Women who have a personal history of breast cancer are also at higher risk for developing a second primary in the contralateral breast and may pursue contralateral prophylactic mastectomy (CPM) as a preventive option. High-risk women who have no personal history of breast cancer may also consider bilateral prophylactic mastectomy (BPM). As a preventive measure, however, PM remains controversial. There are no randomized controlled trials to substantiate the potential benefit or harms of PM. Because PM is an irreversible procedure, both providers and patients must understand its consequences, current evidence for its benefits, limitations, and available alternatives. This article describes the high-risk women in whom PM may be considered, and summarizes data on the efficacy of PM as a treatment for the prevention of breast cancer.

Cancer risk assessment and patient selection

As a preventive measure, PM will achieve maximal absolute risk reduction in women at highest risk for breast cancer. The average lifetime risk of breast cancer for women in the United States is 12.7% with a lifespan of 85 years; the risk is greatest after the sixth decade of life [1]. Most women tend to overestimate their risk of developing breast cancer [2]. Therefore,

---

* Corresponding author.
E-mail address: degnim.amy@mayo.edu (A.C. Degnim).

doi:10.1016/j.suc.2007.01.009
surgical.theclinics.com

providing realistic risk estimates can help women to make informed decisions regarding risk reduction. Although the commonly used Gail model is accurate for predicting breast cancer incidence in populations of women, it does not incorporate information on family history and has limited accuracy of risk prediction in individuals [3]. Despite the lack of a single accurate breast cancer risk prediction model for individualized risk prediction, some high-risk subgroups are identifiable.

In contrast to women of average risk, individuals who have deleterious mutations of BRCA1 or BRCA2 genes are a special subset of women who have strongly elevated risks of developing breast cancer. A recent meta-analysis revealed average cumulative breast cancer risks of 65% and 45% in BRCA1 and BRCA2 mutation carriers by age 70 years, respectively (Fig. 1) [4]. These individuals are also at a higher risk of developing ovarian cancer, with a 40% lifetime risk for BRCA1 and 20% for BRCA2 carriers. Some women who have a strong family history do not undergo BRCA

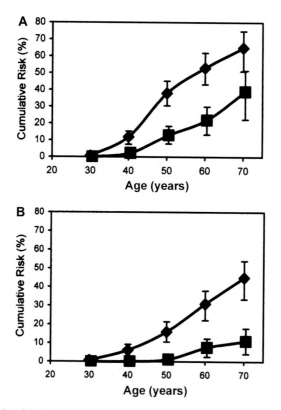

Fig. 1. Cumulative risk of breast (◆) and ovarian (■) cancer in (A) BRCA1-mutation carriers and (B) BRCA2-mutation carriers. (*Adapted from* Antoniou A, Pharoah PD, Narod S, et al. Average risk of breast and ovarian cancer associated with BRCA1 or BRCA2 mutations detected in case series unselected for family history: a combined analysis of 22 studies. Am J Hum Genet 2003;72(5):1124; with permission.)

testing or may test negative for deleterious mutations, however. For such individuals who have a strong family history of breast cancer, Claus tables can provide estimates of breast cancer risk [5].

A personal history of breast cancer is a long-established risk factor for development of a new primary breast cancer [6]. Long term follow-up studies in women who have Stage I and II breast cancer report a contralateral breast cancer risk of approximately 1% per year, with a cumulative risk of 17% at 20 years after diagnosis of the first breast cancer [7,8]. The risk of a second breast cancer is much higher in women who have a strong family history of breast cancer—up to 35% by 16 years after the diagnosis of index cancer [9]. In women who have BRCA1 and BRCA2 mutations, the risk of contralateral breast cancer is dramatically high—12% to 31% at 5 years after the primary cancer diagnosis [10–12], and it reached 39% at 15 years in a study of BRCA carriers who underwent breast-conserving treatment [13].

Other variables associated with an increased risk of contralateral breast cancer include family history [7,14], multicentric primary breast cancer [15], history of radiation therapy for the first breast cancer [16], lobular neoplasia [17,18], and additional ipsilateral high-risk pathology [19]. The relationship of age at diagnosis and risk of contralateral breast cancer is unclear, with two studies demonstrating increased risk in young women [17,20] and one study demonstrating the opposite [19]. Patients newly diagnosed with breast cancer who present with these features are at higher risk for developing cancer in the contralateral breast, and CPM is a reasonable consideration in these patients.

Factors associated with a generalized increased risk of breast cancer (albeit a lower absolute risk than the groups described above) include lobular carcinoma in situ (LCIS), atypical hyperplasia, and increased breast density. Atypical hyperplasia found at surgical breast biopsy (preferably confirmed by a breast pathologist) is associated with a relative breast cancer risk of fourfold to fivefold compared with the general population in retrospectively studied cohorts [21]. Women who have dense, fibroglandular breasts that are mammographically and clinically hard to evaluate present a challenge for clinical evaluation and breast cancer detection. Increasing mammographic breast density is associated with increasing risk of breast cancer [22], as well as identification of interval cancers [23]. Thus women who have dense breast tissue and high-risk histology or a family history of breast cancer may wish to undergo PM because of concerns of inadequate detection with the use of standard imaging modalities.

Efficacy of prophylactic mastectomy

Women who elect bilateral and contralateral PM are different in their characteristics and goals for risk reduction surgery. The efficacy of these two preventive procedures will therefore be discussed separately.

Impact of bilateral prophylactic mastectomy on breast cancer incidence

In BRCA carriers, three studies confirm that BPM reduces the incidence of breast cancer. Meijers-Heijboer and colleagues [24] conducted a prospective study of 139 BRCA1 or BRCA2 mutation carriers. Seventy-six women underwent BPM, and 63 remained under close surveillance. No breast cancers developed (a 100% reduction) in the BPM group with a mean follow-up of 2.9 years; however, the risk reduction effect of BPM in this study cannot be isolated from the risk-reducing effect of prophylactic salpingo-oophorectomy (PSO), which also has proven risk-reducing effect (described below under "Risk reduction alternatives to prophylactic mastectomy"). In the Meijers-Heijboers study, a statistically greater proportion of women in the BPM group underwent premenopausal PSO (58%) compared with those in the surveillance group (38%).

Hartmann and colleagues [25] reported no breast cancers at a median follow-up of 13.4 years in 26 women who had BRCA mutations who underwent BPM. Using various statistical models, the relative risk reduction attributed to BPM was estimated as 85% to 100%. In the more recent Prevention and Observation of Surgical Endpoints (PROSE) study of Rebbeck and colleagues [26], 105 BRCA carriers were followed prospectively after BPM and compared with 378 matched BRCA controls who did not have the procedure. With mean follow-up of 6.4 years, breast cancer was diagnosed in two (1.9%) of those who had BPM versus 184 (48.7%) of those who did not. Cases and controls in this study were matched based on PSO, with a relative breast cancer risk reduction of 95% in those who had PSO and 90% in those who had intact ovaries. Taken together, these studies confirm a 90% to 95% reduction in breast cancer risk after BPM in BRCA carriers.

Several studies provide evidence on the efficacy of BPM for high-risk women regardless of BRCA status. Hartmann and colleagues [27] retrospectively studied BPM among high-risk women based on a positive family history of breast cancer. In their cohort of 639 women from 1960 to 1993, 90% underwent bilateral subcutaneous mastectomy with preservation of the nipple-areolar complex (NAC), whereas it was removed in the remaining 10%. The cohort was divided into high- and moderate-risk groups, and the incidence of breast cancer in these groups was compared with that of a control group consisting of their female siblings who did not undergo BPM [27]. With a median follow-up of 14 years, the incidence of breast cancer was reduced 90% to 94% in the high-risk group and 90% in the moderate-risk group. There was no statistically significant difference in breast cancer incidence based on preservation or removal of the NAC. The efficacy of BPM in community practices was evaluated in a population-based study by Geiger and colleagues [28]. In this retrospective case-cohort study, BPM reduced breast cancer risk by 95%, although the absolute risk of breast cancer in the control population was low (4%). Borgen and colleagues [29] also reported effective risk reduction from BPM, with less than 1% incidence of breast cancer at 14.8 years mean follow-up in 370 women who underwent BPM.

Despite these dramatic reductions in breast cancer incidence after BPM, it is important that both physicians and patients understand that breast cancers can occur after risk reduction surgery. Numerous case reports in the literature add to the small failure rates described above, with intervals to cancer diagnosis ranging from 3 to 42 years after surgery [30–35]. Women considering prophylactic mastectomy must be informed clearly about the persistent long-term possibility of developing breast cancer after PM.

Impact of bilateral prophylactic mastectomy on survival

There are no data confirming an overall survival benefit in patients undergoing BPM for cancer prevention compared with similar risk individuals who do not. Although the studies on BPM in BRCA carriers clearly show reductions in breast cancer occurrence, there is no prospective clinical evidence yet that confirms a statistically significant overall survival advantage attributable to this procedure. Among women who had a family history but unknown BRCA status, the study of Hartmann and colleagues [27] demonstrated reductions in disease-specific mortality after BPM, with an 81% to 94% reduction in mortality from breast cancer for the high-risk group, and 100% reduction in breast cancer mortality for the moderate-risk group.

Despite the very high lifetime breast cancer risk in BRCA carriers, with modern detection methods and successful treatments for breast cancer it is reasonable to question whether breast cancer prevention actually translates into improved survival. In 1997, Schrag and colleagues [36] used theoretical modeling to estimate survival gains in BRCA carriers undergoing risk reduction surgery. The authors calculated that on average, a 30-year old BRCA1 or BRCA2 mutation carrier would gain 2.9 to 5.3 years of life expectancy from PM and from 0.3 to 1.7 years from PSO. More recently, a similar analysis by Grann and colleagues [37] also reported survival gains of 3.5 years for prophylactic mastectomy and 4.9 years with both BPM and PSO. In both studies, gains in life expectancy declined with age and were minimal for women over 60 years of age (Fig. 2). The preponderance of evidence from the prospective clinical cohorts and theoretical modeling described above suggest that in BRCA carriers, BPM reduces the incidence of breast cancer and likely improves longevity.

Surgical morbidity of bilateral prophylactic mastectomy

The frequency of surgical complications after BPM ranges from 30% to 64%, and is more common after simultaneous reconstruction with BPM [38–40]. The most common complications include pain (35%), infection (17%), and seroma formation (17%) [40]. Zion and colleagues [41] evaluated physical morbidity in terms of unanticipated reoperations following BPM and reconstruction. In that review, 49% of patients required second

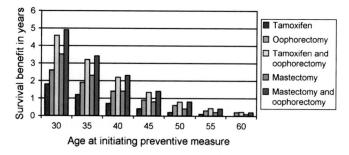

Fig. 2. Effects of timing on benefits of preventive measures, survival. (*Adapted from* Grann VR, Jacobson JS, Thomason D, et al. Effect of prevention strategies on survival and quality-adjusted survival of women with BRCA1/2 mutations: an updated decision analysis. J Clin Oncol 2002;20:2525; with permission.)

operations for one of the following reasons: implant related issues (46%), implant removal (37%), aesthetic concerns (32%), and immediate postoperative complications (22%).

Quality of life after bilateral prophylactic mastectomy

Psychosocial outcomes have been evaluated in patients choosing BPM, including satisfaction with decision, cosmesis, psychological well- being, and issues concerning body image and sexuality; however, there are no studies comparing satisfaction with decision between women who choose BPM and those who undergo close surveillance. Only a small minority of women, approximately 5%, have been dissatisfied with their decision to undergo BPM [29]. The feeling of dissatisfaction was more common among women reporting physician's advice as the primary reason for BPM [29,42]. Dissatisfaction with cosmetic outcomes has been reported in 16% to 40% of patients, mostly pertaining to dissatisfaction with reconstruction [29,42–44]. Cancer-related anxiety, body image concerns, and sexuality are all associated with satisfaction or regret regarding the surgery itself [29,42,45]. On the other hand, women who forego reconstruction following BPM have high levels of satisfaction [42]. Overall, the quality of life among women undergoing BPM appears slightly better than the general population based on Quality of Life Index (QLI) scores [46]. These unexpected results likely reflect the characteristics of women who choose to undergo this preventive surgery rather than an effect of the surgical procedure.

Impact of contralateral prophylactic mastectomy on breast cancer incidence

Similar to BPM, multiple studies have demonstrated a reduction in breast cancer incidence after CPM for both BRCA carriers and other women. Van Sprundel and colleagues [47] retrospectively evaluated 148 BRCA1/2 carriers previously treated for unilateral invasive breast cancer Stages I-IIIA.

In 79 women who underwent CPM, only 1 developed an invasive contralateral breast cancer at mean follow-up of 3.5 years, compared with 6 out of 69 in the surveillance group ($P < .001$). Furthermore, the 91% reduction in contralateral breast cancer was independent of the effect of PSO. Several other studies address incidence of breast cancer after CPM in otherwise high-risk women. McDonnell and colleagues [48] reported a 94% to 96% reduction in breast cancer at a median follow-up of 10 years in 745 women with a first breast cancer and family history of breast or ovarian cancer. In a case control study with 15 years of follow-up, CPM decreased the rate of contralateral breast cancer—4.5% of those treated with CPM versus 27% in controls ($P < .005$) [49]. Finally, a recent retrospective cohort study demonstrated a hazard ratio of 0.03 for contralateral breast cancer in women who underwent CPM [50]. Similar to the data in BPM, the results described here strongly support a dramatic risk reduction in contralateral breast cancer after CPM.

Impact of contralateral prophylactic mastectomy on survival

Despite the reduction in breast cancer occurrences seen after CPM, demonstrating an overall survival advantage for CPM remains as elusive as it is in the setting of BPM. The risk of death from the primary breast cancer is generally higher than that from a second cancer [7,8]; a second cancer is usually early-stage at the time of detection because of close surveillance. This principle is challenged by a recent report that 30% of contralateral breast cancers are node-positive at detection despite close follow-up [49]. In the van Sprundel and coworkers study [47] described above, CPM had no significant effect on overall survival in BRCA1/2 carriers by multivariate analysis adjusting for oophorectomy (known to reduce breast cancer risk by approximately 50%—see "Risk reduction alternatives to prophylactic mastectomy" below). A more recent study of outcomes in an expanded group of the BRCA1 patients treated for breast cancer also showed no survival benefit of CPM [51].

Considering the very high risk of contralateral breast cancer in BRCA patients (in whom a survival advantage of CPM should be greatest), it is somewhat surprising that two studies not limited to BRCA carriers have shown survival advantages for CPM that were not evident in BRCA carriers [49,50]. In the case-control study of Peralta and colleagues [49], CPM resulted in a statistically significant improvement in disease-free survival; overall survival favored the CPM group, but the difference was not statistically significant. These investigators also evaluated disease-specific survival (whether CPM prevented death from breast cancer), stratified by stage. As one might expect, survival was improved for early stage (0–II) patients, although this did not quite meet statistical significance ($P = .06$). Herrinton and colleagues [50] also reported statistically significant improvements in disease-specific survival and overall survival in women who had CPM compared with those who did not.

In the special subgroup of patients who have invasive lobular cancers, two studies evaluated the effect of CPM on survival. In a retrospectively studied cohort of 419 women who had invasive lobular cancer and mean follow-up of 6 years, patients who underwent CPM had a better prognosis than those with unilateral mastectomy [52], but this association may merely reflect the selection of patients who had better overall prognosis from their primary cancer for a contralateral risk-reducing operation. In a comparable study by Babiera and colleagues [53], however, no overall survival advantage was reported at 5 years follow-up for patients who had invasive lobular cancer and who underwent CPM.

Whether the reported possible survival benefits of CPM are attributable to the procedure remains uncertain. The analyses were not uniformly adjusted for adjuvant treatments and other prognostic factors that would be expected to impact survival. Because of the retrospective nature of these studies, they are subject to selection bias [54]. Only the study of Peralta and colleagues [49] controlled for prognostic factors in assessing effects of CPM on survival. Their finding that CPM is associated with improved disease-specific survival in lower-stage patients fits with the following reasoning: prognosis is primarily determined by the stage of the index tumor [17,20], and breast cancer patients who have better-prognosis tumors and a high risk of a second cancer are the most likely to benefit from CPM. Similar to the setting of BPM, a reduction in the incidence of contralateral cancer from CPM does not necessarily translate into survival advantage, and prognosis based on the index tumor should be a factor when considering CPM.

Surgical morbidity and quality of life of contralateral prophylactic mastectomy

There are no studies specifically evaluating the surgical morbidity of CPM, but there are data about the level of satisfaction and quality of life after CPM. A high level of satisfaction with the decision and cosmetic outcome post-CPM has been reported ranging from 83% to 94% [55–57]. Decreased satisfaction with CPM was associated with decreased satisfaction with appearance, complications with reconstruction, and increased level of stress in life [57]. A recent study reporting on quality of life affirmed a high level of contentment with quality of life in 76% of patients responding to the survey questionnaire. Less contentment with quality of life in this study was not associated with CPM, but rather was related to physical and mental health in general and concerns regarding physical appearance [56].

One potential advantage of CPM is attainment of improved symmetry when reconstruction is performed bilaterally. In addition once a patient undergoes transabdominal myocutaneous (TRAM) flap for unilateral reconstruction, it cannot be used for contralateral reconstruction at a later date; however, other sources of autologous tissue transfer and implant based reconstructive options can still be used for this purpose.

Risk reduction alternatives to prophylactic mastectomy

Many high-risk women are not interested in risk reduction mastectomy; only a portion of BRCA mutation carriers express interest in the procedure [58]. Whether or not an individual is considering PM, knowledge of all risk reduction options is necessary for an informed decision. Chemoprevention and prophylactic oophorectomy are the two primary breast cancer risk reduction treatments that leave the breast tissue intact. The use of tamoxifen for prevention of breast cancer in cancer-free BRCA carriers was evaluated in a retrospectively identified subset of the NSABP P-1 study [59]. Of 288 cases that developed in the cohort, 19 were confirmed BRCA mutation carriers. In this very small sample, it appeared that tamoxifen reduced breast cancer risk in BRCA2 carriers, but not in BRCA1 carriers. This finding might be expected because most BRCA1 tumors are estrogen receptor negative [60,61].

A larger study by Narod and colleagues [62] investigated the effect of tamoxifen on contralateral breast cancer rates in BRCA1/2 carriers treated in an era before routine hormone receptor testing. They reported an approximate 50% reduction in contralateral breast cancer rates associated with tamoxifen use. In this study, oophorectomy also reduced contralateral breast cancer risk by approximately 60%. In a recent updated report on this expanded cohort, reductions in breast cancer risk were identified in both BRCA1 and BRCA2 subsets, although the reduction was not statistically significant in the BRCA2 subgroup [63]. The statistically significant reduction seen in the BRCA1 subgroup (likely predominantly estrogen receptor negative tumors) is clinically important, because physicians' recommendations about tamoxifen use in mutation carriers are highly dependent on ER status [64]. These data suggest that tamoxifen is effective in preventing both estrogen receptor-positive and negative second primary cancers in BRCA carriers.

Bilateral oophorectomy also significantly impacts breast cancer risk. In a prospective cohort of 170 BRCA mutation carriers followed for 2 years, Kauff and colleagues [65] reported a 4.3% incidence of breast cancer in BRCA patients who underwent PSO, compared with 12.9% in those followed with close surveillance. In a larger sample with longer follow-up, Rebbeck and colleagues [66] reported on breast cancer rates in 99 women who had undergone PSO compared with 142 matched controls without PSO. With a mean follow-up of 8.8 years, they found a significantly lower breast cancer incidence for BRCA patients treated with PSO (21%) versus surveillance (42%). In a recent expanded report from the same group, an approximate 50% risk reduction for breast cancer was confirmed in both BRCA1 and BRCA2 subgroups, with the greatest risk reduction evident when PSO was performed before age 40 [67]. Outcomes modeling for BRCA carriers based on interventions of tamoxifen, oophorectomy, and mastectomy demonstrate that tamoxifen with oophorectomy yields almost the same survival

gain as mastectomy with oophorectomy (see Fig. 2) [37]. Although the reductions in breast cancer risk from chemoprevention or PSO alone are
not quite as high as those resulting from PM, they are substantial reductions
without the disfiguring effects and morbidity of surgery, and may be preferable approaches for many women.

Surgical technique and use of sentinel lymph node biopsy

Historically total mastectomy has been considered the preferred standard
surgical procedure for prophylaxis, because of the removal of the NAC and
its associated ductal tissue at risk for cancer development. Although subcutaneous mastectomy has been performed for this purpose, it has been criticized because of increased likelihood of retained breast tissue under the skin
flaps and within the NAC. More recent publications on skin-sparing mastectomy (SSM) in breast cancer patients report its oncologic safety and superior aesthetic results [68,69]. It is logical to extrapolate the data from
these studies to the scenario of surgical prophylaxis. In addition to SSM,
NAC-sparing mastectomy (NSM) techniques are also described and currently offered in highly selected patients [70]. It is important to emphasize
that the current techniques of SSM and NSM are different from the classic
subcutaneous mastectomy used in the past. As SSM and NSM are currently
performed, the skin flaps are thinner than the subcutaneous mastectomy of
the past. Furthermore, the core of ductal tissue within the nipple is excised
and evaluated as a separate specimen, making it a reasonably safe option for
patients undergoing PM [71].

The possibility of finding an occult synchronous invasive tumor during
a prophylactic mastectomy is quite low at approximately 5% [17,20,72–74].
Routine use of sentinel lymph node (SLN) biopsy in this setting is therefore not recommended; however, patients older than 60 years of age and those
who have invasive lobular cancer or lobular carcinoma in-situ are at higher
risk for invasive cancer at the time of PM, and should be considered for
SLN biopsy [75].

Future directions

A novel nonsurgical approach to reducing breast cancer risk is linked to
the protective effect of full-term pregnancy at younger ages [76]. Russo and
Russo [77] have shown that treatment of young virgin rats with human cho-
rionic gonadotrophin (hCG), like full term pregnancy, induces permanent
differentiation of the terminal ductal-lobular units (TDLUs), reduces proliferative activity of the mammary epithelium, induces the synthesis of inhibin
(a protein with tumor suppressor activity), and increases the expression of
genes associated with programmed cell death. They also observed that these
genes remained activated even after the cessation of hCG administration,

suggesting long lasting genome imprinting by hCG-induced changes [77]. In theory, hCG treatment of high-risk women at young ages may reduce the long-term risk of breast cancer. Ongoing research into the biology of premalignant change will also hold promise for other novel risk reduction strategies.

Summary

A preponderance of evidence confirms that prophylactic mastectomy reduces the incidence of breast cancer, but the downstream desirable effects on survival are not convincingly proven. Undoubtedly some individuals will benefit from preventing breast cancer, but the challenge remains to accurately identify them in order to minimize morbidity to the remainder. Ironically, prophylactic mastectomy is a preventive procedure that is more radical than the treatment of breast cancer for the majority of women who are eligible for breast conservation. The Society of Surgical Oncology has proposed guidelines for considering PM, but there are no absolute indications for this procedure [78]. Ideally the patient should initiate the discussion, because this has been shown to be highly correlated with long term satisfaction after PM [79]. PM should only be undertaken after careful consideration, with discussion of realistic breast cancer risk estimates in absolute terms. For women with a new diagnosis of breast cancer, prognosis of the primary tumor and risk factors for contralateral breast cancer should be considerations in the risk/benefit discussion. Making a referral to a genetic or psychiatric counselor may be beneficial. Especially in women who have no known breast cancer, the expected outcomes of surgery should be discussed in detail as well as the alternatives of close surveillance, chemoprevention, oophorectomy, and participation in prevention trials. Research holds the promise of better preventive measures in the future.

References

[1] Feuer EJ, Wun LM, Boring CC, et al. The lifetime risk of developing breast cancer. J Natl Cancer Inst 1993;85(11):892–7.
[2] Alexander NE, Ross J, Sumner W, et al. The effect of an educational intervention on the perceived risk of breast cancer. J Gen Intern Med 1996;11(2):92–7.
[3] Rockhill B, Spiegelman D, Byrne C, et al. Validation of the Gail et al. model of breast cancer risk prediction and implications for chemoprevention. J Natl Cancer Inst 2001;93(5): 358–66.
[4] Antoniou A, Pharoah PD, Narod S, et al. Average risk of breast and ovarian cancer associated with BRCA1 or BRCA2 mutations detected in case series unselected for family history: a combined analysis of 22 studies. Am J Hum Genet 2003;72(5):1117–30.
[5] Claus EB, Risch N, Thompson WD. Autosomal dominant inheritance of early-onset breast cancer: implications for risk prediction. Cancer 1994;73(3):643–51.
[6] Foote FW, Stewart FW. Comparative studies of cancerous versus noncancerous breast, I and II. Ann Surg 1945;131:197–222.

[7] Rosen PP, Groshen S, Kinne DW, et al. Contralateral breast carcinoma: an assessment of risk and prognosis in stage I (T1N0M0) and stage II (T1N1M0) patients with 20-year follow-up. Surgery 1989;196(5):904–10.

[8] Rosen PP, Groshen S, Kinne DW. Prognosis in $T_2N_0M_0$ stage I breast carcinoma: a 20-year follow-up study. J Clin Oncol 1991;9(9):1650–61.

[9] Harris RE, Lynch HT, Guirgis HA. Familial breast cancer: risk to the contralateral breast. J Natl Cancer Inst 1978;60(5):955–60.

[10] Verhoog LC, Brekelmans CT, Seynaeve C, et al. Survival and tumour characteristics of breast cancer patients with germline mutations of BRCA1. Lancet 1998;351(9099): 316–21.

[11] Verhoog LC, Brekelmans CT, Seynaeve C, et al. Survival in hereditary breast cancer associated with germline mutations of BRCA2. J Clin Oncol 1999;17(11):3396–402.

[12] Robson M, Gilewski T, Haas B, et al. BRCA-associated breast cancer in young women. J Clin Oncol 1998;16(5):1642–9.

[13] Pierce LJ, Levin AM, Rebbeck TR, et al. Ten-year multi-institutional results of breast conserving surgery and radiotherapy in BRCA1/2-associated stage I/II breast cancer. J Clin Oncol 2006;24:2437–43.

[14] Anderson DE, Badzioch MD. Bilaterality in familial breast cancer patients. Cancer 1985;56: 2092–8.

[15] Lesser ML, Rosen PP, Kinne DW. Multicentricity and bilaterality in invasive breast carcinoma. Surgery 1982;91(2):234–40.

[16] Storm HH, Jensen OM. Risk of contralateral breast cancer in Denmark, 1943-80. Br J Cancer 1986;54(3):483–92.

[17] Healey EA, Cook EF, Oray EJ, et al. Contralateral breast cancer: clinical characteristics and impact on prognosis. J Clin Oncol 1993;11(8):1545–52.

[18] Broet P, de la Rochefordiere A, Scholl SM, et al. Contralateral breast cancer: annual incidence and risk parameters. J Clin Oncol 1995;13(7):1578–83.

[19] Goldflam K, Hunt KK, Gershenwald JE, et al. Contralateral prophylactic mastectomy. Predictors of significant histologic findings. Cancer 2004;101(9):1977–86.

[20] Robinson E, Rennert G, Rennert HS, et al. Survival of first and second primary breast cancer. Cancer 1993;71(1):172–6.

[21] Hartmann LC, Sellers TA, Frost MH, et al. Benign breast disease and the risk of breast cancer. N Engl J Med 2005;353:229–37.

[22] Kerlikowske K, Shepherd J, Creasman J, et al. Are breast density and bone mineral density independent risk factors for breast cancer? J Natl Cancer Inst 2005;97(5):368–74.

[23] Mandelson MT, Oestreicher N, Porter PL, et al. Breast density as a predictor of mammographic detection: comparison of interval- and screen-detected cancers. J Natl Cancer Inst 2000;92(13):1081–7.

[24] Meijers-Heijboer H, van Geel B, van Putten WL, et al. Breast cancer after prophylactic bilateral mastectomy in women with a BRCA1 or BRCA 2 mutation. N Engl J Med 2001; 345(3):159–64.

[25] Hartmann LC, Sellers TA, Schaid DJ, et al. Efficacy of bilateral prophylactic mastectomy in BRCA1 and BRCA2 gene mutation carriers. J Natl Cancer Inst 2001;93(21):1633–7.

[26] Rebbeck TR, Friebel T, Lynch HT, et al. Bilateral prophylactic mastectomy reduces breast cancer risk in BRCA1 and BRCA2 mutation carriers: the PROSE study group. J Clin Oncol 2004;22(6):1055–62.

[27] Hartmann LC, Schaid DJ, Woods JE, et al. Efficacy of bilateral prophylactic mastectomy in women with a family history of breast cancer. N Engl J Med 1999;340(2):77–84.

[28] Geiger AM, Yu O, Herrinton LJ, et al. A population-based study of bilateral prophylactic mastectomy efficacy in women at elevated risk for breast cancer in community practices. Arch Intern Med 2005;165(5):516–20.

[29] Borgen PI, Hill AD, Tran KN, et al. Patient regrets after bilateral prophylactic mastectomy. Ann Surg Oncol 1998;5(7):603–6.

[30] Eldar S, Meguid MM, Beatty JD. Cancer of the breast after prophylactic subcutaneous mastectomy. Am J Surg 1984;148:692–3.

[31] Goodnight JE, Quagliana JM, Morton DL. Failure of subcutaneous mastectomy to prevent the development of breast cancer. J Surg Oncol 1984;26:198–201.

[32] Holleb A, Montgomery R, Farrow JH. The hazard of incomplete simple mastectomy. Surg Gynecol Obstet 1965;121:819–22.

[33] Jameson MB, Roberts E, Nixon J, et al. Metastatic breast cancer 42 years after bilateral subcutaneous mastectomies. Clin Oncol (R Coll Radiol) 1997;9:119–21.

[34] Willemsen HW, Kaas R, Peterse JH, et al. Breast carcinoma in residual breast tissue after prophylactic bilateral subcutaneous mastectomy. Eur J Surg Oncol 1998;24:331–8.

[35] Ziegler LD, Kroll SS. Primary breast cancer after prophylactic mastectomy. Am J Clin Oncol 1991;14:451–4.

[36] Schrag D, Kuntz KM, Garber JE, et al. Decision analysis—effects of prophylactic mastectomy and oophorectomy on life expectancy among women with BRCA1 or BRCA2 mutations. N Engl J Med 1997;336(20):1465–71.

[37] Grann VR, Jacobson JS, Thomason D, et al. Effect of prevention strategies on survival and quality-adjusted survival of women with BRCA1/2 mutations: an updated decision analysis. J Clin Oncol 2002;20(10):2520–9.

[38] Gabriel S, Woods J, O'Fallono M, et al. Complications leading to surgery after breast implantation. N Engl J Med 1997;336(10):677–82.

[39] Contant CM, Menke-Pluijmers MB, Seynaeve C, et al. Clinical experience of prophylactic mastectomy followed by immediate breast reconstruction in women at hereditary risk of breast cancer (HB(O)C) or a proven BRCA1 and BRCA2 germ-line mutation. Eur J Surg Oncol 2002;28(6):627–32.

[40] Barton MB, West CN, Liu I-LA, et al. Complications following bilateral prophylactic mastectomy. J Natl Cancer Inst Monogr 2005;35:61–6.

[41] Zion SM, Slezak JM, Sellers TA, et al. Reoperations after prophylactic mastectomy with or without implant reconstruction. Cancer 2003;98(10):2152–60.

[42] Frost MH, Schaid DJ, Slezak JM, et al. Long-term satisfaction and psychological and social function following bilateral prophylactic mastectomy. JAMA 2000;284:319–24.

[43] Stefanek ME, Helzlsouer KJ, Wilcox PM, et al. Predictors of satisfaction with bilateral prophylactic mastectomy. Prev Med 1995;24(4):412–9.

[44] Bresser PJC, Seynaeve C, Van Gool AR, et al. Satisfaction with prophylactic mastectomy and breast reconstruction in genetically predisposed women. Plast Reconstr Surg 2006; 117(6):1675–82.

[45] Metcalfe KA. Prophylactic bilateral mastectomy for breast cancer prevention. J Womens Health 2004;13(7):822–9.

[46] Metcalfe KA, Esplen MJ, Goel V, et al. Predictors of quality of life in women with a bilateral prophylactic mastectomy. Breast J 2005;11(1):65–9.

[47] van Sprundel TC, Schmidt MK, Rookous MA, et al. Risk reduction of contralateral breast cancer and survival after contralateral mastectomy in BRCA1 and BRCA2 mutation carriers. Br J Cancer 2005;93(3):287–92.

[48] McDonnell SK, Schaid DJ, Myers JL, et al. Efficacy of contralateral prophylactic mastectomy in women with a personal and family history of breast cancer. J Clin Oncol 2001; 19(19):3938–43.

[49] Peralta EA, Ellenhorn JDI, Wagman LD, et al. Contralateral prophylactic mastectomy improves the outcome of selected patients undergoing mastectomy for breast cancer. Am J Surg 2000;180(6):439–45.

[50] Herrinton LJ, Barlow WE, Yu O, et al. Efficacy of prophylactic mastectomy in women with unilateral breast cancer: a cancer research network project. J Clin Oncol 2005;23(19): 4275–86.

[51] Brekelmans CT, Seynaeve C, Menke-Pluymers M, et al. Survival and prognostic factors in BRCA1-associated breast cancer. Ann Oncol 2006;17(3):391–400.

[52] Lee JSY, Grant CS, Donohue JH, et al. Arguments against routine contralateral mastectomy or undirected biopsy for invasive lobular breast cancer. Surgery 1995;118(4):640–8.

[53] Babiera GV, Lowry AM, Davidson BS, et al. The role of contralateral prophylactic mastectomy in invasive lobular carcinoma. Breast J 1997;3(1):2–6.

[54] Lostumbo L, Carbine N, Wallace J, et al. Prophylactic mastectomy in the prevention of breast cancer. Cochrane Database Syst Rev 2004;(4):CD002748. pub2. doi: 10.1002/14651858.

[55] Montgomery LL, Tran KN, Heelan MC, et al. Issues of regret in women with contralateral prophylactic mastectomies. Ann Surg Oncol 1999;6:546–52.

[56] Geiger AM, West CN, Nekhlyudov L, et al. Contentment with quality of life among breast cancer survivors with and without contralateral prophylactic mastectomy. J Clin Oncol 2006;24(9):1350–6.

[57] Frost MH, Slezak JM, Tran NV, et al. Satisfaction after contralateral prophylactic mastectomy: the significance of mastectomy type, reconstructive complications, and body appearance. J Clin Oncol 2005;23(31):7849–56.

[58] Lynch HT, Lemon SJ, Durham ST, et al. A descriptive study of BRCA1 testing and reactions to disclosure of test results. Cancer 1997;79:2219–28.

[59] King MC, Wieand S, Hale K, et al. Tamoxifen and breast cancer incidence among women with inherited mutations in BRCA1 and BRCA2: National Surgical Adjuvant Breast and Bowel Project (NSABBP-P1) Breast Cancer Prevention Trial. JAMA 2001; 286:2251–6.

[60] Loman N, Johansson O, Bendahl P-O, et al. Steroid receptors in hereditary breast carcinomas associated with BRCA1 or BRCA 2 mutations or unknown susceptibility genes. Cancer 1998;83:310–9.

[61] Eisinger F, Jacquemier J, Nogues C, et al. Steroid receptors in hereditary breast carcinomas associated with BRCA1 or BRCA2 mutations or unknown susceptibility genes. Cancer 1999;85:2291–5.

[62] Narod SA, Brunet J, Ghadirian P, et al. Tamoxifen and risk of contralateral breast cancer in BRCA1 and BRCA2 mutation carriers: a case-control study. Lancet 2000;356:1876–81.

[63] Gronwald J, Tung N, Foulkes WD, et al. Tamoxifen and contralateral breast cancer in BRCA1 and BRCA2 carriers: an update. Int J Cancer 2006;118(9):2281–4.

[64] Peshkin BN, Isaacs C, Finch C, et al. Tamoxifen as chemoprevention in BRCA1 and BRCA2 mutation carriers with breast cancer: a pilot survey of physicians. J Clin Oncol 2003;21: 4322–8.

[65] Kauff ND, Satagopan JM, Robson ME, et al. Risk-reducing salpingo-oophorectomy in women with a BRCA1 or BRCA2 mutation. N Eng J Med 2002;346:1609–15.

[66] Rebbeck TR, Lynch HT, Neuhausen SL, et al. Prophylactic oophorectomy in carriers of BRCA1 and BRCA2 mutations. N Eng J Med 2002;346:1616–22.

[67] Eisen A, Lubinski J, Klijn J, et al. Breast cancer risk following bilateral oophorectomy in BRCA1 and BRCA2 mutation carriers: an international case-control study. J Clin Oncol 2005;23(30):7491–6.

[68] Newman LA, Kuerer HM, Hunt KK, et al. Presentation, treatment, and outcome of local recurrence after skin-sparing mastectomy and immediate breast reconstruction. Ann Surg Oncol 1998;5(7):620–6.

[69] Simmons RM, Fish SK, Gayle L, et al. Local and distant recurrence rates in skin-sparing mastectomies compared with non-skin-sparing mastectomies. Ann Surg Oncol 1999;6(7): 676–81.

[70] Crowe JP Jr, Kim JA, Yetman R, et al. Nipple-sparing mastectomy: technique and results of 54 procedures. Arch Surg 2004;139(2):148–50.

[71] Garcia-Etienne CA, Borgen PI. Update on the indications for nipple-sparing mastectomy. J Support Oncol 2006;4(5):225–30.

[72] Bernstein JL, Thomson WD, Risch N, et al. Risk factors predicting the incidence of second primary breast cancer among women diagnosed with a first primary breast cancer. Am J Epidemiol 1992;136(8):925–36.

[73] Fisher ER, Fisher B, Sass R, et al. Pathologic findings from the National Surgical Adjuvant Breast Project (Protocol No. 4). XI. Bilateral breast cancer. Cancer 1984;54(12):3002–11.

[74] Singletary SE, Taylor SH, Guinee VF, et al. Occurrence and prognosis of contralateral carcinoma of the breast. J Am Coll Surg 1994;178(4):390–6.

[75] Boughey JC, Khakpour N, Meric-Bernstam F, et al. Selective use of sentinel lymph node surgery during prophylactic mastectomy. Cancer 2006;107(7):1440–7.

[76] MacMahon B, Cole P, Lin TM, et al. Age at first birth and breast cancer risk. Bulletin of the World Health Organization 1970;43:209–21.

[77] Russo IH, Russo J. Hormonal approach to breast cancer prevention. J Cell Biochem Suppl 2000;34:1–6.

[78] Society of Surgical Oncology. Position statement on prophylactic mastectomy. Available at: http://www.surgonc.org/default.aspx?id=179. Accessed October 2, 2006.

[79] Nckhlyudov L, Bower M, Herrinton LJ, et al. Women's decision-making roles regarding contralateral prophylactic mastectomy. J Natl Cancer Inst Monogr 2005;35:55–60.

ELSEVIER
SAUNDERS

SURGICAL
CLINICS OF
NORTH AMERICA

Surg Clin N Am 87 (2007) 333–351

Ductal Carcinoma In Situ—Current Management

Martin J. O'Sullivan, MD, Monica Morrow, MD*

Department of Surgical Oncology, Fox Chase Cancer Center, 333 Cottman Avenue, Philadelphia, PA 19111-2497, USA

Ductal carcinoma in situ (DCIS) is the proliferation of malignant mammary ductal epithelial cells without evidence of invasion beyond the confines of the basement membrane. Before the widespread use of screening mammography, only 3% to 5% of mammary cancers were DCIS; most were palpable masses [1]. Recently, a marked increase in the incidence (or detection) of DCIS has been observed. The Surveillance, Epidemiology, and End Results (SEER) program of the National Cancer Institute reported that the incidence of DCIS increased by 200% between 1983 and 1992 [2], with similar increases seen for black and white women. Several studies have indicated that DCIS accounts for 15% to 30% of all screen-detected tumors in women participating in large, organized screening mammography programs [3–9]. The increases in the incidence of DCIS have been much more pronounced in women aged 40 to 69 years than in those under 39 or over 70 [2], providing support for the idea that the increased adoption of mammography by American women is responsible for much of the observed increase in the incidence of DCIS, and raising considerable controversy about the biologic significance of mammographically detected DCIS.

It has been proposed that a significant proportion of mammographically identified DCIS is clinically indolent, and its identification results in a costly diagnostic work-up and potentially disfiguring surgical intervention, which is unlikely to benefit the patient [2]. Autopsy studies also have indicated that the incidence of DCIS in asymptomatic women ranges from 0.2% to 18.2% [10–16], indicating that some DCIS does not become evident during a woman's lifetime. Other data refute this, however, indicating that although DCIS is less likely to present as a palpable mass when compared with previous time points, the proportion of patients with grade 3 DCIS

---

* Corresponding author.
E-mail address: monica.morrow@fccc.edu (M. Morrow).

0039-6109/07/$ - see front matter © 2007 Elsevier Inc. All rights reserved.
doi:10.1016/j.suc.2007.01.006
surgical.theclinics.com

is increasing [17,18]. High-grade DCIS is associated with a higher risk of local recurrence after treatment by excision alone than low-grade DCIS [19] and with a shorter time period to the development of invasive recurrence than low-grade DCIS. Such findings do not support the idea that mammographically detected DCIS is unlikely to become clinically significant during a woman's lifetime [18]. Definition of the molecular factors necessary for progression to invasive carcinoma and a better understanding of the time course needed for the development of the fully malignant phenotype are necessary before it will be possible to determine which DCIS lesions are unlikely to become invasive carcinoma during a woman's lifetime and can be observed safely.

Support for the concept that DCIS and invasive cancer are part of the same process comes from the similarity in risk factors predisposing to both conditions. Gapstur and colleagues [20] studied 37,105 women enrolled in the Iowa Women's Health Study who were followed for 11 years. Risk factor information was collected prospectively. During the study, 1520 breast carcinomas were observed, of which 175 were DCIS. Those who developed DCIS or invasive breast cancers had the same risk factor profiles, and the magnitude of risk conveyed by each of the risk factors was similar for both conditions. A similar concordance between risk factors for DCIS and invasive carcinoma was reported by Kerlikowske and colleagues [21] in a study of 39,542 women undergoing screening mammography and by Claus and colleagues [22] in a case control study of 875 Connecticut residents who had DCIS.

Classification

Some of the problem in defining the natural history of DCIS is because of the tendency to classify this heterogeneous lesion as a single entity. In the past, most DCIS presented as a palpable mass, as previously noted. Today, the most common presentation of DCIS is as a mammographic abnormality, usually clustered microcalcifications. Gross DCIS is not uncommon, however. In a series of 202 patients seen between 1988 and 1996, Brenin and Morrow [23] reported that clinical presentations of DCIS accounted for 23% of the cases. What is unclear is whether the biologic behavior of DCIS lesions that become clinically evident is similar to that of lesions detected by mammography. By inference, this raises the question of whether the results of older studies with long-term follow-up, primarily involving patients who had clinical DCIS, should be applied to patients being treated today.

A similar problem exists with pathologic classifications of DCIS. The traditional pathologic classification of DCIS was based on the morphology of the lesion and recognized five subtypes: comedo, papillary, micropapillary, solid, and cribriform [24]. This was at a time when the main management strategy was mastectomy, and such classification was largely an academic exercise. More recently, some authors have grouped DCIS lesions into two groups, comedo and noncomedo, based on the observations that the cells of comedo DCIS have a more malignant appearance cytologically [24,25] and that invasive carcinoma is more likely to be associated with the comedo subtype than with the other DCIS variants [18,26]. A major problem with classification systems based on architecture alone is that as many as 30% to 62% of DCIS lesions, particularly those that are larger in size, display more than one pattern [27,28]. Perhaps in part because of the variability of architectural patterns, interobserver correlation in the categorization of DCIS lesions using even the simple comedo/noncomedo classification is poor [29].

Classification with nuclear grade and necrosis has been advocated in an effort to avoid the problems seen with architectural classifications. Silverstein and colleagues [30] have proposed three groups of DCIS patients based on the presence or absence of comedo necrosis and high nuclear grade: high-grade, nonhigh-grade with comedo necrosis, and nonhigh-grade without comedo necrosis. One study, however, found only fair-to-moderate concordance among 23 pathologists for each of five classification systems, including the Silverstein system, studied [29]. An international consensus conference on the classification of ductal carcinoma in situ failed to endorse any single classification schema, but recommended that the pathology report should include information on nuclear grade, necrosis, polarization, and architectural pattern [31]. At present, the most important fact regarding classification systems is that none of them have been demonstrated prospectively to predict the risk of invasive breast cancer development or local recurrence in the preserved breast.

Studies of molecular markers also have been performed in an effort to identify DCIS that is likely to progress to invasive carcinoma. Detailed discussion is outside the scope of this article, but such studies indicate that although there are differences in marker expression across DCIS lesions of different degrees of differentiation, these markers are insufficient to identify those cases of DCIS that will become invasive from those that will not [32–46].

Investigation and diagnosis

A careful clinical examination is mandatory in all cases. Such examination is usually normal, but coexisting pathology may be found in the ipsilateral or contralateral breast. Mammographic magnification views help to delineate the extent of the calcifications. Fine needle aspiration cannot distinguish between DCIS and invasive ductal cancer reliably. Therefore, definitive diagnosis is with core biopsy. Vacuum-assisted biopsy has higher sensitivity and specificity than core biopsy, but may miss invasive cancer in up to 18% of cases because of sampling errors [47]. The greater the number of core biopsies, the less likely one is to miss invasive cancer. This has implications in management of the axilla. Needle localization-guided biopsy is required in rare cases, but diagnosis by needle biopsy increases the likelihood of completion of local therapy with a single surgical procedure [48] and is more cost-effective than surgical biopsy [49].

Treatment of ductal carcinoma in situ

Local therapy for DCIS may consist of mastectomy, excision and radiation therapy (RT), or excision alone. Systemic therapy is limited to hormonal manipulation. This wide range of surgical therapies reflects the heterogeneity of DCIS and the uncertainty about its natural history. Prevention of local recurrence (invasive and noninvasive) is the major goal DCIS treatment. In patients who have pure DCIS, there is essentially no risk of metastases at diagnosis, so an invasive local recurrence has the potential to impact upon survival. When considering treatment options in DCIS, however, it is worth remembering that cause-specific survival rates exceed 95% regardless of the type of local therapy employed [50–58].

Mastectomy

Mastectomy is a curative treatment for approximately 98% of patients who have DCIS [59–67]. This is true whether the DICS is gross or mammographic and regardless of the grade or subtype of DCIS. Recurrent carcinoma after a mastectomy for DCIS may occur in two ways. First, undetected invasive carcinoma may be present in the breast at the time of mastectomy. This is particularly likely in older studies in which histologic sampling of the mastectomy specimen was often less extensive than that which is performed today. An alternate explanation for postmastectomy recurrence is the development of a new carcinoma in residual breast tissue left behind on the skin flaps. The failure of recurrence rates to increase with longer follow-up intervals after mastectomy suggests that most cases of recurrence are caused by undiagnosed invasive carcinoma rather than carcinogenesis in residual breast tissue.

Breast-conserving surgery

Although mastectomy is an extremely effective DICS therapy for which all patients are eligible, a large body of evidence indicates that most patients who have DCIS do not require a mastectomy. Multiple prospective randomized trials comparing mastectomy and breast-conserving surgery (BCS) in invasive carcinoma have shown no survival differences between these procedures. There has been no direct comparison between mastectomy and BCS for DCIS, and there is unlikely to be one at this stage. The concern that invasive local recurrence in DCIS patients treated with BCS might result in increased breast cancer mortality has not been demonstrated. Solin and colleagues

[53] reported a 15-year, cause-specific actuarial survival rate of 98% in 1003 women with mammographically detected DCIS treated with excision and RT between 1973 and 1995. This indicates that the overall risk of breast cancer death is quite low, even in a time period when the extent of surgery, quality of mammography, and extent of histologic evaluation were quite different than they are today. In addition, this study predated the era of adjuvant tamoxifen. Those patients who develop invasive recurrence, however, have a risk of developing distant metastases reported to range from 11% to 27% [68,69]. The potential for breast cancer death after invasive recurrence emphasizes the importance of both careful patient selection for BCS and the need for regular surveillance for the detection of recurrence.

If the extent of the DCIS relative to the patient's breast size suggests that a cosmetically acceptable resection can be done, an attempt should be made to estimate the risk of local recurrence with a breast-conserving approach. There is controversy over which factors predict an increased risk of local recurrence, and factors that place a patient at risk for an invasive local recurrence have not been reproducibly identified. In addition, there is no agreement on what is an unacceptably high risk of local failure. Failure to obtain a negative margin and young patient age both have been shown to increase the risk of local recurrence in patients treated with excision and RT. Tumor touching ink is accepted universally as an inadequate margin. Beyond that, it is unclear whether larger negative margin widths are associated with a reduction in the risk of local recurrence. In the study of Neuschatz and colleagues [70], 31% of patients with margins of 1 to 2 mm were found to have residual DCIS at re-excision, a finding very similar to the 30% incidence observed in those with focally positive margins. When excision margins were greater than 2 mm, residual DCIS was not observed, supporting the observation of Faverly and colleagues [71] that gaps between DCIS lesions are usually 1 mm or less in size. The discontinuous growth pattern of low- and intermediate-grade DCIS mandates the use of postexcision mammography in patients who have calcification lesions and small negative margins (usually defined as <2 mm) to exclude the presence of residual calcifications. Ultimately, the determination of what constitutes an adequate margin of resection will consider which margin is approximated by tumor, the extent of tumor approaching the margin, and other factors that may impact upon the risk of local recurrence such as patient age. Patient age has emerged as an important predictor of local recurrence (LR) in DCIS. In the National Surgical Adjuvant Breast And Bowel Project (NSABP) B-17 trial [50], LR rates decreased from 15% in women aged no more than 49 years to 10% for those in theirs 50s and 9% for those aged 60 and older, although this difference did not reach statistical significance. A 57% reduction in the risk of local recurrence was observed for patients over the age of 49 in the NSABP B-24 trial [52]. The European Organisation for Research and Treatment of Cancer (EORTC) study also found that women aged 40 and younger had a relative risk of 1.89 (95% confidence interval [CI],

1.12 to 3.19; $P = .026$) for local recurrence in multivariate analysis [51]. These findings do not indicate that all younger women need to be treated with mastectomy. Instead they suggest that careful attention to the completeness of excision and the use of radiation and tamoxifen are appropriate in this age group to minimize the risk of local failure.

The impact of grade and histology of DCIS on local recurrence is less clear. It initially was suggested that high-grade and/or comedo DCIS lesions had a higher risk of breast recurrence after treatment with excision and RT than low-grade lesions [72,73]. Studies with longer follow-up [64,74–76], however, demonstrated that high histologic grade or comedo necrosis were associated with a shorter interval to recurrence but no difference in the incidence of recurrence after 10 years of follow-up. The NSABP B-17 [50] and EORTC 10853 [51] trials found high- and intermediate-grade DCIS to be more commonly associated with local failure after treatment with excision and RT than low-grade DCIS. In the EORTC study [51], histologic subtypes cribriform and solid/comedo were associated with a 2.25- and 2.39-fold increase in the risk of recurrence, respectively, when compared with clinging or micropapillary histology. Both the NSABP B-24 trial [52] and the EORTC study [51] found that clinical presentations of DCIS were associated with a higher rate of local failure than mammographic ones, but they did not distinguish between nipple discharge and mass lesions.

In both prospective and retrospective series, BCS attains breast cancer survivals of 96% to 100% [50–58,77–79], a result that is comparable with mastectomy. Local recurrence rates are higher than with mastectomy, however, even if whole-breast radiation is administered (Table 1).

The benefit of radiation treatment

Retrospective studies have suggested that highly selected subgroups of patients with DCIS may be treated with excision alone [79–82]. The benefit

Table 1
Modern series of local recurrence and cause-specific survival in patients with ductal carcinoma in situ undergoing breast-conserving surgery and radiotherapy

Author	Year	Number of patients	Follow-up (years)	Local recurrence with radiotherapy	Cause-specific survival
Solin [53]	2005	1003	15	19%	98% (15 years)
Mirza [54]	2000	87	11	13.0%	97% (10 years)
Cutuli [77]	2002	515	10	18.2%	—
Rodrigues [55]	2002	239	10	13.0%	97% (10 years)
Hiramatsu [56]	1995	76	10	15.0%	96% (10 years)
Silverstein [79]	1999	213	7.6	17.3%	—
Vargas [57]	2005	313	7.5	9.4%	98.8% (10 years)
Amichetti [58]	1997	139	6.8	9.0%	100% (6.8 years)

of RT in women undergoing BCS for DCIS has been studied directly in three large randomized trials involving more than 3500 patients:

NSABP protocol B-17 [50]
EORTC protocol 10853 [51]
The United Kingdom, Australia, New Zealand (UK/ANZ) DCIS trial [83]

In all three studies, 50 Gy of radiation was administered to the whole breast in 25 fractions. A boost to the tumor bed was employed in 9% of patients in the B17 trial and 5% in the EORTC 10853 trial. These studies are summarized in Table 2. All found a significant reduction in ipsilateral recurrence following radiation treatment. No survival differences have been demonstrated in any of the randomized trials. In NSABP B-17, with 12 years of follow-up, the use of postoperative RT was associated with a 50% proportional decrease in the odds of an in-breast recurrence (cumulative local recurrence rate 31.7% [no RT] versus 15.7%; $P < .00005$) [50]. This effect was observed for both noninvasive and invasive local recurrences, although the rate of invasive recurrence was reduced to a slightly greater extent than noninvasive recurrence (16.8% versus 7.7%, and 14.6% versus 8%, respectively). It is worth noting that a negative margin in this trial was defined as no tumor cells touching the inked margin, without requirement for a particular margin width.

The EORTC trial 10853 reported a 10-year local recurrence-free survival of 74% in the BCS group alone compared with 85% in the BCS and RT group [51]. The risk of recurrent DCIS and invasive cancer was reduced by

Table 2
Summary of the three randomized trials of breast-conserving surgery with or without radiotherapy postoperatively for ductal carcinoma in situ

| | Number of patients | Ipsilateral local recurrence | | | | Overall survival | | |
		Without radiotherapy (RT)	With RT	Risk reduction	p-value	Without RT	With RT	p-value
NSABP B-17 12-year follow-up	813	31.7%	15.7%	50%	$<.00005$	86%	87%	0.8
EORTC 10853 10.5-year follow-up	1010	26%	15%	47%	$<.0001$	95%	95%	0.53
UK/ANZ Crude incidence	1030	14%	6%	62%	$<.0001$	Too few deaths to analyze		

Abbreviations: EORTC, European Organization for Treatment and Research of Cancer; NSABP, National Surgical Adjuvant Breast and Bowel Project; UK/ANZ, United Kingdom/ Australia New Zealand.

RT from 14% to 7% and from 13% to 8%, respectively. All patient subgroups benefited from RT. In subgroups with a very low risk of recurrence (ie, well-differentiated DCIS with a clinging or micropapillary pattern), the relative benefit of RT was similar to that in other groups. The absolute benefit, however, was small because of the overall low rate of recurrence.

The UK/ANZ DCIS Trial examined 1701 women with mammographically detected DCIS who underwent excision of DCIS with clear margins who were assigned randomly to RT and/or to tamoxifen versus placebo, using a two-by-two factorial design [83]. This trial had four subgroups: BCS alone, BCS and RT, BCS and tamoxifen, and BCS with both RT and tamoxifen. With a median follow-up of 53 months, those who underwent RT had a significantly lower risk of ipsilateral invasive (hazard ratio 0.45) and intraductal recurrence (hazard ratio 0.36), findings which were comparable with the NSABP and EORTC trials.

Considerable interest exists in identifying patients with DCIS who may not require RT, because of its inconvenience, expense, and impact upon future therapy should recurrence occur. Subsets of patients who do not benefit from RT, however, have not been reproducibly identified. In a nonrandomized study, Silverstein and colleagues [79] compared outcomes of patients who had DCIS treated with and without RT and suggested that if a negative margin width of greater than 1 cm was obtained, RT was not beneficial in reducing local recurrences, an issue not addressed in the randomized trials described previously. In a recent prospective study , Wong and colleagues [84] attempted to duplicate the findings of Silverstein and colleagues [79] that excision to a margin of greater than 1 cm results in a low rate of local recurrence in the absence of RT. In this study, 158 patients with a mean age of 51 and with predominantly grade 1 and 2 DCIS underwent excision of DCIS to a negative margin of greater than 1 cm. There was a 12% 5-year local recurrence rate, and 31% of the recurrences were invasive. This study was stopped before its planned accrual of 200 patients because of this high rate of local failure [84].

To date, no subgroup had been identified that does not benefit from RT. The absolute magnitude of benefit, however, varies and this should be discussed with patients at the time that local therapy is selected.

Axillary surgery/sentinel lymph node biopsy

DCIS is noninvasive; therefore, intuitively, no axillary procedure should be required. The NSABP B-17 and B-24 studies document that the risk of axillary recurrence in patients treated with BCS with or without RT and with or without tamoxifen is extremely low. In long-term follow-up of the NSABP B-17 and B-24 studies, the rates of axillary recurrence in both the control and treatment arms were less than 0.1% [85]. These low rates of axillary failure do not provide justification for the routine use of sentinel lymph node biopsy (SLNB) in DCIS.

Most investigators argue that the selective use of SLNB in patients with DCIS who are at significant risk for having coexistent invasive carcinoma is appropriate. Patients diagnosed as having DCIS with large bore vacuum-assisted biopsy devices are found to have invasive cancer in approximately 5% to 18% of cases [47,86–90]. In patients requiring mastectomy, the opportunity for SLNB is lost if it is not performed at the same time as the mastectomy, and the authors consider this an indication for SLNB. Gross or clinically evident DCIS, and DCIS that is suspicious for microinvasion are also circumstances in which invasive cancer is found frequently and where SLNB should be considered. When microinvasion is identified definitely at the time of biopsy, SLNB should be performed, because axillary metastases have been reported in 3% to 20% of such patients [91–95].

SLNB is not warranted in all patients who have DCIS because of the small but real morbidity of the procedure. The American College of Surgeons Oncology Group recently published data from the Z0010 trial in which 198 surgeons in 126 institutions performed SLNB in 5327 patients [96]. At 6-month follow-up, the mean incidences of axillary paresthesia, arm lymphedema, and decreased range-of-shoulder movement were 8.6%, 7.0%, and 3.8% respectively. Seromas occurred in 7.1% of patients. Other less common complications included hematoma (1.4%), infection (1%), and brachial plexus injury (0.2%) [96].

The use of immunohistochemistry (IHC) is not recommended for evaluation of the sentinel node in DCIS. [97–99]. The prognostic significance of the micrometastases identified by sentinel lymph node mapping, especially those seen only on IHC staining, is uncertain. Some have suggested that the small clusters of cells observed in the SLNs of patients who have DCIS represent artifacts of the procedure rather than true clonogens capable of distant spread and growth [100]. It is clear that displacement of breast epithelial cells can occur after breast biopsy [101–103] and can result in a falsely positive SLNB [104]. In a long-term clinico–pathologic study by Lara and colleagues [105], although 13% of patients who had DCIS were found to have involved SLNs by IHC staining, this information had no prognostic value with regard to their risk of local, regional, or distant recurrence. One must remember that the emphasis should be on the avoidance of local recurrence rather than analyzing small cell clusters in lymph nodes of very uncertain significance.

Use of endocrine therapy in ductal carcinoma in situ

Endocrine therapy has two potential benefits in DCIS. First, it may be therapeutic in the prevention of local recurrence, and second, it may prevent the development of new primary breast cancers. Solin and colleagues [53] have demonstrated that the risk of new ipsilateral and contralateral breast cancers in women who have DCIS is equal to the risk of true local recurrence at the primary tumor site for 15 years after diagnosis.

Two trials have studied the use of tamoxifen directly in women who have DCIS, with somewhat conflicting results (Table 3). The NSABP B-24 trial [52] randomized 1804 patients with DCIS who were treated with excision and RT to 20 mg tamoxifen daily or a placebo for 5 years. At a median follow-up of 74 months in 1798 patients, the patients in the tamoxifen arm had an 8.2% incidence of breast cancer events compared with 13.4% for the placebo group ($P = .0009$). Tamoxifen reduced the rate of ipsilateral invasive recurrences by 44%, but did not significantly reduce the risk of recurrent DCIS in the ipsilateral breast. Although the incidence of contralateral breast cancers was low (3.4% invasive and noninvasive in the placebo group), a 52% reduction was noted in the tamoxifen group. Tamoxifen was observed to reduce breast cancer events in those over and under age 50, with or without positive margins, and in patients with comedo necrosis.

In contrast, no benefit for tamoxifen was demonstrated in the UK/ANZ trial, described previously [83]. With a median follow-up of 52.6 months, there was no significant benefit from tamoxifen in preventing invasive ipsilateral or contralateral events after BCS. The only advantage of tamoxifen was a 3.4% reduction in ipsilateral in situ recurrence. It is possible that a longer duration of follow-up, may, in fact demonstrate a more significant benefit for tamoxifen. This study's outcome, however, is of some concern, because the benefit of tamoxifen in reducing contralateral breast cancer recurrence is documented well, and its two-by-two design allowed participating institutions to select the study arms to which they would randomize patients.

What is clear, however, is that the benefit from tamoxifen is restricted to women with ER-positive DCIS. Allred and colleagues [106] determined the ER status in a subset of 628 patients (327 placebo, 301 tamoxifen) in the NSABP B-24 study. In women who had ER-positive tumors, the effectiveness of tamoxifen versus placebo in reducing all breast cancer events was clear (relative risk = 0.41, 95% CI = .25-0.65, $P = .0002$). Significant reductions in incidence were seen in both the ipsilateral and the contralateral breast. In women who had ER-negative tumors, little benefit was seen (RR = .80, $P = .51$). Approximately 80% of cases of DCIS are reported to

Table 3
Randomized trials of tamoxifen for ductal carcinoma in situ

	Number of patients	Median follow-up (months)	All breast cancer events			
			No tamoxifen	Tamoxifen	Hazard ratio	p-value
NSABP B-24	1798	74	13.4%	8.2%	0.63	0.0009
UK/ANZ	1576	52.6	18.0%	14.0%	0.83	0.13

Abbreviations: NSABP, National Surgical Adjuvant Breast and Bowel Project; UK/ANZ, United Kingdom/Australia New Zealand.

be ER-positive [106], with comedo DCIS being less frequently ER-positive than other subtypes [107,108]. There are no data to support the use of aromatase inhibitors (AIs) in DCIS currently. The greater efficacy of AIs in reducing contralateral breast cancer [109] has stimulated studies of the role of AIs in DCIS. The increase of osteoporosis seen with AIs, however, is of concern in a population with a low risk of breast cancer death such as women who have DCIS. At present, AIs should not be used outside of a clinical trial.

Selection of treatment for the individual patient

The appropriate therapy for DCIS depends on the extent of the DCIS lesion, the risk of local recurrence, and the patient's attitude toward risk and benefit. Guidelines for the selection of local therapy in patients who have DCIS have been developed by a joint committee of the American College of Surgeons, American College of Radiology, and the College of American Pathologists and are summarized in Box 1. The evaluation begins with an assessment of the extent of the DCIS lesion. Magnification mammography is essential for this evaluation, even if the calcifications clearly require biopsy based on the screening mammogram. Holland and colleagues [110,111] noted that conventional two-view mammography (craniocaudal and

---

Box 1. Indications for mastectomy in ductal carcinoma in situ

Absolute indications
Women with two or more primary tumors in the breast
Diffuse malignant-appearing calcifications
Persistent positive margins after reasonable surgical attempts
Inability to give radiation when needed for local control because
    of a history of prior breast irradiation or active systemic lupus
    erythematosus
Patient choice

Relative indications
Extensive DCIS that can only be removed with a small negative
    margin, particularly in a young woman
Tumor size to breast size ratio would result in a poor cosmetic
    result
Pregnancy—the long natural history of DCIS suggests that for
    some women, excision during pregnancy and with radiation
    delivered post-partum may be reasonable. In the absence of
    definitive data, such decisions should be made on an individual
    case basis.

mediolateral oblique views only) underestimates the extent of well-differentiated DCIS by 2 cm in 47% of cases. The use of magnification views reduces this discrepancy to only approximately 14% of cases. An accurate
determination of lesion size allows preoperative selection of those patients
who are appropriate candidates for breast preservation and minimizes the
number of surgical procedures that are needed to achieve an adequate negative margin. Morrow and colleagues [112] reported the results of magnification mammography in 263 patients who were clinical candidates for
breast conservation, including 51 who had DCIS. Breast preservation was
performed successfully in 97% of patients found to have localized tumors
by magnification mammography. Kearney and Morrow [113] reported
173 patients evaluated with magnification mammography in whom a diagnostic excision to negative margins was attempted. Negative margins were
obtained in 161 patients (93%) with a single surgical procedure. These
data indicate that the extent of DCIS can be identified preoperatively in
most patients, avoiding attempts at breast preservation in those with extensive disease. One study recently examined the role of MRI in 33 patients diagnosed histologically with DCIS. The overall sensitivity of MRI for
diagnosing DCIS in the presence of microcalcifications was .79 (95% CI,
.61 to .91) [114]. For calcifications alone, sensitivity was .68 (.45 to .86)
and 1.00 (.72 to 1) for calcifications associated with masses. That study concluded that the not-perfect sensitivity of MRI was a crucial point that prevents the clinical use of MRI in the diagnosis of mammographically detected
calcifications. Another study of 45 patients who had biopsy-proven DCIS
demonstrated a wide variety in the appearance of DCIS on MRI. Although
imaging features may provide information about the underlying biology
(density and inflammation) of the DCIS, MRI was most likely to overestimate the size of less dense, diffuse DCIS lesions [115]. One other study of
22 patients who had DCIS indicated that MRI overestimated or underesti-
mated the size of the DCIS in 62% of patients [116]. At present, there is no
clear role for MRI in the routine evaluation of patients who have DCIS.

In the absence of contraindications to BCT, patient preference should
play a major role in treatment selection. Long-term survival in DCIS is excellent regardless of the therapeutic strategy selected. Patient attitudes
toward local recurrence, radiation, cosmetic outcome, and potentially toward tamoxifen may be major factors in treatment selection. Bordeleau
and colleagues [117] used a decision analysis model to determine optimal
treatment for DCIS based on the risk of recurrence and the impact of therapy on health-related quality of life (HRQOL). Wide local excision alone
was the preferred therapy when the 10-year risk of local recurrence was
less than 15%. For those estimated to have a 10-year risk of recurrence of
15% to 38%, excision and RT were preferred except when mastectomy
was associated with a minimal decrease in HRQOL. For those with a risk
of recurrence greater than 38%, and for those who had a 10-year risk of
contralateral breast cancer of greater than 10%, the addition of tamoxifen

to excision and RT was supported. The results of this model were influenced by the individual's perception of the impact of mastectomy on HRQOL, emphasizing the importance of patient participation in the decision-making process for the disease.

Katz and colleagues [118,119] examined a population-based cohort of 659 women from the Detroit and Los Angeles SEER areas diagnosed with DCIS in 2002 to directly examine the role of patients in the therapeutic decision-making process. Mastectomy was more common in those women with larger high-grade DCIS lesions, but BCS was the most common treatment recommendation for all women in the absence of specific medical contraindications to BCS. Not surprisingly, surgeon discussion and recommendation were powerful factors contributing to this practice pattern. Patient attitudes, however, were also important in determining surgical treatment. Greater patient involvement in the decision-making process was associated with higher rates of mastectomy, primarily because of concerns about recurrence. Only 13.1% of women who were not influenced or slightly influenced by concerns about recurrence underwent mastectomy, compared with 48.8% of women who were greatly influenced by this concern ($P < .001$). Similar findings were observed for concerns about radiation. Previous data indicated that patients who perceived that they had a choice of therapy and participated in the decision-making process were more satisfied with the outcome of their care, independent of age, education, or the type of treatment received [120].

Summary

DCIS is a heterogeneous disease whose natural history is defined poorly. Screening mammography has increased the detection rate of DCIS, but physicians remain unable to identify cases of DCIS that will not progress to invasive carcinoma during an individual's lifetime. Genomics holds great promise in this regard, but prospective studies with long-term follow-up will be needed before concluding that a subset of DCIS is clinically insignificant. The varying intensity of treatment options for DCIS, ranging from mastectomy to excision, RT, and tamoxifen, to excision alone, reflects the uncertainty about the natural history of DCIS and differing physician values regarding the impact of local recurrence. The extent of DCIS within the breast is the major determinant of whether the patient is a candidate for a breast-conserving approach, and contraindications to the use of breast conservation treatment and to the use of irradiation have been defined. In discussing therapy with patients, it is important to emphasize that the risk of breast cancer death is extremely low, regardless of the type of local therapy chosen. The clinical decision-making process in DCIS would benefit greatly from improvements in the ability to convey information about the long-term risks and benefits of therapy, and the tradeoffs in HRQOL, to patients, and to incorporate their preferences into the decision-making process.

References

[1] Rosner D, Bedwani RN, Vana J, et al. Noninvasive breast carcinoma: results of a national survey by the American College of Surgeons. Ann Surg 1980;192(2):139–47.

[2] Ernster VL, Barclay J, Kerlikowske K, et al. Incidence and treatment for ductal carcinoma in situ of the breast. JAMA 1996;275(12):913–8.

[3] Seidman H, Gelb SK, Silverberg E, et al. Survival experience in the Breast Cancer Detection Demonstration Project. CA Cancer J Clin 1987;37:258–90.

[4] Rosenberg RD, Lando JF, Hunt WC, et al. The New Mexico Mammography Project: screening mammography performance in Albuquerque, New Mexico, 1991 to 1993. Cancer 1996;78:1731–9.

[5] Olivotto IA, Kan L, d'Yachkova Y, et al. Ten years of breast screening in the screening mammography program of British Columbia. J Med Screen 2000;7:152–9.

[6] May DS, Lee NC, Nadel MR, et al. The National Breast And Cervical Cancer Early Detection Program: report on the first 4 years of mammography provided to medically underserved women. AJR Am J Roentgenol 1998;170:97–104.

[7] May DS, Lee NC, Richardson LC, et al. Mammography and breast cancer detection by race and Hispanic ethnicity: results from a national program (United States). Cancer Causes Control 2000;11:697–705.

[8] Canada H. Organized breast cancer screening programs in Canada: 1996 report. Laboratory Centre for Disease Control, Health Canada. Minister of Public Works and Government Services Canada; 1999.

[9] UK Trial of Early Detection of Breast Cancer Group. 16-year mortality from breast cancer in the UK Trial of Early Detection of Breast Cancer. Lancet 1999;353:1909–14.

[10] Alpers C, Wellings S. The prevalence of carcinoma in situ in normal and cancer-associated breast. Hum Pathol 1985;16(8):796–807.

[11] Bartow S, Pathak D, Black W, et al. Prevalence of benign, atypical, and malignant breast lesions in populations at different risk for breast cancer. Cancer 1987;60(11):2751–60.

[12] Bhatal PS, Brown RW, Lesueur GC, et al. Frequency of benign and malignant breast lesions in 207 consecutive autopsies in Australian women. Br J Cancer 1985;51(2):271–8.

[13] Kramer WM, Rush BF Jr. Mammary duct proliferation in the elderly. Cancer 1973;31(1):130–7.

[14] Nielsen M, Jensen J, Anderson J. Precancerous and cancerous breast lesions during lifetime and at autopsy: a study of 83 women. Cancer 1984;54(4):612–5.

[15] Nielsen M, Thomsen JL, Primdahl S, et al. Breast cancer and atypia among young and middle-aged women: a study of 110 medicolegal autopsies. Br J Cancer 1987;56(6):814–9.

[16] Wellings SR, Jensen HM. On the origin and progression of ductal carcinoma in the human breast. J Natl Cancer Inst 1973;50(5):1111–8.

[17] Pandya S, Mackarem G, Lee AKC, et al. Ductal carcinoma in situ: the impact of screening on clinical presentation and pathologic features. Breast J 1998;4:146–51.

[18] Silverstein MJ, Waisman JR, Gamagami P, et al. Intraductal carcinoma of the breast (208 cases). Clinical factors influencing treatment choice. Cancer 1990;66(1):102–8.

[19] Fisher ER, Dignam J, Tan-Chiu E, et al. Pathologic findings from the National Surgical Adjuvant Breast Project (NSABP) eight-year update of protocol B-17: intraductal carcinoma. Cancer 1999;86(3):429–38.

[20] Gapstur SM, Morrow M, Sellers TA. Hormone replacement therapy and risk of breast cancer with a favorable histology: results of the Iowa Women's Health Study. JAMA 1999;281(22):2091–7.

[21] Kerlikowske K, Barclay J, Grady D, et al. Risk factors for ductal carcinoma in situ. J Natl Cancer Inst 1997;89(1):76–82.

[22] Claus EB, Stowe M, Carter D. Breast carcinoma in situ: risk factors and screening patterns. J Natl Cancer Inst 2001;93(23):1811–7.

[23] Brenin D, Morrow M. Is mastectomy overtreatment for ductal carcinoma in situ? Breast Cancer Res Treat 1998;50:28.

[24] Rosen PP, Oberman H. Tumors of the mammary gland. Washington, DC: Armed Forces Institute of Pathology; 1993.

[25] Page DL, Anderson TJ. Diagnostic histopathology of the breast. Edinburgh, Scotland: Churchill Livingstone; 1987.

[26] Moriya T, Silverbert SG. Intraductal carcinoma (ductal carcinoma in situ) of the breast. A comparison of pure noninvasive tumors with those including different proportions of infiltrating carcinoma. Cancer 1994;74(11):2972–8.

[27] Lennington WJ, Jensen RA, Dalton LW, et al. Ductal carcinoma in situ of the breast. Heterogeneity of individual lesions. Cancer 1994;73(1):118–24.

[28] Quinn CM, Ostrowski JL, Parkin GJS, et al. Ductal carcinoma in situ of the breast: the clinical significance of histological classification. Histopathology 1997;30(2):113–9.

[29] Sloane JP, Amendoeira I, Apostolikas N, et al. Consistency achieved by 23 European pathologists in categorizing ductal carcinoma in situ of the breast using five classifications. European Commission Working Group on Breast Screening Pathology. Hum Pathol 1998; 29(10):1056–62.

[30] Silverstein MJ, Poller DN, Waisman JR, et al. Prognostic classification of breast ductal carcinoma in situ. Lancet 1995;345(8958):1154–7.

[31] The Consensus Conference Committee. Consensus conference of the classification of ductal carcinoma in situ. Cancer 1997;80(9):1798–802.

[32] Guidi AJ, Fischer L, Harris JR, et al. Microvessel density and distribution in ductal carcinoma in situ of the breast. J Natl Cancer Inst 1994;86(8):614–9.

[33] Bobrow LG, Happerfield LC, Gregory WM, et al. The classification of ductal carcinoma in situ and its association with biological markers. Semin Diagn Pathol 1994;11(3):199–207.

[34] Evans AJ, Pinder SE, Ellis IO, et al. Correlations between the mammographic features of ductal carcinoma in situ (DCIS) and C-erbB2 oncogene expression. Clin Radiol 1994;49(8): 559–62.

[35] Otteson GL, Christensen IJ, Larsen JK, et al. Carcinoma in situ of the breast: correlation of histopathology to immunohistochemical markers and DNA ploidy. Breast Cancer Res Treat 2000;60(3):219–26.

[36] Siziopikou KP, Prioleau JE, Harris JR, et al. bcl-2 expression in the spectrum of preinvasive breast lesions. Cancer 1996;77(3):499–506.

[37] Zafrani B, Leroyer A, Fourquet A, et al. Mammographically detected ductal in situ carcinoma of the breast analyzed with a new classification. A study of 127 cases: correlation with estrogen and progesterone receptors, p53 and c-erbB-2 proteins, and proliferative activity. Semin Diagn Pathol 1994;11(3):208–14.

[38] Nofech-Mozes S, Spayne J, Rakovitch E, et al. Prognostic and predictive molecular markers in DCIS: a review. Adv Anat Pathol 2005;12(5):256–64.

[39] Bircan S, Kapucuoglu N, Baspinar S, et al. CD24 expression in ductal carcinoma in situ and invasive ductal carcinoma of breast: an immunohistochemistry-based pilot study. Pathol Res Pract 2006;202(8):569–76.

[40] Schuetz CS, Bonin M, Clare SE, et al. Progression-specific genes identified by expression profiling of matched ductal carcinomas in situ and invasive breast tumors, combining laser capture microdissection and oligonucleotide microarray analysis. Cancer Res 2006;66(10): 5278–86.

[41] Vogl G, Dietze O, Hauser-Kronberger C. Angiogenic potential of ductal carcinoma in situ (DCIS) of human breast. Histopathology 2005;47(6):617–24.

[42] Oliveira VM, Piato S, Silva MA. Correlation of cyclooxygenase-2 and aromatase immunohistochemical expression in invasive ductal carcinoma, ductal carcinoma in situ, and adjacent normal epithelium. Breast Cancer Res Treat 2006;95(3):235–41.

[43] Mylonas I, Makovitzky J, Jeschke U, et al. Expression of Her2/neu, steroid receptors (ER and PR), Ki67 and p53 in invasive mammary ductal carcinoma associated with ductal carcinoma in situ (DCIS) versus invasive breast cancer alone. Anticancer Res 2005;25(3A): 1719–23.

[44] Lebrecht A, Grimm C, Euller G, et al. Transforming growth factor beta 1 serum levels in patients with preinvasive and invasive lesions of the breast. Int J Biol Markers 2004; 19(3):236–9.

[45] Emberley ED, Alowami S, Snell L, et al. S100A7 (psoriasin) expression is associated with aggressive features and alteration of Jab1 in ductal carcinoma in situ of the breast. Breast Cancer Res 2004;6(4):R308–15.

[46] Schmid BC, Rudas M, Rezniczek GA, et al. CXCR4 is expressed in ductal carcinoma in situ of the breast and in atypical ductal hyperplasia. Breast Cancer Res Treat 2004;84(3): 247–50.

[47] Lee CH, Carter D, Philpotts LE, et al. Ductal carcinoma in situ diagnosed with stereotactic core needle biopsy: can invasion be predicted? Radiology 2000;217(2):466–70.

[48] Morrow M, Venta L, Stinson T, et al. Prospective comparison of stereotactic core biopsy and surgical excision as diagnostic procedures for breast cancer patients. Ann Surg 2001; 233(4):537–41.

[49] Golub RM, Bennett CL, Stinson T, et al. Cost minimization study of image-guided core biopsy versus surgical excisional biopsy for women with abnormal mammograms. J Clin Oncol 2004;22(12):2430–7.

[50] Fisher B, Land S, Mamounas E, et al. Prevention of invasive breast cancer in women with ductal carcinoma in situ: an update of the National Surgical Adjuvant Breast And Bowel Project experience. Semin Oncol 2001;28(4):400–18.

[51] EORTC Breast Cancer Cooperative Group; EORTC Radiotherapy Group; Bijker N, Meijnen P, Peterse JL, et al. Breast-conserving treatment with or without radiotherapy in ductal carcinoma in situ. Ten-year results of European Organisation for Research and Treatment of Cancer randomized phase III trial 10853—a study by the EORTC Breast Cancer Cooperative Group and EORTC Radiotherapy Group. J Clin Oncol 2006; 24(21):3381–7.

[52] Fisher B, Dignam J, Wolmark N, et al. Tamoxifen in treatment of intraductal breast cancer: National Surgical Adjuvant Breast and Bowel Project B-24 randomised controlled trial. Lancet 1999;353(9169):1993–2000.

[53] Solin LJ, Fourquet A, Vicini FA, et al. Long-term outcome after breast-conservation treatment with radiation for mammographically detected ductal carcinoma in situ of the breast. Cancer 2005;103(6):1137–46.

[54] Mirza NQ, Vlastos G, Meric F, et al. Ductal carcinoma in situ: long-term results of breast-conserving therapy. Ann Surg Oncol 2000;7(9):656–64.

[55] Rodrigues N, Carter D, Dillon D, et al. Correlation of clinical and pathologic features with outcome in patients with ductal carcinoma in situ of the breast treated with breast-conserving surgery and radiotherapy. Int J Radiat Oncol Biol Phys 2002;54(5):1331–5.

[56] Hiramatsu H, Bornstein BA, Recht A, et al. Local recurrence after conservative surgery and radiation therapy for ductal carcinoma in situ: possible importance of family history. Cancer J Sci Am 1995;1(1):55–61.

[57] Vargas C, Kestin L, Go N, et al. Factors associated with local recurrence and cause-specific survival in patients with ductal carcinoma in situ of the breast treated with breast-conserving therapy or mastectomy. Int J Radiat Oncol Biol Phys 2005;63(5):1514–21.

[58] Amichetti M, Caffo O, Richetti A, et al. Ten-year results of treatment of ductal carcinoma in situ (DCIS) of the breast with conservative surgery and radiotherapy. Eur J Cancer 1997; 33(10):1559–65.

[59] Arnesson LG, Smeds S, Fagerberg G, et al. Follow-up of two treatment modalities for ductal carcinoma in situ of the breast. Br J Surg 1989;76(7):672–5.

[60] Ashikari R, Huvos AG, Snyder RE. Prospective study of noninfiltrating carcinoma of the breast. Cancer 1977;39(2):435–9.

[61] Jha MK, Avlonitis VS, Griffith CD, et al. Aggressive local treatment for screen-detected DCIS results in very low rates of recurrence. Eur J Surg Oncol 2001;27(5):454–8.

[62] Kinne DW, Petrek JA, Osborne MP, et al. Breast carcinoma in situ. Arch Surg 1989;124(1): 33–6.

[63] Schuh ME, Nemoto T, Penetrante R, et al. Intraductal carcinoma. Analysis of presentation, pathologic findings, and outcome of disease. Arch Surg 1986;121(11):1303–7.

[64] Silverstein MJ. Van Nuys experience by treatment. In: Silverstein MJ, editor. Ductal carcinoma in situ of the breast. Baltimore (MD): Williams and Wilkins; 1997. p. 443–8.

[65] Sunshine JA, Moseley MS, Fletcher WS, et al. Breast carcinoma in situ: a retrospective review of 112 cases with a minimum 10-year follow-up. Am J Surg 1985;150(1):44–51.

[66] Von Rueden DG, Wilson RE. Intraductal carcinoma of the breast. Surg Gynecol Obstet 1984;158(2):105–11.

[67] Ward BA, McKhann CF, Ravikumar TS. Ten-year follow-up of breast carcinoma in situ in Connecticut. Arch Surg 1992;127:1392–5.

[68] Silverstein MJ, Lagios MD, Martino S, et al. Outcome after invasive local recurrence in patients with ductal carcinoma in situ of the breast. J Clin Oncol 1998;16(4):1367–73.

[69] Solin LJ, Fourquet A, Vicini FA, et al. Salvage treatment for local recurrence after breast-conserving surgery and radiation as initial treatment for mammographically detected ductal carcinoma in situ of the breast. Cancer 2001;91(6):1090–7.

[70] Neuschatz AC, DiPetrillo T, Steinhoff M, et al. The value of breast lumpectomy margin assessment as a predictor of residual tumor burden in ductal carcinoma in situ of the breast. Cancer 2002;94(7):1917–24.

[71] Faverly DRG, Burgers L, Bult P, et al. Three-dimensional imaging of mammary ductal carcinoma in situ: clinical implications. Semin Diagn Pathol 1994;11(3):193–8.

[72] Kuske RR, Bean JM, Garcia DM, et al. Breast conservation therapy for intraductal carcinoma of the breast. Int J Radiat Oncol Biol Phys 1993;26(3):391–6.

[73] Solin LJ, Recht A, Fourquet A, et al. Ten-year results of breast-conserving surgery and definitive irradiation for intraductal carcinoma (ductal carcinoma in situ) of the breast. Cancer 1991;68(11):2337–44.

[74] Solin LJ, Kurtz J, Fourquet A, et al. Fifteen-year results of breast-conserving surgery and definitive breast irradiation for the treatment of ductal carcinoma in situ of the breast. J Clin Oncol 1996;14(3):754–63.

[75] McCormick B, Rosen PP, Kinne D, et al. Duct carcinoma in situ of the breast: an analysis of local control after conservation surgery and radiotherapy. Int J Radiat Oncol Biol Phys 1991;21(2):289–92.

[76] Ray GR, Adelson J, Hayhurst E, et al. Ductal carcinoma in situ of the breast: results of treatment by conservative surgery and definitive irradiation. Int J Radiat Oncol Biol Phys 1994;28(1):105–11.

[77] Cutuli B, Cohen-Solal-le Nir C, de Lafontan B, et al. Breast-conserving therapy for ductal carcinoma in situ of the breast: the French Cancer Centers' experience. Int J Radiat Oncol Biol Phys 2002;53(4):868–79.

[78] Solin LJ, Fourquet A, Vicini FA, et al. Mammographically detected ductal carcinoma in situ of the breast treated with breast-conserving surgery and definitive breast irradiation: long-term outcome and prognostic significance of patient age and margin status. Int J Radiat Oncol Biol Phys 2001;50(4):991–1002.

[79] Silverstein MJ, Lagios MD, Groshen S, et al. The influence of margin width on local control of ductal carcinoma in situ of the breast. N Engl J Med 1999;340(19):1455–61.

[80] Schwartz GF, Finkel GC, Garcia JC, et al. Subclinical ductal carcinoma in situ of the breast. Treatment by local excision and surveillance alone. Cancer 1992;70(10): 2468–74.

[81] Lagios MD, Margolin FR, Westdahl PR, et al. Mammographically detected duct carcinoma in situ. Frequency of local recurrence following tylectomy and prognostic effect of nuclear grade on local recurrence. Cancer 1989;63(4):618–24.

[82] Lagios MD, Silverstein MJ. Ductal carcinoma in situ. The success of breast conservation therapy: a shared experience of two single institutional nonrandomized prospective studies. Surg Oncol Clin N Am 1997;6(2):385–92.

[83] Houghton J, George WD, Cuzick J, et al. Radiotherapy and tamoxifen in women with completely excised ductal carcinoma in situ of the breast in the UK, Australia, and New Zealand: randomised controlled trial. Lancet 2003;362:95–103.

[84] Wong JS, Kaelin CM, Troyan SL, et al. Prospective study of wide excision alone for ductal carcinoma in situ of the breast. J Clin Oncol 2006;24(7):1031–6.

[85] Julian TB, Land S, Haile S, et al. Is sentinel node biopsy in DCIS necessary? Ann Surg Oncol 2006;135:11.

[86] Kettritz U, Rotter K, Schreer I, et al. Stereotactic vacuum-assisted breast biopsy in 2874 patients: a multicenter study. Cancer 2004;100(2):245–51.

[87] Liberman L, Smolkin JH, Dershaw DD, et al. Calcification retrieval at stereotactic, 11-gauge, directional, vacuum-assisted breast biopsy. Radiology 1998;208:251–60.

[88] Brem RF, Schoonjans JM, Sanow L, et al. Reliability of histologic diagnosis of breast cancer with stereotactic vacuum-assisted biopsy. Am Surg 2001;67:388–92.

[89] Won B, Reynolds HE, Lazaridis CL, et al. Stereotactic biopsy of ductal carcinoma in situ of the breast using an 11-gauge vacuum-assisted device: persistent underestimation of disease. AJR Am J Roentgenol 1999;173:227–9.

[90] Jackman RJ, Burbank F, Parker SH, et al. Stereotactic breast biopsy of nonpalpable lesions: determinants of ductal carcinoma in situ underestimation rates. Radiology 2001; 218:497–502.

[91] Klauber-DeMore N, Tan LK, Liberman L, et al. Sentinel lymph node biopsy: is it indicated in patients with high-risk ductal carcinoma in situ and ductal carcinoma in situ with micro-invasion? Ann Surg Oncol 2000;7(9):636–42.

[92] Cox CE, Nguyen K, Gray RJ, et al. Importance of lymphatic mapping in ductal carcinoma in situ (DCIS): why map DCIS? Am Surg 2001;67(6):513–9.

[93] Mittendorf EA, Arciero CA, Gutchell V, et al. Core biopsy diagnosis of ductal carcinoma in situ: an indication for sentinel lymph node biopsy. Curr Surg 2005;62(2):253–7.

[94] Camp R, Feezor R, Kasraeian A, et al. Sentinel lymph node biopsy for ductal carcinoma in situ: an evolving approach at the University of Florida. Breast J 2005;11(6):394–7.

[95] Sakr R, Barranger E, Antoine M, et al. Ductal carcinoma in situ: value of sentinel lymph node biopsy. J Surg Oncol 2006;94(5):426–30.

[96] Wilke LG, McCall LM, Posther KE, et al. Surgical complications associated with sentinel lymph node biopsy: results from a prospective international cooperative group trial. Ann Surg Oncol 2006;13(4):491–500.

[97] Fitzgibbons PL, Page DL, Weaver D, et al. Prognostic factors in breast cancer. College of American pathologists consensus statement 1999. Arch Pathol Lab Med 2000; 124:966–78.

[98] Lyman GH, Giuliano AE, Somerfield MR, et al. American Society of Clinical Oncology guideline recommendations for sentinel lymph node biopsy in early-stage breast cancer. J Clin Oncol 2005;23:7703–20.

[99] Schwartz GF, Giuliano AE, Veronesi U. Proceedings of the consensus conference on the role of sentinel lymph node biopsy in carcinoma of the breast, April 19–22, 2001, Philadelphia, (PA). Cancer 2002;94:2542–51.

[100] Cote RJ, Peterson HF, Chaiwun B, et al. and International Breast Cancer Study Group. Role of immunohistochemical detection of lymph node metastases in management of breast cancer. Lancet 1999;354:896–900.

[101] Carter BA, Jensen RA, Simpson JF, et al. Benign transport of breast epithelium into axillary lymph nodes after biopsy. Am J Clin Pathol 2000;113:259–65.

[102] Youngson BJ, Liberman L, Rosen PP. Displacement of carcinomatous epithelium in surgical breast specimens following stereotactic core biopsy. Am J Clin Pathol 1995;103: 598–602.

[103] Douglas-Jones AG, Verghese A. Diagnostic difficulty arising from displaced epithelium after core biopsy in intracystic papillary lesions of the breast. J Clin Pathol 2002;55:780–3.

[104] Bleiweiss IJ, Nagi CS, Jaffer S. Axillary sentinel lymph nodes can be falsely positive due to iatrogenic displacement and transport of benign epithelial cells in patients with breast carcinoma. J Clin Oncol 2006;24(13):2013–8.

[105] Lara JF, Young SM, Velilla RE, et al. The relevance of occult axillary micrometastasis in ductal carcinoma in situ: a clinicopathologic study with long-term follow-up. Cancer 2003; 98:2105–13.

[106] Allred DC, Bryant J, Land S, et al. Estrogen receptor expression as a predictive marker of the effectiveness of tamoxifen in the treatment of DCIS: findings from NSABP Protocol B-24 [abstract]. Presented at 25th Annual San Antonio Breast Cancer Symposium. San Antonio (TX), December 11–14, 2002.

[107] Bur ME, Zimarowski MJ, Schnitt SJ, et al. Estrogen receptor immunohistochemistry in carcinoma in situ of the breast. Cancer 1992;69(5):1174–81.

[108] Poller DN, Snead DR, Roberts EC, et al. Oestrogen receptor expression in ductal carcinoma in situ of the breast: relationship to flow cytometric analysis of DNA and expression of the c-erbB-2 oncoprotein. Br J Cancer 1993;68(1):156–61.

[109] Howell A, Cuzick J, Baum M, et al. Results of the ATAC (arimidex, tamoxifen, alone or in combination) trial after completion of 5 years' adjuvant treatment for breast cancer. Lancet 2005;365(9453):60–2.

[110] Holland R, Hendriks J. Microcalcifications associated with ductal carcinoma in situ: mammographic—pathologic correlation. Semin Diagn Pathol 1994;11(3):181–92.

[111] Holland R, Hendriks JH, Verbeek AL, et al. Extent, distribution, and mammographic/histological correlations of breast ductal carcinoma in situ. Lancet 1990;335(8688):519–22.

[112] Morrow M, Schmidt R, Hassett C. Patient selection for breast-conserving surgery with magnification mammography. Surgery 1995;118(4):621–6.

[113] Kearney T, Morrow M. Effect of re-excision on the success of breast conserving surgery. Ann Surg Oncol 1995;2(4):303–7.

[114] Bazzocchi M, Zuiani C, Panizza P, et al. Contrast-enhanced breast MRI in patients with suspicious microcalcifications on mammography: results of a multicenter trial. AJR Am J Roentgenol 2006;186(6):1723–32.

[115] Esserman LJ, Kumar AS, Herrera AF, et al. Magnetic resonance imaging captures the biology of ductal carcinoma in situ. J Clin Oncol 2006;24(28):4603–10.

[116] Schouten van der Velden AP, Boetes C, Bult P, et al. The value of magnetic resonance imaging in diagnosis and size assessment of in situ and small invasive breast carcinoma. Am J Surg 2006;192(2):172–8.

[117] Bordeleau L, Rakovitch E, Naimark DM, et al. A comparison of four treatment strategies for ductal carcinoma in situ using decision analysis. Cancer 2001;92(1):23–9.

[118] Katz SJ, Lantz PM, Janz NK, et al. Patient involvement in surgery treatment decisions for breast cancer. J Clin Oncol 2005;23(24):5526–33.

[119] Katz SJ, Lantz PM, Janz NK. Patterns and correlates of local therapy for women with ductal carcinoma in situ. J Clin Oncol 2005;23(13):3001–7.

[120] Katz SJ, Lantz PM, Zemencuk JK. Correlates of surgical treatment type for women with noninvasive and invasive breast cancer. J Womens Health Gend Based Med 2001;10(7): 659–70.

ELSEVIER
SAUNDERS

SURGICAL
CLINICS OF
NORTH AMERICA

Surg Clin N Am 87 (2007) 353–364

Lymphatic Mapping Techniques and Sentinel Lymph Node Biopsy in Breast Cancer

Erika A. Newman, MD[a],
Lisa A. Newman, MD, MPH, FACS[b],*

[a]Department of Surgery, University of Michigan, 1500 East Medical Center Drive,
Ann Arbor, MI 48109-0932, USA
[b]Breast Center, University of Michigan Comprehensive Cancer Center, 1500 East Medical
Center Drive, Ann Arbor, MI 48109-0932, USA

The axillary nodal status is accepted universally as the most powerful prognostic tool available for early stage breast cancer. Breast cancer patients routinely undergo surgical staging of the axilla because other primary tumor features are inadequate in predicting the presence versus absence of nodal positivity [1–3]. The status of the axillary lymph nodes also guides treatment options and adjuvant therapies. The removal of level I and level II lymph nodes at axillary node dissection (ALND) is the most accurate method to assess nodal status, and it is the universal standard. ALND is associated with several adverse long-term sequelae including lymphedema, the disruption of nerves in the axilla, chronic shoulder pain, weakness, and joint dysfunction. Additionally, the survival advantage of ALND has been challenged, and less morbid methods of evaluating the axillary nodal basin have been sought.

Breast cancer spreads from the tumor bed to one or a few lymph nodes before it spreads to other axillary nodes. These sentinel nodes can be identified and surgically excised for histological analysis. Lymphatic mapping with sentinel lymph node biopsy (SLNB) has emerged as an effective method of detecting axillary metastases. Veronesi and colleagues [4] randomly assigned 516 women with early stage breast cancer to either SLNB and ALND or SLNB alone (ALND was performed only for axillary metastases in the SLNB-alone arm). The authors demonstrated that SLNB was

---

* Corresponding author.
E-mail address: lanewman@umich.edu (L.A. Newman).

0039-6109/07/$ - see front matter © 2007 Published by Elsevier Inc.
doi:10.1016/j.suc.2007.01.013

accurate and reliable with a false-negative rate of 8%. There was less pain and better arm mobility in those who underwent SLNB only. Additionally, there were no differences in local recurrence or survival at follow-up. The NSABP-32 trial is the largest multicenter trial to date examining the safety and accuracy of SLNB [5]. The trial randomly assigned women with clinically negative axillae to receive SLNB with an ALND or SLNB alone. Early results have demonstrated that SLNB is safe and reliable, with false-negative rates of 8% to 10%, and lower morbidity than ALND. Although the long-term results are forthcoming, the clinical advantages of SLNB are apparent, and the procedure is becoming the preferred standard by patients and breast cancer surgeons.

Given the rapid growth of lymphatic mapping and SLNB, surgical groups have developed several variations in practice, and many technical aspects of the procedure are evolving. These variations have included the choice of mapping label, radioisotope quantity and processing, label injection site, timing of radioisotope injection, and the use of preoperative lymphoscintigraphy scanning. Because these controversies have not been studied extensively in clinical trials, the method of lymphatic mapping ultimately should be selected based on those methods that have been proven safe, and on the services and resources of a given breast care program. Table 1 summarizes the results of various studies that have analyzed SLNB accuracy as a function of mapping technique [6–18].

Choice mapping label

Radioisotope alone

Krag and colleagues [19] first described the use of radioisotope alone for breast cancer in 1993, using technetium-99m sulfur colloid and a hand-held gamma probe. The sentinel node identification rate was 98%, with a false-negative rate of 11%. Technetium-99m sulfur colloid is the most widely used radioisotope for lymphatic mapping in the United States. In Europe, technetium 99m-colloidal albumin is used most. The specific radioisotope selected for the mapping process is determined largely by availability and by the center's nuclear medicine practices [20]. The doses of radioactive technetium vary by institution and range from 0.1 to 4 mCi.

Blue dye

Isosulfan blue dye (Lymphazurin 1%, US Surgical Corp, Norwalk, CT) initially was studied extensively in lymphatic mapping for melanoma. The use of isosulfan blue dye as a single agent in SLNB for breast cancer initially was reported by Giuliano and colleagues [6], with sentinel node identification rates of 98%, without false-negative nodes. The major disadvantage of isosulfan blue dye is the risk of life-threatening allergic and anaphylactic

Table 1
Selected studies evaluating accuracy of sentinel lymph node biopsy as a function of lymphatic mapping technique

Study	Total # cases	Sentinel lymph node (SLN) identification rate (%)	SLN FN rate (%)	Factors associated with SLN nonidentification						Factors associated with SLN FN risk					
				Learning curve	Tumor location (medial worse)	Older-age patient	Prior excisional biopsy	Single versus dual mapping agent	Larger-sized tumor	Learning curve	Tumor location (upper outer quadrant worse)	Older-aged patient	Prior excisional biopsy	Single versus dual mapping agent	Larger-sized tumor
Canavese [9]	212	97.1%	6.5%	No	NR	NR	NR	Yes	No	No	NR	NR	NR	No	Yes
Albertini [7]	62	92%	0%	NR	NR	NR	NA[a]	Yes	NR	No	No	No	No	No	No
McMasters [10]	806	88%	7.2%	No	No	Yes	No	Yes	No	No	Yes	No	No	Yes	No
Veronesi [8]	163	98%	4.7%	No	No	No	No	NA (Tc only used)	Yes	No	Yes	No	No	NA	Yes
Veronesi [11]	376	98.7%	6.7%	No	No	NR	NR	No	No	No	No	No	NR	No	No
Cox [12]	465	94.4%	UK	Yes	NR	NR	No	Yes	NR	Yes	NR	NR	NR	NR	NR
Giuliano [6]	174	65.5%	8.1%	Yes	NR	NR	NR	NA (dye only used)	NR	Yes	NR	NR	NR	NR	NR
Bedrosian [13]	104[b]	99%	3.3%	NR	NR	NR	NR	NR	No	NR	NR	NR	NR	NR	No
Haigh [14]	284[c]	81.0%	3.2%	NR	No	NR	No	NR	No	Yes	No	NR	No	NR	No
Wong [15]	2206	92.5%	8.0%	NR	No	NR	No	NR	Yes	NR	No	NR	No	NR	No
Krag [16]	443	93%	12.8%	NR	Yes	Yes	Yes	NA (isotope-only used)	No	NR	Yes	No	No	NA (isotope-only used)	No
O'Hea [17]	59	93%	15%	NR	No	NR	No	Yes	No	Yes	No[d]	NR	No	No	Yes
Guenther [18]	260	81.9%	NR[d]	Yes	Yes	NR	No	NA (dye only used)	NA[e]	NA[e]	NA[e]	NA[e]	NA[e]	NA[e]	NA[e]

Abbreviations: NR, not reported; NA, not applicable.
[a] Patients with prior excisional biopsy excluded from study.
[b] All T2 and T3 tumors.
[c] Including 181 lymphatic mapping cases with prior excisional biopsy.
[d] Medial location worse.
[e] Analyses limited to 47 patients with unsuccessful mapping procedures.

reactions. The reported allergic reaction rate ranges from 1% to 3% [21,22]. Most reactions consist of urticaria, rash, blue hives, and pruritus [23]. Although rare, anaphylaxis and hypotension also have been reported. Overall, isosulfan blue dye has excellent results for lymphatic mapping in breast cancer, and is the blue dye most commonly used.

Methylene blue also has been successful in SLNB for breast cancer. Simmons and colleagues [24,25] identified the sentinel node in approximately 93% of patients studied in a cohort of more than 100 patients; concordance with radioisotope was observed in 95%.

Additionally, methylene blue was compared with Isosulfan blue dye by Blessing and colleagues [26] in 2002. The authors found that all patients had high concomitant isotope mapping and similar sentinel node identification rates. Methylene blue is preferred by some authors because of its lower costs, and also because of its lower risk of allergic reactions. Methylene blue must be injected in the subcutaneous tissues; inadvertent injection into the dermis has resulted in severe skin reactions including necrosis and dermolysis.

Combination of blue dye and radioisotope

Several authors have demonstrated that the combination of radioisotope and blue dye for lymphatic mapping improves the sentinel lymph node (SLN) identification rate. Albertini and colleagues [7] first reported the successful use of lymphatic mapping with both blue dye and radioisotopes prospectively. The results have been confirmed with several studies demonstrating that the combination method improves the sentinel node identification rate, and dual-agent lymphatic mapping has been accepted universally [27]. Some centers have elected to rely on radioisotope mapping alone, given the potentially life-threatening allergic reactions of isosulfan blue dye.

Filtered versus unfiltered radioisotope

Identification of a radioactive lymph node depends upon adequate uptake of the radioisotope from the breast parenchyma by intramammary lymphatics. The radioisotope must travel from the breast to the sentinel node in a timely fashion. Radioisotope uptake and travel times ultimately depend on the size of the labeled carrier and on the amount of carrier fluid used. Large particles may not migrate to regional nodes at all (those greater than 400 nm), and those too small may migrate too quickly to the entire nodal basin, making identification of single sentinel nodes difficult. The size of technitium-99 sulfur colloid may be altered by the selective use of filters and the pore size of filters used. Filtration through 100 or 220 nm filters has been studied, with goals of particle sizes ranging from 50 to 200 nm. Filtered preparations resulting in smaller particles travel more quickly and may potentially reach more SLNs, including the higher echelon nodes, if there is a prolonged interval between injection of radioisotope and surgery [19]. The unfiltered colloid may be less likely to travel to higher echelon nodes, given its larger size and slower transit time. Linehan and colleagues [28] compared the success of SLNB using filtered versus unfiltered technetium-99m sulfur colloid combined with blue dye mapping. Although the authors found no difference in the overall SLN identification rate, there were significantly more SLNs that were radioactive in the unfiltered group versus the filtered group (88% versus 73%; $P = .03$). These results suggest that filtered smaller particles may pass too quickly from the injection site through the nodal basin before the sentinel nodes are removed.

There has been no consensus on the use of filtered versus unfiltered radioisotopes for lymphatic mapping in breast cancer. The various features may be considered advantages or disadvantages, and selection depends upon the timing of surgery in relation to injection times.

Injection site for mapping agents

Peri-tumoral injection

In efforts to replicate the intramammary lymphatic pathways that may have been traversed by metastases, the initial data regarding SLNB used peri-tumoral injections of the mapping agents [5,6]. For patients who have nonpalpable tumors, this method has proven difficult and time-consuming, because it requires the use of additional imaging modalities to guide the peri-tumoral injection of radioisotopes. Peri-tumoral injections also have a higher potential for shinethrough, where residual radioactivity from the peri-tumoral injection site creates misleading background activity detected by the gamma probe from the axilla. It is for these reasons that alternate injection sites have been pursued.

Subareolar and dermal injection

Mammary lymphatics develop as radial extensions from the nipple breast bud. Nearly all breast tissue lymphatic drainage passes through the subareolar plexus of Sappey and then into the axillary nodal basin; hence dermal and subareolar injections are potential approaches for the injection of mapping agents. The sites are particularly advantageous for patients who have nonpalpable or multicentric tumors; they also eliminate the shinethrough effect.

A potential disadvantage to subareolar and dermal injections is that up to 10% of breast cancers may demonstrate nonaxillary lymphatic drainage with sentinel nodes found in the internal mammary or supraclavicular nodal basins; hence not all breast tumors will have the same drainage patterns as the overlying skin and nipple areas. Additionally, subareolar and dermal injection of blue dye may cause considerable postoperative discoloration of the breast (blue breast), which may last for several months.

Veronesi and colleagues [8] first described subdermal injections of technetium-99m labeled albumin into the dermis overlying the tumor of 163 patients undergoing SLNB and ALND. The authors found that the SLN identification rate was 98%, with a false-negative rate of 4.7%. Several authors have confirmed the reliability of dermal injections by direct comparisons between peri-tumoral and skin radioisotope injections. Borgstein and colleagues [29] studied 33 breast cancer patients undergoing lymphatic mapping, consisting of dermal injections of blue dye and peri-tumoral injections of radioisotope. The authors found 100% concordance between blue and radioactive SLNs in 30 of the 33 patients studied, without any false negatives. Linehan and colleagues studied 200 patients undergoing SLNB with peri-tumoral or excisional biopsy site blue dye injections. In the study, half of the patients also received Tc99-sulfur colloid injected peri-tumorally, and the other half received radioisotopes by means of dermal injections. The SLN identification rates were 92% for those patients receiving intraparenchymal injections of both blue dye and radioisotopes. For those patients receiving intraparenchymal injection of blue dye and dermal injection of radioisotopes, the SLN identification rate was 100%. In both subsets of patients, the concordance between blue-stained and radioactive sentinel nodes was also high (97% and 95%, respectively). Those patients receiving dermal injections of radioisotopes had a greater proportion of sentinel nodes radioactive when compared with the group receiving peri-tumoral injections of radioisotopes (97% versus 78%; $P < .001$). A subsequent report compared 134 patients receiving intraparenchymal lymphatic mapping with 164 patients with mapping using intraparenchymal blue dye and dermal injection of radioisotopes [30]. The SLN identification rate was significantly higher in the group receiving dermal injections of radioisotopes (98% versus 89%). There was no difference in the false-negative rates (4.4% and 4.8%).

Several authors have studied the differences between lymphatic drainage pathways of intradermal versus intraparenchymal injections of radioisotopes. Shen and colleagues [31] studied the preoperative lymphoscintigraphy scans of 30 patients undergoing lymphatic mapping for cutaneous breast melanomas and 97 patients undergoing lymphatic mapping with peri-tumoral injection for breast cancer. The authors found that there were a higher percentage of nonaxillary SLNs in the melanoma/dermal injection group (26% versus 5%). In the melanoma cases, there were bilateral axillary and supraclavicular drainage sites detected, whereas the breast cancer cases mapped to the ipsilateral axillae. The results demonstrated that axillary drainage patterns varied between peri-tumoral and dermal lymphatics. Additionally, given the importance of the ipsilateral axillary, mammary, and supraclavicular nodal basins in the staging of breast cancer, if drainage to these sites can be detected with dermal injection, the dermal route may be adequate for the staging of breast cancer.

Klimberg and colleagues [32] compared lymphatic mapping using subareolar injections of radioisotope to peri-tumorally injected blue dye. The authors found successful mapping in 64 of 68 patients studied (94%). The SLN identification rate for blue dye was 89.9% versus an identification rate of 94.2% for radioisotope. In the study, all blue nodes were also radio-active, indicating that subareolar injection did not miss any axillary SLNs using this method of mapping.

Subareolar and dermal injection sites also have been examined using various areas of the breast for injection. Beitsch and colleagues [33] studied subareolar radioisotope injected into the mirror-image quadrant of the nipple–areolar tissue and peri-tumoral blue dye injections. The SLN identi-fication for blue dye and radioisotopes were 94% and 99%, respectively, and 99% of the blue SLNs were also radioactive. Kern [34,35] reported suc-cessful results of lymphatic mapping using subareolar injections of blue dye and radioisotopes at the upper, outer aspect of the nipple–areolar tissue.

Although SLNB has proven reliable in women who have unifocal disease, the studies examining the ideal injection site have set the stage for the con-sideration of SLNB in multicentric and multifocal disease. Tousimis and colleagues [36] reported results from the largest series examining lymphatic mapping in multicentric and multifocal breast cancer. The authors examined 70 patients who underwent mapping using a combination of radioisotopes and blue dye. In the study, 63 patients received a single intradermal injection of radioisotopes directly over the largest tumor, and five patients received radioisotope peri-tumoral radioisotope injections. Additionally, 67 patients received a single intraparenchymal blue dye injection adjacent to the supero–lateral side of the largest invasive tumor or biopsy cavity. The au-thors found that the accuracy (SLN identification rate of 96%) and false-negative rate (8%) of SLNB in patients who had multicentric and multifocal breast cancers were comparable to those with unifocal tumors. Though con-firmatory studies are warranted, these results demonstrate the feasibility of SLNB in patients who have multicentric and multifocal breast cancer.

Preoperative lymphoscintigraphy

Patients undergoing lymphatic mapping with radioisotopes most often receive a preoperative lymphoscintigram (PL) to aid in SLN identification. PL typically consists of anterior and lateral views and specific patient posi-tioning to optimize transit time and radioisotope drainage [37]. Scanning routinely is initiated 20 minutes after radioisotope injection, and images are repeated until the primary SLN basin is identified and there is adequate uptake. The patient then is taken to the operating room for SLNB.

It is controversial whether preoperative scanning is of diagnostic value. Many authors have examined the accuracy of the PL, and given the addi-tional time and cost, question its value in improving the identification of sentinel lymph nodes. Proponents of the technique have argued that the scan may guide the timing of surgery when radioisotope injection is performed on the same day as the operation. Additionally, PL will identify the primary drainage pattern, and also internal mammary (IM) sentinel nodes. There is no consensus regarding the management IM SLNs that have been identified by PL, and current recommendations for adjuvant therapies have been defined mostly by axillary nodal metastases. McMasters and colleagues [38] evaluated the role of PL in breast cancer. In the study, a PL was performed in 348 of 588 patients (59%), and 240 patients did not receive scans. The SLN was identified in 221 of the 240 (92%) patients who did not undergo preoperative scanning. In these patients, the false-negative rate was 1.6%. In those patients receiving a preoperative lymphoscintigram, the SLN was identified in 310 of the 348 (89.1%) patients, with a false-negative rate of 8.7%. The authors found no significant difference in the SLN identification rate, false-negative rate, or number of SLNs removed between patients receiving PL and those proceeding to operation without scanning. Borgstein and colleagues [39] also studied the role of PL in breast cancer patients. The authors found that the intraoperative gamma probe was more sensitive in detecting radioactive nodes in the axilla than the PL, even when delayed images were obtained. In the study, axillary accumulation was absent in 14 of 130 patients receiving PL. The intraoperative gamma probe was unsuccessful in detecting radioactivity in 8 of 130 cases (seven of these patients also had negative PL).

Data have continued to emerge questioning the ability of PL to improve the accuracy of SLNB, and some centers have abandoned the technique, focusing only on resecting SLNs in the axilla, and relying on the intraoperative gamma probe to detect radioactive SLNs. Until there are definitive data regarding the treatment and importance of nonaxillary drainage, the decision to use PL is ultimately the decision of the surgeon and the multidisciplinary breast team.

Timing of radioisotope injection

Lymphatic mapping with radioisotopes is performed either as a 1- or 2-day procedure. The half-life of technitium-99 is approximately 6 hours and must be taken into account when planning SLNB.

The single-day procedure requires breast injection on the morning of surgery, followed by serial imaging at 1 to several hours after injection until the SLN is identified. In some cases, the process can take several hours and may significantly delay the operation. The effect of delay on patients and on operating room scheduling has led some centers to use a 2-day mapping procedure, with injection of radioisotopes 1 day before operation. The 2-day procedure has been criticized because of the concern that it may require higher doses of radioisotopes, or that with prolonged exposure, radioisotopes may move into higher-echelon nonsentinel lymph nodes. Winchester and colleagues [40] evaluated lymphatic mapping with radioisotope injection

1 day before operation. The study consisted of 180 patients receiving lymphatic mapping and SLNB, with technitium-99 sulfur colloid injected 1 day preoperatively. The authors found that the SLN identification rate was 90%, and was influenced largely by the surgeon's learning curve. Additionally, mapping was improved when 1.0 mCi-filtered radioisotope was used (versus 0.5 to 1.0 mCi unfiltered radioisotope). McCarter and colleagues [41] also had successful outcomes using the 2-day procedure. The authors studied 933 patients who received 0.1 mCi of dermal technitium-99 sulfur colloid in 0.05 cc normal saline on the day of surgery, and 387 patients who received 0.5 mCi technitium-99 sulfur colloid dermal injections on the day before operation. All of the patients had peri-tumoral blue dye injections intraoperatively. The median number of SLNs identified in the 2-day group was slightly higher than in the 1-day group, and the mean level of isotope counts was similar between the two groups. Likewise, Solorzano and colleagues [42] reported success with the 2-day lymphatic mapping technique. The authors found that injection of 2.5 mCi technetium sulfur colloid (filtered) peri-tumorally on the day before surgery with lymphoscintigraphy to track drainage resulted in an overall SLN identification of 97.5%. All positive SLNs with blue dye staining were also radioactive. Based on the current literature, a 2-day lymphatic mapping procedure is safe and reliable for SLNB in breast cancer.

The future and controversies

In addition to those previously mentioned controversial areas, the prognostic value of axillary nodal micrometastases identified by immunohistochemistry (IHC) analysis for cytokeratin is unknown, although the topic is the subject of ongoing clinical trials. Because it is not proven that micrometastases have any effect on breast cancer treatment, recurrences, or survival, IHC is generally not included as a routine component of SLNB [43].

Patients who have negative sentinel lymph nodes are safely spared an ALND. The question remains if patients who have positive SLNs gain a survival advantage from completion node dissection. The American College of Surgeons Oncology Group sought to answer this question with a prospective randomized controlled trial of ALND in women with early stage breast cancer and a positive SLNB [44]. The trial was terminated early because of poor patient accrual. Until data from clinical trials are available, completion of ALND remains the standard treatment for patients who have positive SLNs.

Finally, although SLNB is becoming standard for early stage breast cancer, the role of SLNB in patients who have locally advanced disease, and those receiving neoadjuvant chemotherapy (NCTX) is not well established. Breast cancer patients receiving neoadjuvant chemotherapy may undergo pre-chemotherapy sentinel lymph node biopsy (as a definitive staging procedure at presentation) or post-chemotherapy (to document the post-treatment nodal status). The pre-chemotherapy strategy commits many patients to a completion ALND on the basis of pre-treatment nodal positivity, thereby negating some of the neoadjuvant chemotherapy downstaging benefits. Several groups have studied the performance of SLNB after NCTX [45–47]. This sequence has been criticized for wide variations in the false-negative rates. The optimal strategy for incorporating lymphatic mapping into neoadjuvant chemotherapy regimens has yet to be determined and is the subject of ongoing research.

Summary

The value of SLNB in the staging and prognosis of breast cancer patients with early stage disease is defined clearly, and lymphatic mapping is becoming the standard of care for most centers. It is projected that SLNB will soon replace ALND completely as the initial evaluation procedure of the axillary nodal basin for metastases. As the specifics of lymphatic mapping evolve, the process should be individualized and tailored to institutional capabilities and the practice preferences of the entire multidisciplinary team to yield the most consistent and reliable results.

References

[1] Carter CL, Allen C, Henson DE. Relation of tumor size, lymph node status, and survival in 24,740 breast cancer cases. Cancer 1989;63:181–7.

[2] Rivadeneira DE, Simmons RM, Christos PJ, et al. Predictive factors associated with axillary lymph node metastases in T1a and T1b breast carcinomas: analysis in more than 900 patients. J Am Coll Surg 2000;191:1–8.

[3] Gann PH, Colilla SA, Gapstur SM, et al. Factors associated with axillary lymph node metastasis from breast carcinoma: descriptive and predictive analyses. Cancer 1999;86: 1511–9.

[4] Veronesi U, Paganelli G, Giuseppe V, et al. A randomized comparison of sentinel node biopsy with routine axillary dissection in breast cancer. N Engl J Med 2003;349:546–53.

[5] Krag DN, Julian TB, Harlow SP, et al. NSABP-32: phase III, randomized trial comparing axillary resection with sentinel lymph node resection: a description of the trial. Ann Surg Oncol 2004;11S:208–10.

[6] Giuliano AE, Kirgan DM, Guenther JM, et al. Lymphatic mapping and sentinel lymphadenectomy for breast cancer. Ann Surg 1994;220(3):391–8 [discussion: 398–401].

[7] Albertini JJ, Lyman GH, Cox C, et al. Lymphatic mapping and sentinel node biopsy in the patient with breast cancer. JAMA 1996;276(22):1818–22.

[8] Veronesi U, Paganelli G, Galimberti V, et al. Sentinel-node biopsy to avoid axillary dissection in breast cancer with clinically negative lymph nodes. Lancet 1997;349(9069):1864–7.

[9] Canavese G, Gipponi M, Catturich A. Technical issues and pathologic implications of sentinel lymph node biopsy in early-stage breast cancer patients. J Surg Oncol 2001;77:81–7.

[10] McMasters KM, et al. Sentinel lymph node biopsy for breast cancer: a suitable alternative to routine axillary dissection in multi-institutional practice when optimal technique is used. J Clin Oncol 2000;18(13):2560–6.

[11] Veronesi U, Paganelli G, Viale G, et al. Sentinel lymph node biopsy and axillary dissection in breast cancer: results in a large series. J Natl Cancer Inst 1999;91(4):368–73.

[12] Cox CE, Pendas S, Cox JM, et al. Guidelines for sentinel node biopsy and lymphatic mapping of patients with breast cancer. Ann Surg 1998;227(5):645–51 [discussion: 651–3].

[13] Bedrosian I, Reynolds C, Mick R, et al. Accuracy of sentinel lymph node biopsy in patients with large primary tumors. Cancer 2000;88:2540–5.

[14] Haigh PI, Hansen NM, Qi K, et al. Biopsy method and excision volume do not affect success rate of subsequent sentinel lymph node dissection in breast cancer. Ann Surg Oncol 2000; 7(1):21–7.

[15] Wong SL, Edwards MJ, Chao C, et al. The effect of prior breast biopsy method and concurrent definitive breast procedure on success and accuracy of sentinel lymph node biopsy. Ann Surg Oncol 2002;9(3):272–7.

[16] Krag D, Weaver D, Ashikaga T, et al. The sentinel node in breast cancer—a multicenter validation study. N Engl J Med 1998;339(14):941–6.

[17] O'Hea BJ, Hill AD, El-Shirbiny AM, et al. Sentinel lymph node biopsy in breast cancer: initial experience at Memorial Sloan-Kettering Cancer Center. J Am Coll Surg 1998;186(4):423–7.

[18] Guenther JM. Axillary dissection after unsuccessful sentinel lymphadenectomy for breast cancer. Am Surg 1999;65(10):991–4.

[19] Krag DN, et al. Surgical resection and radiolocalization of the sentinel lymph node in breast cancer using a gamma probe. Surg Oncol 1993;2(6):335–9.

[20] Newman LA. Lymphatic mapping and sentinel lymph node biopsy in breast cancer patients: a comprehensive review of variations in performance and technique. J Am Coll Surg 2004; 199(5):804–16.

[21] Lyew MA, Gamblin TC, Ayoub M. Systemic anaphylaxis associated with intramammary isosulfan blue injection used for sentinel node detection under general anesthesia. Anesthesiology 2000;93:1145–6.

[22] Kuerer HM, Wayne JD, Ross MI. Anaphylaxis during breast cancer lymphatic mapping. Surgery 2001;129:119–20.

[23] Montgomery LL, Thorne AC, Van Zee KJ, et al. Isosulfan blue dye reactions during sentinel lymph node mapping for breast cancer. Anesth Analg 2002;95:385–8.

[24] Simmons RM, Smith SM, Osborne MP. Methylene blue dye as an alternative to isosulfan blue dye for sentinel lymph node localization. Breast J 2001;7(3):181–3.

[25] Simmons R, Thevarajah S, Brennan M, et al. Methylene blue dye as an alternative to isosulfan blue dye for sentinel node localization. Ann Surg Oncol 2003;10(3):242–7.

[26] Blessing W, Stolier A, Teng S, et al. A comparison of methylene blue and lymphazurin in breast cancer sentinel node mapping. Am J Surg 2002;184:341–5.

[27] Kim T, Agboola O, Lyman G. Lymphatic mapping and sentinel lymph node sampling in breast cancer. Presented at the Proceedings of the American Society of Clinical Oncology 2002 Annual Symposium. 2002.

[28] Linehan DC, Hill AD, Tran KN, et al. Sentinel lymph node biopsy in breast cancer: unfiltered radioisotope is superior to filtered. J Am Coll Surg 1999;188(4):377–81.

[29] Borgstein PJ, Meijer S, Pijpers R. Intradermal blue dye to identify sentinel lymph node in breast cancer. Lancet 1997;349(9066):1668–9.

[30] Martin RC, Derossis AM, Fey J, et al. Intradermal isotope injection is superior to intramammary in sentinel node biopsy for breast cancer. Surgery 2001;130(3):432–8.

[31] Shen P, Glass EC, DiFronzo LA, et al. Dermal versus intraparenchymal lymphoscintigraphy of the breast. Ann Surg Oncol 2001;8(3):241–8.

[32] Klimberg VS, Rubio IT, Henry R, et al. Subareolar versus peri-tumoral injection for location of the sentinel lymph node. Ann Surg 1999;229(6):860–4 [discussion: 64–5].

[33] Beitsch PD, Clifford E, Whitworth P, et al. Improved lymphatic mapping technique for breast cancer. Breast J 2001;7(4):219–23.

[34] Kern KA. Sentinel lymph node mapping in breast cancer using subareolar injection of blue dye. J Am Coll Surg 1999;189:539–45.

[35] Kern KA. Breast lymphatic mapping using subareolar injections of blue dye and radiocolloid: illustrated technique. J Am Coll Surg 2001;192:545–50.

[36] Tousimis E, Van Zee KJ, Fey JV, et al. The accuracy of sentinel lymph node biopsy in multicentric and multifocal invasive breast cancers. J Am Coll Surg 2003;197(4):529–35.

[37] Haigh PI, Hansen NM, Giuliano AE, et al. Factors affecting sentinel node localization during preoperative breast lymphoscintigraphy. J Nucl Med 2000;41(10):1682–8.

[38] McMasters KM, Wong SL, Tuttle TM, et al. Preoperative lymphoscintigraphy for breast cancer does not improve the ability to identify axillary sentinel lymph nodes. Ann Surg 2000;231(5):724–31.

[39] Borgstein PJ, Pijpers R, Comans EF, et al. Sentinel lymph node biopsy in breast cancer: guidelines and pitfalls of lymphoscintigraphy and gamma probe detection. J Am Coll Surg 1998;186(3):275–83.

[40] Winchester DJ, Sener SF, Winchester DP, et al. Sentinel lymphadenectomy for breast cancer: experience with 180 consecutive patients: efficacy of filtered technetium 99m sulphur colloid with overnight migration time. J Am Coll Surg 1999;188(6):597–603.

[41] McCarter MD, Yeung H, Yeh S, et al. Localization of the sentinel node in breast cancer: identical results with same-day and day-before isotope injection. Ann Surg Oncol 2001; 8(8):682–6.

[42] Solorzano CC, Ross MI, Delpassand E, et al. Utility of breast sentinel lymph node biopsy using day-before-surgery injection of high-dose 99mTc-labeled sulfur colloid. Ann Surg Oncol 2001;8:821–7.

[43] Wilke LG, Giuliano A. Sentinel lymph node biopsy in patients with early-stage breast cancer: status of the national clinical trials. Surg Clin North Am 2003;83(4):901–10.

[44] American College of Surgeons Oncology Group. ACOSOG Z11 protocol. Available at: https://www.acosog.org/studies/organ_site/breast/archives/2004.jsp. Accessed April 3, 2007.

[45] Mamounas EP, Cohen L, Cohen A. Sentinel lymph node biopsy after neoadjuvant systemic therapy for breast cancer. Surg Clin North Am 2003;83(4):931–42.

[46] Breslin TM, Cohen L, Sahin A, et al. Sentinel lymph node biopsy is accurate after neoadjuvant chemotherapy for breast cancer. J Clin Oncol 2000;18(20):3480–6.

[47] Balch GC, Mithani SK, Richards KR, et al. Lymphatic mapping and sentinel lymphadenectomy after preoperative therapy for stage II and III breast cancer. Ann Surg Oncol 2003; 10(6):616–21.

ELSEVIER
SAUNDERS

SURGICAL
CLINICS OF
NORTH AMERICA

Surg Clin N Am 87 (2007) 365–377

Axillary Management After Sentinel Lymph Node Biopsy in Breast Cancer Patients

Aeisha Rivers, MD, Nora Hansen, MD*

Lynn Sage Comprehensive Breast Center/Northwestern University, 675 North St. Clair Street, Galter 13-174, Chicago, IL 60611, USA

The standard level I/II axillary lymph node dissection (ALND) has been a routine component of the surgical care of breast cancer patients over the past century, by providing the prognostically powerful definitive proof of axillary node-negative versus node-positive disease. Historically, ALND with surgical removal of nodal metastases in levels I and II of the axilla was thought to aid in achieving excellent local–regional control of disease in breast cancer patients. The extent to which an ALND contributes to breast cancer survival, however, is uncertain. The prognostic and staging benefits of the ALND must be weighed against the acknowledged morbidity associated with the procedure.

When suitable alternatives to ALND were considered, clinical examination and imaging modalities failed to consistently stage the axilla with accuracy [1,2]. As a result, intraoperative lymphatic mapping (IOLM) rapidly emerged as a primary approach to staging the axilla. Sentinel lymph node (SLN) biopsy has proven to be an accurate and less morbid, minimally invasive approach to evaluating the status of axillary lymph nodes. Guiliano and colleagues [3] reported greater identification of axillary metastases with the addition of SLN biopsy owing to the more detailed pathologic examination of the SLN. Many institutions have come to accept a negative SLN as an accurate means of identifying the node-negative patient for whom the ALND can be avoided. A completion ALND remains the standard of

* Corresponding author.
E-mail address: nhansen@nmh.org (N. Hansen).

0039-6109/07/$ - see front matter © 2007 Published by Elsevier Inc.
doi:10.1016/j.suc.2007.01.014

surgical.theclinics.com

care for a patient who has a positive SLN; however, this practice has been questioned in recent years for various reasons, including:

Postsurgical morbidity
Futility in removing negative nonsentinel nodes
Questionable survival benefit
The infrequency of axillary recurrence

Should axillary dissection remain the standard of care in patients with positive sentinel lymph nodes?

Morbidity associated with axillary lymph node dissection

ALND has been associated with a significant risk of lymphedema, sensory disturbances, shoulder dysfunction, wound infection, and incisional pain [4–6]. ALND patients face a lifelong risk of lymphedema that ranges from 10% to 50% [7], depending on other risk factors, duration of follow-up, and method of detection. Recent data from two very large multicenter trials provide initial reports on the morbidity associated with SLN biopsy as opposed to ALND. Among all examined variables, patients undergoing SLN biopsy fair better than patients undergoing complete axillary evaluation.

Nonsentinel node metastases

With improvements in breast cancer screening and increased public awareness, an earlier stage distribution for breast cancer and a lower incidence of axillary metastases are starting to be seen. Recent estimates suggest that only 30% of patients have evidence of axillary metastases at the time of diagnosis [8]. Studies of patients undergoing SLN biopsy with a concomitant ALND have demonstrated that axillary metastases will be limited to the SLN in 30% to 67% of cases [9–13]. Several other authors have confirmed that roughly 50% of patients who have positive SLNs subsequently are found to have no evidence of further axillary disease [9,14,15]. Removal of negative nodes does not provide any significant benefit, yet a fair number of patients with metastases isolated to the SLN still will be subjected to ALND and all of its associated morbidity to have definitive proof of their node-negative status. There is clearly no benefit to removing negative axillary nodes, and when residual metastases do extend beyond the SLN, chemotherapy has been shown to sterilize 23% of axillary metastases [16,17].

From 1995 to 1999, Calhoun and colleagues [18] identified 634 breast cancer patients who underwent SLN biopsy. SLNs were scrutinized further using immunohistochemistry if hematoxylin and eosin evaluation was negative, and ALND was recommended for patients who had SLN biopsies positive by immunohistochemistry (IHC). Seventy-eight patients (12.3%) with IHC-positive SLNs were offered ALND. Sixty-one consented, whereas 17 refused. Fifty-eight (95.1%) had negative non-SLNs. Three (4.9%) had non-SLN metastases; one (1.6%) had macrometastatic disease, whereas two (3.3%) had micrometastases. Among patients with SLNs positive by IHC only, there were no axillary recurrences after a mean of 80.5 months. When ALND was performed in the setting of an IHC-positive SLN, 1.6% of non-SLNs harbored macrometastases, and 3.3% had micrometastases. When ALND was not performed, axillary recurrence was not seen. The reported low risk of non-SLN disease in this setting provides further evidence in support of avoiding ALND for SLNs positive by IHC only.

On the contrary, according to Menes and colleagues [19], who examined the nonsentinel nodes in 124 SLN-positive patients, nonsentinel node metastases were found in 19% of patients who had sentinel node metastases less than 0.2 mm, 20% of patients who had SLN metastases measuring 0.2 mm to 2 mm, and 46% of patients who had metastases greater than 2 mm. This dataset demonstrates that in patients who are considered SLN-negative (metastases <.2 mm) and in those who have micrometastases, omitting an axillary dissection may leave residual axillary disease in 20% of cases.

The discordant findings noted in these two studies provide further evidence that conclusive, prospective, long term data from multicenter trials evaluating issues specific to SLN biopsy is well awaited.

Survival impact

Other data to support avoiding ALND in SLN-positive patients comes from important clinical trials. During the 1970s, as part of the NSABP B-04 study, clinically node-negative patients were randomized to three treatment arms: radical mastectomy, total mastectomy with radiation, and total mastectomy with axillary observation. Regardless of the type of axillary management received (axillary lymph node dissection in the radical mastectomy group, radiation alone in the second group, or observation with delayed intervention in the third group), the overall survival was equivalent. This outcome equivalence has persisted on 25-year follow-up [20]. These historical data from NSABP B-04 suggest that prophylactic resection of occult axillary metastases is comparable, in terms of survival, to axillary observation and delayed therapeutic ALND in cases of regional failure. NSABP B-04 suggests that ALND is unlikely to confer a survival benefit. Despite these findings, ALND has remained an essential component of breast cancer management.

Accrual to this phase III clinical trial was completed in an era of surgical treatment alone for breast cancer management, before the advent of effective systemic therapy for breast cancer. Subsequently, axillary nodal status became the most powerful determinant of magnitude of benefit from adjuvant systemic therapy. This remained true for several years while the adjuvant therapies for breast disease have continued to evolve. Decisions regarding additional therapy are now less dependent on the status of the axilla. Unfortunately, the B-04 study was not powered statistically to address the survival benefits of ALND; it was designed to evaluate the overall safety of modified surgical strategies (radical mastectomy versus total mastectomy versus total mastectomy and locoregional irradiation) as treatment for operable breast cancer. Thus critics continue to argue that locoregional control may provide some benefit in terms of survival.

Local recurrence

When scrutinized further, NSABP B-04 data provide information regarding axillary recurrence. In the radical mastectomy group, 40% of the patients were found to have positive axillary lymph nodes, with the axillary recurrence rate approaching approximately 1%. Assuming equal randomization between the three treatment arms, one can deduce that approximately 40% of the patients in each group possessed axillary metastases. Within the group of patients treated with total mastectomy alone, without a specific axillary intervention, however, only 18.6% developed an axillary relapse as an initial treatment failure. As suggested by the NSABP B-04 study, clinically occult and untreated axillary metastases will progress into clinically evident disease requiring a delayed/therapeutic ALND in approximately half of cases, and this outcome does not appear to adversely affect survival when compared with patients whose axillary disease was detected by a staging ALND at the time of diagnosis [20].

Axillary recurrence after a level I or II axillary dissection is unusual, occurring in 0.5% to 3% of patients in the literature [21–23]. More recently, several investigators have explored the rate of axillary recurrence after SLN biopsy. Since its introduction, the technique of SLN biopsy has evolved to optimize detection of axillary disease with false-negative rates approaching 5% [3,9,10,24–28]. Given this, one might expect a rate of axillary relapse or distant recurrence greater than or equal to 5%. This is not the case, however, according to contemporary reports.

Jeruss and colleagues [15] presented follow-up data on 864 patients. Of the 633 SLN-negative patients, 4.7% underwent completion ALND, while the remaining patients were observed. Only two (0.32%) SLN-negative patients developed recurrence within the axilla; one of which had undergone completion ALND. Sixty-eight percent of the SLN-positive patients were managed with ALND, while 32% were observed over a median follow-up of 27.4 months. There were no recurrences among the SLN-positive group. None of the study participants received radiation therapy with additional fields to include the axilla. They compiled 10 published reports of axillary relapse after sentinel node biopsy and calculated an overall recurrence rate of 0.4%, suggesting that axillary observation may be a feasible alternative in cases of both negative and positive SLNs [15]. Similarly, a pooled analysis by Smidt and colleagues [29] evaluated over 3000 patients with a median follow-up of 25 months resulting in an axillary recurrence rate of 0.25% in SLN-negative patients. This included information from their own dataset, in which they encountered two patients who had axillary recurrence, representing 0.46% of the study population.

The Memorial Sloan Kettering group reported an overall rate of axillary recurrence of 0.25% after SLN biopsy [30]. Only 10 axillary relapses were identified among all 4008 patients. Among 2340 SLN-negative patients treated without ALND, only three recurrences were seen, corresponding to a 0.12% axillary recurrence rate, providing further evidence that it is safe to omit ALND after a negative SLN. The local recurrence rates after positive SLN biopsy treated with and without ALND were 0.35% and 1.4%, respectively. In their opinion, the rarity of axillary recurrence after SLN biopsy confirms that SLN biopsy is at least equivalent to ALND in regards to staging the axilla and achieving local control of axillary disease.

Badgwell and colleagues [31] at Ohio State University retrospectively reviewed patterns of recurrence after SLN biopsy in 222 patients with a minimum of 24-month follow-up. Of 159 SLN-negative patients, five (3%) developed recurrences. One had local (breast) recurrence, and four had distant recurrences. There were no isolated regional (axillary) recurrences within the SLN-negative group. Among SLN-positive patients, the overall recurrence rate was 9.5%, with three local, one regional, and two distant recurrences. The complete absence of axillary relapse among the SLN-negative patients is comparable to an early prospective observational study by Giuliano and colleagues [32], in which no local, regional, or distant recurrences were noted among 67 SLN-negative patients, with a median follow-up of 39 months. After an extensive review if the literature, Newman [33] reported upon 10 studies evaluating patients with negative SLNs treated without ALND. This report yielded results from 10 studies published between 2000 and 2005 in which the rate of axillary recurrence ranged from 0% to 1.4% over the course of 26 to 39 months.

Fewer studies have focused their evaluation on the rates of axillary and systemic failures after positive SLN biopsy. Published results from the John Wayne Cancer Institute in 2003 describe the outcome of 46 SLN-positive patients treated without completion ALND based on patient preference or increased operative risk [34]. The degree of sentinel node disease ranged from cellular metastases in 50%, micrometastases in 35%, to macrometastases in the remaining 15% of study patients. After a mean follow-up of 32 months, zero axillary recurrences were identified, and one systemic recurrence was identified. Again, Newman [33] reported the results of five separate studies evaluating the axillary recurrence rates among SLN-positive patients treated without ALND published between 2003 and 2005. The axillary recurrence rate ranged from 0% to 2.6%, with average follow-up ranging from 25 to 32 months.

Again, this is further evidence in favor of the SLN's ability to accurately stage the axilla. The results of several major clinical trials evaluating multiple long term outcome variables after SLN biopsy are anticipated, however.

Contemporary considerations

Contemporary considerations include the advent of adjuvant therapy, the American College of Surgeons Oncology Group (ACOSOG) Z0010 trial, the American College of Surgeons Oncology Group (ACOSOG) Z0011 trial, the National Surgical Adjuvant Breast Project (NSABP) B-32 trial, and the Axillary Lymphatic Mapping Against Nodal Axillary Clearance (ALMANAC) trial.

Adjuvant therapy

In the context of contemporary guidelines for the administration of adjuvant systemic therapy, more frequently decisions regarding systemic treatment are being based on primary tumor features such as tumor size, hormone receptor status, and the presence or absence of adverse histologic features. Less focus is being placed on the status of axillary nodes [35]. Oftentimes, a combination of doxorubicin and cyclophosphamide with or without a taxane will be recommended on the basis of age or adverse histopathologic features noted within the primary tumor. Endocrine therapy may be offered to hormone receptor-positive patients in the setting of extreme patient age without much regard for lymph node status [36]. Also, the tangents used in standard whole breast radiation usually will reach the level I and II axillary nodes incidentally, so that those nodal basins will receive some radiation therapy automatically.

American College of Surgeons Oncology Group Z0010 trial

The American College of Surgeons Oncology Group Z0010 trial [37–39] was designed to evaluate the prevalence and significance of micrometastases within the sentinel node and bone marrow of T1 and T2 breast cancer patients, and determine the rate of regional recurrence in patients with negative SLNs by hematoxylin and eosin staining. Between 1999 and 2003, over 5500 patients were enrolled. In this prospective, single-arm, observational study, clinically node-negative patients undergoing breast conservation therapy and SLN biopsy also were subjected to bilateral bone marrow biopsy. ALND was performed in cases of SLN failure. SLNs deemed negative by hematoxylin and eosin (H&E) were sent to a core laboratory for immunohistochemical evaluation along with bilateral bone marrow aspirates. Patients who had one or two positive SLNs were then eligible for randomization in ACOSOG Z0011. Completion ALND was required for patients who had three or more positive SLNs, and for patients with one to two positive SLNs who did not consent to ACOSOG Z0011. Postoperatively, these patients were to receive whole-breast radiation without additional fields to include the supraclavicular lymph nodes. Adjuvant systemic therapy was recommended for all patients with SLNs positive by H&E. Primary and secondary endpoints included overall survival, disease-free survival, and axillary recurrence. In addition to determining the prevalence and prognostic significance of micrometastases detected by IHC, investigators also hope to glean some evidence regarding the rate of axillary recurrence in patients whose nodes are negative by H&E staining.

The first available published data from this trial report the surgical complications associated with SLN biopsy in 5327 patients. SLN metastases were identified by H&E staining in 24% of the study population. Patients who subsequently underwent ALND were excluded from the analysis. Early complications such as anaphylaxis (0.1%), brachial plexus injury (0.2%), wound infection (1%), hematoma (1.4%), and seroma (7.1%) were relatively uncommon and much lower than seen with traditional ALND. It was noted, however, that patients who had five or more SLNs removed experienced increased rates of wound infection and seroma when compared with patients with fewer SLNs removed. Lymphedema was defined as an increase of 2 cm from the presurgical arm measurement when compared with the contralateral arm. Six-month follow-up data reported axillary paresthesia (8.6%), decreased upper extremity range of motion (3.8%), and lymphedema (6.9%). Increasing age and body mass index (BMI) were associated with an increased incidence of lymphedema after SLN biopsy. Interestingly, postoperative adjuvant radiation therapy was not associated significantly with an increased risk of upper extremity lymphedema. In their report of the ACOSOG Z0010 data, Wilke and colleagues [40] presented an extensive review of the literature regarding complications after SLN biopsy versus ALND. According to their analysis of all available data, the incidence of lymphedema after ALND ranges from 7% to 20% as opposed to the low incidence of lymphedema noted among the Z0010 patients.

American College of Surgeons Oncology Group Z0011 trial

The American College of Surgeons Oncology Group Z0011 trial [37–39] was a phase III clinical trial for clinically node-negative patients with T1 or T2 tumors treated with breast conservation therapy and found to be SLN positive. Eligible patients who had a maximum of two positive SLNs were randomized to either completion ALND or axillary observation. The objectives of this study included assessing for the possible survival impact of ALND and comparing the morbidity associated with SLN biopsy alone versus SLN biopsy with completion ALND. Unfortunately, after 5 1/2 years, Z0011 was closed because of poor accrual rates. A total of 891 patients were enrolled instead of the desired 1900. Very few adverse events were reported in either group, requiring a substantial increase in the number of patients enrolled in the study.

According to an abstract presented at the 2006 meeting of the American Society of Clinical Oncology [41], 1003 patients from the Z0010 trial were eligible for randomization on Z0011. Of these, only 37% were entered in Z0011. Z0010 participants accounted for 42% of patients in Z0011. Sixteen percent of patients not randomized refused ALND. Sixty-nine percent of those not randomized had ALND. Sixty-seven percent of these had no additional positive nodes. Only 14% had more than four positive nodes. In the opinion of the authors, clinical bias in favor of the standard of care, completion ALND, likely played a role in the failure to accrue. Despite this, the data suggest that most patients were without additional nodal disease upon completion ALND. Long-term follow-up data are not yet available.

The American College of Surgeons Oncology Group (ACOSOG) attempted to define the value of the ALND in node-positive breast cancer by comparing disease-free survival, overall survival, postsurgical morbidity, and local control in sentinel node-positive patients randomized to axillary observation versus the standard completion axillary surgery [42]. The inability to complete this important trial likely will strengthen interest in use of statistical models that can identify patients likely to harbor additional metastatic nodes following resection of at least one metastatic sentinel node [43,44]. The goal of these prediction tools is to refine the selection of SLN-positive patients who require completion ALND.

Axillary Lymphatic Mapping Against Nodal Axillary Clearance trial

The ALMANAC trial [45] was a multicenter randomized study that compared postsurgical morbidities and quality-of-life outcomes associated with SLN biopsy versus ALND. Between 1999 and 2003, 1031 clinically node-negative breast cancer patients were randomized to SLN biopsy or standard axillary surgery. In 2003, the trial was terminated early after it became apparent that patients randomized to the SLN arm experienced far less postsurgical morbidity. Follow-up data are available at 1, 3, 6, and 12 months after surgery. Initial reports indicate that the rates of lymphedema and sensory deficit were higher in the ALND group at all time points ($P < .001$). Shoulder abduction and flexion were also worse in the ALND group during initial follow-up assessment. As mobility improved, these differences persisted at subsequent time points, but were no longer statistically significant. Other advantages associated with SLN biopsy included shorter hospital stay, less axillary drain usage, and faster return to normal activities of daily living ($P < .001$ for all three variables). The authors' conclusion that SLN was associated with less arm and shoulder morbidity than ALND is consistent with evidence previously reported in the literature [32]. The authors admit that 25% of patients in the standard axillary therapy arm underwent four-node sampling, a less extensive method of nodal evaluation. Thus, the benefits of SLN biopsy over true axillary lymph node dissection are likely to be greater than reported. Quality-of-life assessments were based upon subjective responses to validated quality-of-life instruments detailing physical, social, emotional, and functional well-being, and arm function. In all aspects, patients in the SLN arm reported better quality-of-life scores than the ALND patients at all time points ($P < .003$).

At 12-month follow-up, there were four local recurrences: one in the SLN biopsy group and three in the standard treatment arm. Additional information regarding local recurrence rates and survival effects will be available in the future in conjunction with results from the ACOSOG trials and NSABP B-32.

NSABP B-32

NSABP B-32 was a large multicenter randomized phase III clinical trial comparing SLND with ALND [38,39]. With the help of over 230 surgeons at 75 participating institutions, over 5600 clinically node-negative patients were accrued over a 4.5-year period between May 1999 and February 2004. Eligible patients with T1-T3 invasive cancer were randomized to SLN biopsy followed by ALND versus SLN biopsy with ALND only in cases with failed SLN identification or positive SLN. All patients who had negative SLNs will have further nodal evaluation with immunohisto-chemistry at a central laboratory. The investigators hope to demonstrate that patients who have a histologically negative SLN with no further axillary surgery will have the same long-term outcomes, with less morbidity, and better functional outcomes than those patients who subsequently receive a completion ALND. Comparisons will be made in regards to survival, locoregional control, and postsurgical morbidity. It is also hoped that this study will provide insight as to whether there is prognostic value associated with completion ALND after a positive SLN biopsy. Other secondary goals include confirming the success rate and accuracy of the SLN procedure, evaluating the sensitivity and specificity of frozen section evaluation, and determining the significance of immunohistochemically detected metastases.

Preliminary data are available regarding technical results in over 5200 patients [46]. Consistent with previous reports in the literature, the overall rate of SLN identification was 97%. Allergic reactions were rare (0.7%). Twenty-six percent of patients possessed positive SLNs, and similar to results from Z0011, in 61.5% of the SN-positive patients, no additional positive nodes were found on completion ALND. There was no significant difference in SLN identification rates between the two groups of patients. Further results from this trial are forthcoming.

Predicting the status of nonsentinel nodes

Given the uncertainties regarding the survival benefits associated with the completion ALND, a valid argument can be made that the critical issue is to identify the subset of high-risk SLN-positive patients who are likely to have metastases beyond the SLN node. As mentioned previously, Menes and colleagues [19] identified nonsentinel node metastases in 19% of patients with sentinel node metastases less than 0.2 mm, 20% of patients with SLN metastases measuring 0.2 mm to 2 mm, 46% of patients with metastases greater than 2 mm. This dataset demonstrates that in patients who are considered SLN-negative (metastases less than 0.2 mm) and those with micrometastases, omitting an axillary dissection may leave residual axillary disease in 20% of patients. So the logical question arises: Can we identify patients with positive SLNs who can avoid a completion ALND safely?

Van Zee and colleagues [43] therefore developed a nomogram that estimates the likelihood that an individual SLN-positive patient will have additional metastatic nodes in the completion ALND specimen. Degnim and colleagues [44] conducted a meta-analysis of studies involving SLN biopsy with concomitant ALND, and this pooled analysis provides a robust assessment of clinicopathologic features associated with likelihood of detecting metastatic disease in nonsentinel nodes. Chu and colleagues [47] also evaluated clinicopathologic features of 157 patients who underwent SLN biopsy followed by ALND to determine risk factors for nonsentinel node involvement. All of these investigators have found primary tumor size and extent of SLN pathology to be strong predictors of non-SLN disease. Despite the fact that the nomogram does not offer treatment recommendations, it often is employed in clinical practice.

Viale and colleagues [48] examined the SLNs and non-SLNs of over 1200 patients in a similar fashion to also produce a predictive model. According to their data, the size and number of SLN metastases and lymphovascular invasion were significant predictors of further axillary involvement. In their opinion, even SLN-positive patients with the lowest possible predicted risk of additional disease (13%) should be offered completion axillary lymph node dissection. Similarly, other investigators have weighed in on this issue with concordant results. Katz and colleagues [49] conducted a retrospective evaluation of the records of over 1133 patients undergoing SLN biopsy, which yielded information on 367 SLN-positive patients. Increasing number of positive SLNs, decreasing number of negative SLNs, increasing size of the SLN metastasis, and the presence of lymphovascular invasion were associated with the likelihood of finding additional nodal disease on completion ALND. The lowest calculated risk of additional disease in their study cohort was still 14%. Interestingly, according to their extensive review of the literature, the rate of non-SLN metastases in patients with sentinel lymph node micrometastases ranged from 0% to 34%. In this study, Katz and colleagues offered that they also recommend completion axillary lymph node dissection in the setting of a positive SLN until definitive clinical trial data stating the contrary are available.

Is there still a role for axillary lymph node dissection?

According to the available data, SLN biopsy is proving to be an accurate staging technique with less postsurgical morbidity than standard ALND. Survival benefits associated with SLN biopsy and ALND, and the significance of IHC-detected micrometastases have yet to be determined. The long-term results of several multicenter trials are pending, yet preliminary results are in favor of abandoning ALND in favor of the less-invasive alternative.

Despite this, ALND remains the standard of care in breast cancer patients who have clinically palpable axillary lymph nodes that are suspicious for metastatic disease. Although controversial, many clinicians believe that axillary metastases will precede systemic spread of disease. Therefore, axillary clearance of clinically palpable nodes could quell the progression of metastases. Regardless of whether this theory is true, not many would argue against debulking suspicious nodal disease.

References

[1] Fisher B, Wolmark N, Bauer M, et al. The accuracy of clinical nodal staging and of limited axillary dissection as a determinant of histologic nodal status in carcinoma of the breast. Surg Gynecol Obstet 1981;152:765–72.

[2] Dees EC, Shulman LN, Souba WW, et al. Does information from axillary dissection change treatment in clinically node-negative patients with breast cancer? Ann Surg 1997;226:279–87.

[3] Guiliano AE, Dale PS, Turner RR, et al. Improved axillary staging of breast cancer with sentinel lymphadenectomy. Ann Surg 1995;222:394–401.

[4] Engel J, Kerr J, Schlesinger-Raab A, et al. Axilla surgery severely affects quality of life: results of a 5-year prospective study in breast cancer patients. Breast Cancer Res Treat 2003;79: 47–57.

[5] Kissen MW, Querci della Rovere G, Easton D, et al. Risk of lymphoedema following the treatment of breast cancer. Br J Surg 1986;73:580–4.

[6] Ivens D, Hoe AL, Podd TJ, et al. Assessment of morbidity from complete axillary dissection. Br J Cancer 1992;66:136–8.

[7] Erickson VS, Pearson ML, Ganz PA, et al. Arm edema in breast cancer patients. J Natl Cancer Inst 2001;93:96–111.

[8] Cady B. The need to re-examine axillary lymph node dissection in invasive breast cancer. J Clin Oncol 1997;15:2345–50.

[9] Krag D, Weaver D, Ashikaga T, et al. The sentinel node in breast cancer—a multicenter validation study. N Engl J Med 1998;339(14):941–6.

[10] Giuliano AE, Kirgan DM, Guenther JM, et al. Lymphatic mapping and sentinel lymphadenectomy for breast cancer. Ann Surg 1994;220:391–8 [discussion: 398–401].

[11] Giuliano AE, Jones RC, Brennan M, et al. Sentinel lymphadenectomy in breast cancer. J Clin Oncol 1997;15:2345–50.

[12] Borgstein PJ, Pijpers R, Comans EF, et al. Sentinel lymph node biopsy in breast cancer: guidelines and pitfalls of lymphoscintigraphy and gamma probe detection. J Am Coll Surg 1998;186:275–83.

[13] Albertini JJ, Lyman GH, Cox C, et al. Lymphatic mapping and sentinel node biopsy in the patient with breast cancer. JAMA 1996;276:1818–22.

[14] Abdessalam SF, Zervos EE, Prasad M, et al. Predictors of positive axillary lymph nodes after sentinel lymph node biopsy in breast cancer. Am J Surg 2001;182:316–20.

[15] Jeruss JS, Winchester DJ, Sener SF, et al. Axillary recurrence after sentinel node biopsy. Ann Surg Oncol 2005;12:34–40.

[16] Rouzier R, Extra JM, Klijanienko J, et al. Incidence and prognostic significance of complete axillary downstaging in breast cancer patients with T1 to T3 tumors and cytologically proven axillary metastatic lymph nodes. J Clin Oncol 2002;20:5–10.

[17] Kuerer HM, Sahin AA, Hunt KK, et al. Incidence and impact of documented eradication of breast cancer axillary lymph node metastases before surgery in patients treated with neoadjuvant chemotherapy. Ann Surg 1999;230:72–8.

[18] Calhoun KE, Hansen NM, Turner RR, et al. Nonsentinel node metastases in breast cancer patients with isolated tumor cells in the sentinel node: implications for completion axillary dissection. Am J Surg 2005;190:588–91.

[19] Menes TS, Tartter PI, Mizrachi H, et al. Breast cancer patients with pN0(i+) and pN1(mi) sentinel nodes have high rate of nonsentinel node metastases. J Am Coll Surg 2005;200(3): 323–7.

[20] Fisher B, Jeong JH, Anderson S, et al. Twenty-five year follow-up of a randomized trial comparing radical mastectomy, total mastectomy, and total mastectomy followed by irradiation. N Engl J Med 2002;347:567–75.

[21] Fisher B, Montague E, Redmind C, et al. Findings from NSABP Protocol No. B-04. Comparison of radical mastectomy with alternative treatments for primary breast cancer. Cancer 1980;46:1–13.

[22] Wright FC, Walker J, Law L, et al. Outcomes after localized axillary node recurrence in breast cancer. Ann Surg Oncol 2003;10:1054–8.

[23] Clemons M, Danson S, Hamilton T, et al. Locoregionally recurrent breast cancer: incidence, risk factors, and survival. Cancer Treat Rev 2001;27:67–82.

[24] Morton DL, Wen DR, Wong JH, et al. Technical details of intraoperative lymphatic mapping for early stage melanoma. Arch Surg 1992;127(4):392–9.

[25] Krag DN, Weaver DL, Alex JC, et al. Surgical resection and radiolocalization of the sentinel node in breast cancer using gamma probe. Surg Oncol 1993;2:335–40.

[26] Veronesi U, Paganelli G, Galimberti V, et al. Sentinel node biopsy to avoid axillary dissection in breast cancer with clinically negative lymph nodes. Lancet 1997;349:1864–7.

[27] McMasters KM, Wong SL, Tuttle TM, et al. Preoperative lymphoscintigraphy for breast cancer does not improve the ability to identify axillary sentinel lymph nodes. Ann Surg 2000;231(5):724–31.

[28] Miltenberg DM, Miller C, Karamlou TB, et al. Meta-analysis of sentinel lymph node biopsy in breast cancer. J Surg Res 1999;84(2):138–42.

[29] Smidt ML, Janssen CM, Kuster DM, et al. Axillary recurrence after a negative sentinel node biopsy for breast cancer: incidence and clinical significance. Ann Surg Oncol 2004;12(1): 29–33.

[30] Naik AM, Fey J, Gemignani M, et al. The risk of axillary relapse after sentinel lymph node biopsy for breast cancer is comparable with that of axillary lymph node dissection. Ann Surg 2004;240(3):462–71.

[31] Badgwell BD, Povoski SP, Abdessalam SF, et al. Patterns of recurrence after sentinel lymph node biopsy for breast cancer. Ann Surg Oncol 2003;10(4):376–80.

[32] Giuliano AE, Haigh PI, Brennan MB, et al. Prospective observational study of sentinel lymphadenectomy without further axillary dissection in patients with sentinel node-negative breast cancer. J Clin Oncol 2000;18:2553–9.

[33] Newman LA. The practice of lymphatic mapping and sentinel lymph node biopsy for breast cancer patients. J Oncology Practice; in press.

[34] Guenther JM, Hansen NM, Difronzo LA, et al. Axillary dissection is not required for all patients with breast cancer and positive sentinel nodes. Arch Surg 2003;138:52–6.

[35] Marschall J, Nechala P, Colquhoun P, et al. Reassessing the role of axillary lymph node dissection in patients with early stage breast cancer. Can J Surg 2003;46:285–9.

[36] Hughes KS, Schnaper L, Berry D, et al. Lumpectomy plus tamoxifen with and without irradiation in women 70 years of age or older with early breast cancer. N Engl J Med 2004; 351(10):971–7.

[37] American College of Surgeons Oncology Group, home page. Available at: www.acosog.org/. Accessed September 1, 2006.

[38] White RL, Wilke LG. Update on the NSABP and ACOSOG breast cancer sentinel node trials. Am Surg 2004;70:420–4.

[39] Posther KE, Wilke LG, Guiliano AE. Sentinel lymph node dissection and the current status of American trials on breast lymphatic mapping. Semin Oncol 2004;31(3):426–36.

[40] Wilke LG, Mccall LM, Posther KE, et al. Surgical complications associated with sentinel lymph node biopsy: results from a prospective international cooperative group trial. Ann Surg Oncol 2006;13(4):491–500.

[41] Leitch AM, McCall L, Beitsch P, et al. Factors influencing accrual to ACOSOG Z0011, a randomized phase III trial of axillary dissection vs. observation for sentinel node-positive breast cancer. J Clin Oncol 2006;24(18S):601 [2006 ASCO Annual Meeting Proceedings Part I].

[42] Wilke LG, Giuliano A. Sentinel lymph node biopsy in patients with early stage breast cancer: status of the National Clinical Trials. Surg Clin North Am 2003;83:901–10.

[43] Van Zee KJ, Manasseh DM, Bevilacqua JL, et al. A nomogram for predicting the likelihood of additional nodal metastases in breast cancer patients with a positive sentinel node biopsy. Ann Surg Oncol 2003;10:1140–51.

[44] Degnim AC, Griffith KA, Sabel MS, et al. Clinicopathologic features of metastasis in non-sentinel lymph nodes of breast carcinoma patients. Cancer 2003;98:2307–15.

[45] Mansel RE, Fallowfeld L, Kissin M, et al. Randomized multicenter trial of sentinel node biopsy versus standard axillary treatment in operable breast cancer: the ALMANAC trial. J Natl Cancer Inst 2006;98(9):599–609.

[46] Julian TB, Krag D, Brown A, et al. Preliminary technical results of NSABP B-32, a randomized phase III clinical trial to compare sentinel node resection to conventional axillary dissection in clinically node-negative breast cancer patients. Breast Cancer Res Treat 2004;88:S11.

[47] Chu KU, Turner RR, Hansen NM, et al. Sentinel node metastasis in patients with breast carcinoma accurately predicts immunohistochemically detectable nonsentinel node metastasis. Ann Surg Oncol 1999;6:756–61, 24.

[48] Viale G, Maiorano E, Pruneri G, et al. Predicting the risk for additional axillary metastases in patients with breast carcinoma and positive sentinel lymph node biopsy. Ann Surg 2005; 241(2):319–25.

[49] Katz A, Niemierko A, Gage I, et al. Can axillary dissection be avoided in patients with sentinel lymph node metastasis? J Surg Oncol 2006;93:550–8.

ELSEVIER
SAUNDERS

SURGICAL
CLINICS OF
NORTH AMERICA

Surg Clin N Am 87 (2007) 379–398

Management of Patients with Locally Advanced Breast Cancer

Marie Catherine Lee, MD[a],
Lisa A. Newman, MD, MPH, FACS[b],*

[a]Department of Surgery, University of Michigan, 1500 East Medical Center Drive,
3216A Cancer Center/Box 0932, Ann Arbor, MI 48109, USA
[b]University of Michigan Comprehensive Cancer Center, Breast Care Center,
1500 East Medical Center Drive, Ann Arbor, MI 48167, USA

Locally advanced breast cancer (LABC) continues to be a significant problem in the United States and a common breast cancer presentation worldwide. LABC generally is defined by bulky primary chest wall tumors and/or extensive adenopathy. This includes patients with T3 (> 5 cm) or T4 tumors (chest wall fixation or skin ulceration and/or satellitosis) and N2/N3 disease (matted axillary and/or internal mammary metastases) [1]. Of note, recent studies demonstrate that prolonged survival can be achieved in patients with metastatic disease limited to the supraclavicular nodes after appropriate multimodality breast cancer treatment [1,2]. As a result, the sixth edition of the American Joint Committee on Cancer (AJCC) staging system now includes isolated supraclavicular metastases in the stage III/LABC disease category [3]. According to the American College of Surgeons National Cancer Data Base, approximately 6% of breast cancers in the United States present as stage III breast cancer disease [4]. Five-year survival for stage III breast cancer is approximately 50%, compared with 87% for stage I.

The extent to which LABC represents neglect and delayed diagnosis versus aggressive tumor biology is unclear. Data from the Surveillance, Epidemiology, and End Results (SEER) program reveal that the proportion of LABC is notably higher among women of African, Hispanic, and Native American descent compared with white and Asian Americans, contributing to increased mortality in these populations. These disparities partly reflect socioeconomic and health care access inequalities, but parallel variations in the incidence of breast cancer based on country of origin also suggest

* Corresponding author.
  E-mail address: lanewman@umich.edu (L.A. Newman).

0039-6109/07/$ - see front matter © 2007 Published by Elsevier Inc.
doi:10.1016/j.suc.2007.01.012

surgical.theclinics.com

the existence of environmental and genetic factors. This article discusses the history of LABC treatment and the preferred diagnostic–therapeutic management sequence. The evolving subjects of breast conservation, immediate breast reconstruction, optimal neoadjuvant treatment, and lymphatic mapping in patients who have LABC also are addressed.

Evolution of treatment options in locally advanced breast cancer

Surgeons historically have been at the forefront of investigating LABC treatment. Haagensen and Stout [5] at Columbia University provided early data regarding the dismal results of radical mastectomy alone as treatment for LABC over 60 years ago, reporting 5-year local recurrence and survival rates of 46% and 6%, respectively. This experience led to the definition of inoperable LABC when patients presented with extensive breast skin edema or satellitosis, intercostal/parasternal nodules, arm edema, supraclavicular metastases, or inflammatory breast cancer. In contrast, grave local signs of LABC were poor prognostic features, but not contraindications to resection. These included ulceration, limited skin edema, fixation to the pectoralis muscle, and bulky axillary adenopathy.

Therapeutic doses of chest wall radiation were similarly inadequate in controlling LABC. Studies from the 1970s and 1980s by the Joint Center for Radiation Therapy, Guy's Hospital, and the Mallincrodt Institute of Radiology all revealed excessively high failure rates, with 5-year local recurrence rates ranging from 46% to 72%, and survival rates of 16% to 30% [6–8]. Combined treatment with radiation plus surgery was also attempted in this era [9–11], but yielded no significant improvement in disease control.

Preoperative chemotherapy protocols (also known as neoadjuvant or induction chemotherapy) revolutionized LABC care; this approach is now standard for patients with bulky breast and/or axillary disease. Early concerns regarding this approach were based on the potentially negative effects of preoperative chemotherapy on: surgical complication rates, the prognostic value of the axillary staging, and overall survival after delayed surgery. Clinical investigations reported during the 1980s and 1990s addressed and alleviated these concerns.

Comparable operative morbidity was demonstrated in a study of nearly 200 LABC patients treated with mastectomy, approximately half of whom received preoperative chemotherapy; neoadjuvant patients actually had a lower rate of postoperative seroma formation [12]. Danforth and colleagues [13] similarly reported that preoperative chemotherapy neither adversely affects surgical complication rates nor delays postoperative treatment. Most patients are ready for surgery 3 to 4 weeks after the last chemotherapy cycle, when absolute neutrophil and platelet counts are greater than 1500 and 100,000, respectively.

The prognostic value of axillary staging in LABC patients that have received neoadjuvant chemotherapy followed by axillary lymph node dissection was confirmed by McCready and colleagues [14]. A study of 136 LABC cases undergoing modified radical mastectomy following induction chemotherapy revealed that patients with no axillary metastases in the post-chemotherapy mastectomy specimen had a nearly 80% 5-year survival rate. In contrast, fewer than 10% of patients who had 10 or more positive nodes survived 5 years, and patients who had an intermediate number of residual nodes had intermediate survival rates.

The issue of whether neoadjuvant chemotherapy can improve survival in LABC patients remains controversial. However several prospective trials conducted internationally have clearly demonstrated that delaying surgery while systemic therapy is being delivered does not compromise outcome when compared to the sequence of surgery first, followed by postoperative chemotherapy. It has been shown that neoadjuvant therapy does not worsen survival but it does improve resectability. Approximately 80% of patients have significant primary tumor shrinkage; only 2% to 3% have signs of pro-gression [15–17]. Fears of a missed window of opportunity to resect chest wall disease therefore are unfounded, and preoperatively treated patients of-ten are improved operative candidates. Resection is essential for document-ing chemotherapy response and achieving locoregional control, as clinical assessment is notoriously unreliable [18,19]. Table 1 [20–22] summarizes re-sults of various LABC treatment strategies over the past several decades.

Currently, optimal control is achieved with preoperative chemotherapy followed by surgery and radiation. Preoperative versus postoperative che-motherapy have been directly compared in women with LABC and also in women with early stage breast cancer. These prospective clinical trials have demonstrated overall survival equivalence for the two sequences, confirming the oncologic safety of the neoadjuvant approach [23–30]. Since patients with LABC benefit from the tumor downstaging and improved resectability that can be achieved with neoadjuvant chemotherapy, this se-quence has become the preferred approach for patients with bulky, locally advanced disease at time of diagnosis.

Diagnostic and therapeutic management sequence

Establishing a tissue diagnosis is the initial priority on presentation of LABC. In many patients, core biopsy of the tumor, either freehand or under ultrasound guidance, is diagnostic. Core needle is preferred over fine needle aspiration, as cytology is insufficient to confirm invasion. Additionally, mul-tiple cores should be extracted both to confirm invasive cancer and to eval-uate hormone receptor status and HER2/neu expression. This is critical, because palpable ductal carcinoma in situ (DCIS) does exist, and induction chemotherapy is inappropriate for DCIS, even with microinvasion. A neg-ative or nondiagnostic needle biopsy with a clinically suspicious lesion is an indication to proceed to diagnostic open biopsy; cases characterized by skin involvement may be amenable to punch biopsy. If matted, fixed,

Table 1
Locally advanced breast cancer outcome based on treatment delivered and sequence of multimodality therapy

Treatment approach	Components and sequence of treatment	Study	Sample size	5-year local recurrence rate(%)	5-year survival (%)
Single modality	Surgery only	Haagensen and Stout, 1943 [5]	35	46%	6%
		Arnold and Lesnick, 1979 [10]	50	50%	33%
	Radiation (XRT) only	Rubens, 1977 [8]	184	72%	18%
		Harris, 1983 [6]	137	46%	30%
Dual modality	XRT → surgery	Arnold and Lesnick, 1979 [10]	54	70%	30%
	Surgery → XRT	Townsend, 1985 [9]	53	11%	47%
		Arnold and Lesnick, 1979 [10]	122	70%	32%
		Montague and Fletcher, 1985 [11]	132	13%	43% (at 10 years)
	Chemotherapy → surgery	Valagussa, 1983 [20]	205	18%	49%
	Chemotherapy → XRT	Perloff, 1988 [16]	43	19%	Median survival 39 months
		Valagussa, 1983 [20]	198	36%	35%
Triple modality	Surgery → chemotherapy → XRT	Perloff, 1988 [16]	44	27%	Median survival 39 months
		Olson, 1997 [21]	148	20%	65% (estimated from graph)
	Chemotherapy → surgery → XRT	Kuerer, 1999 [38]	372; pCR; n = 43	5%	89%
			<pCR; n = 329	9%	64%
	Surgery → chemotherapy → XRT	Cance, 2002 [22]	62	14%	76%
		Olson, 1997 [21]	164	9%	66% (estimated from graph)

axillary, or supraclavicular adenopathy is present, fine needle aspiration of the nodes may be performed for staging.

Prompt bilateral mammography in this setting is essential, regardless of patient age and date of her most recent study. Diffuse, suspicious microcalcifications or multiple lesions in different quadrants indicate multicentric disease, and are a contraindication to breast conservation therapy (BCT). Patients who have these findings should be informed that they will require mastectomy regardless of their neoadjuvant therapy response [31]. If BCT is a consideration, a microclip placed at the primary tumor is essential before the initiation of induction therapy, unless the primary tumor is associated with a cluster of microcalcifications. Up to 50% of patients may have a complete clinical response, and an unmarked primary site eliminates the possibility of breast preservation in these cases, as the lumpectomy site will no longer be adequately defined.

Breast and axillary ultrasound frequently yield valuable information regarding the extent of disease. In particular, axillary ultrasound can be used for image-guided FNA [32,33]; ultrasound detection of apical axillary/infraclavicular nodal metastases has been shown to provide important prognostic information [34]. Unfortunately, ultrasound has an approximately 20% false-negative rate, as metastases smaller than 5 mm in size are undetectable.

Once a tissue diagnosis is established, LABC patients should undergo multidisciplinary review before treatment. The multidisciplinary team should include surgical, medical and radiation oncologists, pathologists, radiologists, and plastic surgeons, creating a unified treatment proposal and thereby minimizing the possibility that inconsistent messages will be delivered to the patient by the various specialists involved with the management plan. A baseline bone scan, and chest, abdominal, and pelvic CT scans are recommended for detection of metastatic disease. Directed radiographs to sites of new bone pain, or a head CT scan for new neurologic symptoms are also appropriate in selected cases. The yield of a metastatic work-up in an asymptomatic, early breast cancer patient is approximately 2% to 3%, but this risk rises to 30% in LABC [35]. With radiologic evidence of metastatic disease, the role of surgery is controversial. Some data suggest a survival benefit with aggressive breast surgery despite the presence of distant organ metastases. However, these retrospective analyses are limited by an inability to control for inherent selection biases [36].

Patients receiving preoperative chemotherapy should be reassessed after one or two cycles and again at the completion of therapy to document response and explore surgical options. Repeat imaging may be useful at the interim evaluation. If minimal or no response is observed after the initial cycles, a decision should be made to either proceed with surgery or to cross over to a different systemic therapy. Salvage surgery allows for a full pathologic evaluation, facilitating decisions on adjuvant therapy. If an alternative regimen is selected, then reassessment after two cycles of the crossover treatment is necessary. Follow-up imaging is essential after complete delivery of neoadjuvant therapy for final preoperative surgical planning. Occasional patients that appeared to have a unicentric cancer density at presentation will experience unmasking of extensive microcalcifications or multicentric satellite tumors after chemotherapy response, and these findings may convert them to mandatory mastectomy cases.

Subset analyses of the phase III studies reveal that patients who have a complete pathologic response (pCR) have a statistically significant survival benefit, substantiating the concept that primary tumor response is a reliable surrogate for chemotherapy effect on micrometastases. In the NSABP B-18 trial [37], patients with stage I to III breast cancer randomized to receive preoperative doxorubicin and Cytoxan and who experienced a pCR had a 5-year overall survival of 86%, statistically superior to the outcome seen in all other study participants. Predictors of a pCR include relatively smaller size primary breast tumors, estrogen receptor negativity, and high-grade lesions [38].

Controversies in the management of locally advanced breast cancer patients

Breast conservation therapy versus mastectomy

The magnitude of the clinical response to neoadjuvant chemotherapy in LABC prompted investigations of breast conservation for selected patients. Initially, whether the clinical response correlated with either a concentric diminution of the initial mass or a primary tumor that left foci of malignant cells in the remaining parenchyma was unclear. Singletary and colleagues [39] conducted a feasibility study to evaluate the pathologic extent of residual disease in 136 LABC patients treated with induction chemotherapy. Extensive scrutiny of the postchemotherapy mastectomy specimens revealed that the residual tumor would have been amenable to lumpectomy in approximately 25% of patients.

From this and other studies [31], several criteria for BCT in postneoadjuvant LABC have been adopted widely:

- Patient desire for breast preservation
- Absence of multicentric disease (tumors in different quadrants of the breast)
- Absence of diffuse microcalcifications on mammogram
- Absence of skin involvement consistent with inflammatory breast cancer
- Residual tumor mass amenable to a margin-negative lumpectomy resection

Prospective, randomized controlled clinical trial data have confirmed acceptable rates of local control among LABC patients undergoing breast-conserving surgery after neoadjuvant therapy. Several prospective, randomized controlled trials of neoadjuvant versus adjuvant/postoperative chemotherapy have included cohorts of patients with Stage III disease/ LABC. Data from these studies have documented acceptably low rates of local recurrence in LABC patients undergoing breast-conserving surgery after neoadjuvant chemotherapy (Table 2) [40,41]. The NSABP B-18 investigators did note a trend toward higher local recurrence rates among patients requiring preoperative downstaging in order to become lumpectomy eligible (15% versus 7%). This is not necessarily surprising, however, as postlumpectomy local recurrence is one manifestation of aggressive tumor biology, and larger tumors are more likely to demonstrate aggressive behavior, even after mastectomy. Postmastectomy radiation (PMRT) is recommended for patients with T3 tumors because of this concept [42]. Of note, the NSABP defines a negative margin as the absence of tumor cells at the cut, inked specimen margin; wider margins are probably preferable in patients receiving neoadjuvant chemotherapy.

Optimal preoperative systemic therapy regimen

Currently, doxorubicin-based chemotherapy is the most widely-studied induction regimen, and it results in at least 50% tumor shrinkage in more than 75% of cases. The NSABP B-27 protocol randomized patients with resectable breast cancer to one of three neoadjuvant treatment arms: (1) doxorubicin and Cytoxan alone; (2) doxorubicin, Cytoxan, and docetaxel; or (3) preoperative doxorubicin and Cytoxan followed by postoperative docetaxel. Preliminary data [43] reveal a pCR rate of 26% associated with the addition of docetaxel to the preoperative regimen. Similarly, the University of Texas M.D. Anderson Cancer Center [44] has reported a pCR rate of nearly 30% in patients treated with preoperative doxorubicin, Cytoxan, 5-fluorouracil, and weekly Taxol.

The Aberdeen trial investigated whether the number of chemotherapy cycles is a stronger predictor of tumor response compared with chemotherapy type [45,46]. One hundred sixty-two patients with primary tumors of at least 3 cm were given four cycles of doxorubicin-based chemotherapy. Responders then were randomized to either four more cycles of doxorubicin, or crossed over to four cycles of docetaxel, so that all patients received eight preoperative cycles of chemotherapy. Among the responders, the pCR rate for the doxorubicin-only group was 16%, compared with 34% for the responders randomized to the crossover docetaxel regimen (P = .04), demonstrating that the nature of the agent is more important than the quantity. They also showed that poor responders may benefit from crossover to an alternative regimen. Survival analyses at 3 years also suggest improved outcomes for patients on docetaxel plus doxorubicin [46].

Neoadjuvant endocrine therapy for estrogen receptor-positive LABC also holds great promise. Three-to-four months of therapy are preferred for an adequate response assessment, and preliminary studies suggest that aromatase inhibitors such as letrozole are more effective than tamoxifen [47,48]. Other neoadjuvant regimens currently being evaluated include trastuzumab, Navelbine, capecitabine, and gemcitabine. Microarray technology

Table 2
Randomized studies of neoadjuvant versus adjuvant chemotherapy for breast cancer

Study	N	Stages	Treatment	Median follow-up	BCT rate		Local recurrence after BCT		Overall survival at median follow-up	
					Preoperative chemotherapy	Postoperative chemotherapy	Preoperative chemotherapy	Postoperative chemotherapy	Preoperative chemotherapy	Postoperative chemotherapy
Institut Curie [25,26,40,41]	414	IIA-IIIA	FAC×4→XRT ± S versus XRT ± S→ FAC×4 (S reserved for incomplete responders)	66 mo	82%	77%	24%	18%	86%	78%
Royal Marsden [27,28]	309	I-IIIB	Tam + MM±M×4→ S→Tam + MM±M×4 Versus S→MM±M×8 + Tam	48 mo	89%	78%	3%[b]	4%[b]	80%[a]	80%[a]
NSABP [29,30]	1523	I-IIIA	AC×4→S Versus S→ AC×4	72 mo	68%	60%	7.9%	5.8%	80%[c]	80%[c]

Abbreviations: BCT, breast conservation therapy; EVM, epirubicin vincristine methotrexate; FAC 5, -fluorouracil doxorubicin cyclophosphamide; MM ± M, mitoxantrone methotrexate with or without mitomycin-C; MRM, modified radical mastectomy; MTV, mitomycin C thiotepa vindesine; NA, not applicable; S, surgery; Tam, Tamoxifen; XRT, radiation.

[a] Rate estimated from graph.

[b] Local recurrence rates reported for lumpectomy and mastectomy patients combined.

[c] Overall survival rate at 5 years.

and gene expression profiling are also being explored to optimize selection of neoadjuvant therapy [49].

Monitoring response to neoadjuvant chemotherapy

A significant response to the primary chemotherapy regimen is observed in about 80% of cases; however, accurate prediction of a pCR is challenging. Conventional modalities for assessing chemotherapy response, including clinical examination, mammogram, and breast ultrasound, are incorrect in identifying pCR patients in nearly half of cases. The addition of imaging is clearly more useful than physical examination alone [31,50]. Breast MRI [51,52], positron emission tomography [53], and nuclear medicine sestamibi uptake scans [54,55] have been reported in small series as monitoring strategies with encouraging results.

Immediate breast reconstruction

LABC traditionally has been perceived as a contraindication to immediate breast reconstruction (IBR), because of concerns regarding adjuvant treatment delays and the cosmetic effects of PMRT to breast reconstruction. Newman and colleagues [56] studied 50 patients with stage IIB to IIIA breast cancer who underwent mastectomy with IBR and found no adverse effect on surgical complication rates compared with 72 mastectomy patients who had LABC without IBR. There was a slightly prolonged interval for adjuvant chemotherapy among reconstructed patients; this did not affect recurrence rates. IBR with implants, however, was associated with more radiation-related complications; nearly half of the irradiated patients developed contractures or recurrent infections, necessitating implant removal. Other investigators report favorable outcomes for LABC patients undergoing mastectomy and transverse rectus abdominus myocutaneous (TRAM) flap IBR [57], although at least one recent study suggests that radiated TRAM flaps exhibit late-onset fibrosis and contracture [58]. Delayed reconstruction is therefore, usually preferred in LABC patients undergoing mastectomy, because of the substantial likelihood that PMRT will be necessary, and the potential damaging effects of radiating the reconstructed breast. Occasionally, LABC patients will require soft tissue coverage of an extensive chest wall defect at mastectomy. In these cases, a latissimus dorsi flap is the most common approach, as this flap is a technically straightforward and provides durable, radiation-tolerant coverage. A latissimus dorsi flap used for chest wall coverage however, will usually not have the appearance of a reconstructed breast.

Locoregional irradiation for locally advanced breast cancer patients treated with neoadjuvant chemotherapy

The American Society of Clinical Oncology recommends PMRT for all patients who have four or more metastatic axillary lymph nodes based upon axillary surgical findings at presentation (without neoadjuvant chemotherapy), and that PMRT should be considered for any case of operable LABC [42]. In the setting of neoadjuvant therapy, the precise initial pathologic staging is unknown. Because PMRT appears to provide an outcome advantage as adjuvant treatment for surgically resected high-risk disease, a valid question arises regarding the possibility that neoadjuvant chemotherapy might impair the ability to identify these patients.

Patients who have at least four metastatic lymph nodes or 5 cm of residual disease in the breast after chemotherapy clearly benefit from locoregional irradiation, and all lumpectomy patients require breast irradiation. A conservative (and aggressive) approach would be to recommend radiation to all patients that present with LABC, regardless of chemotherapy response. However, patients with little or no residual breast/axillary disease after chemotherapy may not derive a significant benefit from regional nodal irradiation. Existing data are limited regarding whether or not comprehensive irradiation is absolutely necessary to achieve optimal locoregional control of disease in patients presenting with LABC, but in whom a substantial degree of downstaging occurred with neoadjuvant chemotherapy.

Mamounas and colleagues [59] reported patterns of locoregional failure among NSABP B-18 participants, where stage I to III breast cancer patients were randomized to either preoperative or postoperative chemotherapy. Study design prohibited postmastectomy irradiation, and lumpectomy patients received breast irradiation only (ie, without any regional irradiation). Predictors of locoregional failure were the same in both arms of the study, with four or more metastatic axillary nodes identifying patients who clearly benefit from chest wall irradiation regardless of whether or not the patient received chemotherapy prior to surgery. Thus, the NSABP B-18 data suggest that surgical pathology indications for locoregional irradiation are the same for patients that receive neoadjuvant chemotherapy and those that receive postoperative chemotherapy. In contrast, data from the M.D. Anderson Cancer Center suggest that even among patients with a complete response to neoadjuvant chemotherapy, the presenting stage of disease is predictive for risk of locoregional failure, and that this feature should also be taken into account when deciding on radiation needs. In clinical practice, the oncology team should review each patient in a multidisciplinary fashion, and discussions regarding the complete multimodality management (including final radiation planning) should begin at presentation [60].

Integration of lymphatic mapping/sentinel lymph node biopsy into neoadjuvant chemotherapy protocols

Sentinel node biopsy in cases of LABC has been approached with concerns that tumor embolization from a tumor might obstruct and alter lymphatic drainage, resulting in either misidentification of the SLN or an altogether failed mapping. Bedrosian and colleagues [61] and Chung and colleagues

[62] reported excellent SLN identification rates (99% and 100%, respectively), and low false-negative rates (3% for both studies) in their respective series of LABC. Standard axillary lymph node dissection (ALND) however, remains recommended as definitive axillary staging in surgical programs that are still in the learning curve phase of lymphatic mapping for breast cancer.

Most LABC patients are treated with neoadjuvant chemotherapy, and the issue of whether sentinel node staging should be performed before or after neoadjuvant chemotherapy is widely-debated. The earliest studies of SLN biopsy in LABC were performed after delivery of the neoadjuvant chemotherapy, concurrent with the definitive breast surgery. Table 3 [63–76] tabulates the findings of multiple studies where a SLN biopsy was performed with a concomitant ALND after neoadjuvant chemotherapy. The false negative rates range from 0% to 40%, and are influenced by institutional learning curve, sample size of node-positive cases (which serves as the denominator in the false negative fraction), and primary histopathology (with inflammatory breast cancers having the highest false negative rate). The largest series was reported by the multi-institutional NSABP B-27 study, where more than 400 patients underwent lymphatic mapping and SLN after preoperative chemotherapy. In this study, the SLN identification rate was 85%, and the false-negative rate 11%. Although these rates are similar to reported multi-center results of lymphatic mapping performed in the primary surgery setting, the broad variation in single-institution results have left many oncology teams skeptical regarding the accuracy of a post-neoadjuvant chemotherapy sentinel lymph node biopsy in cases of LABC.

Because of ongoing uncertainty regarding the accuracy of SLN biopsy after neoadjuvant chemotherapy, several oncology teams have opted to routinely perform the staging SLN biopsy prior to delivery of the neoadjuvant chemotherapy. Some of these studies are summarized in Table 4 [77–79]. As shown by Olilla and colleagues [79], in a study where all patients underwent a pre-neoadjuvant chemotherapy sentinel lymph node biopsy and a post-neoadjuvant chemotherapy ALND (regardless of initial sentinel node results), patients that are node-negative at presentation uniformly remain node-negative after chemotherapy. Although this approach subjects patients to an additional operation, it does help to stratify the initial extent of disease. Nodal status is important in planning chemotherapy and for determining regional radiation benefit. Practice standards mandate that preinduction SLN-positive patients undergo completion ALND after neoadjuvant chemotherapy, but a significant proportion of these procedures will be negative for residual axillary nodal disease, as preoperative chemotherapy sterilizes axillary metastases in about 25% of cases. The advantages and disadvantages of performing a sentinel lymph node biopsy before versus after neoadjuvant chemotherapy are discussed further in the chapter that focuses on neoadjuvant chemotherapy for breast cancer. Furthermore, axillary metastases are limited to the sentinel node(s) in 25–60% of cases, and these patients will also have a negative post-neoadjuvant chemotherapy ALND.

Table 3
Studies of sentinel lymph node biopsy performed after neoadjuvant chemotherapy

Study	T status	Sample size	Sentinel node identification rate	False-negative rate	Metastases limited to sentinel node(s)
Breslin, 2000 [63]	2,3	51	85% (42/51)	12% (3/25)	40% (10/25)
Nason, 2000 [64]	2,3	15	87% (13/15)	33% (3/9)	≥11%* (≥1/9)
Haid, 2001 [65]	1–3	33	88% (29/33)	0% (0/22)	50% (11/22)
Fernandez, 2001 [66]	1–4	40	90% (36/40)	20% (4/20)	20% (4/20)
Tafra, 2001 [67]	1,2	29	93% (27/29)	0% (0/15)	NR
Stearns, 2002 [68]	3,4	T4d (inflammatory) 8	75% (6/8)	40% (2/5)	24% (5/21)
		Noninflammatory 26	88% (23/26)	6% (1/16)	
Julian, 2002 [69]	1–3	34	91% (31/34)	0% (0/12)	42% (5/12)
Miller, 2002 [70]	1–3	35	86% (30/35)	0% (0/9)	44% (4/9)
Brady, 2002 [71]	1–3	14	93% (13/14)	0% (0/10)	60% (6/10)
Piato, 2003 [72]	1,2	42	98% (41/42)	17% (3/18)	0% (0/18)
Balch, 2003 [73]	2–4	32	97% (31/32)	5% (1/19)	56% (10/18)
Schwartz, 2003 [74]	1–3	21	100% (21/21)	9% (1/11)	64% (7/11)
Reitsamer, 2003 [75]	2,3	30	87% (26/30)	7% (1/15)	53% (8/15)
Mamounas, 2005 [76]	1–3	428	85% (363/428)	11% (15/140)	50% (70/140)

At the University of Michigan, staging of LABC patients undergo a comprehensive evaluation of the axilla at presentation and after devlivery of the neoadjuvant chemotherapy [80]. Fig. 1 summarizes the current University of Michigan Breast Care Center treatment algorithm for the local, regional, and systemic management of patients presenting with LABC. Axillary ultrasound is obtained at presentation, and morphologically suspicious nodes undergo FNA; a negative ultrasound prompts a SLN biopsy before neoadjuvant chemotherapy. Upon completion of chemotherapy, patients with a negative prechemotherapy axillary work-up do not undergo ALND. Patients with documented prechemotherapy nodal disease (by either axillary FNA or sentinel lymph node biopsy) axillary disease undergo SLN biopsy and concomitant ALND at the time of their definitive surgery. This approach stratifies patients into three categories: node-negative, node-positive down-staged to

Table 4
Results of sentinel lymph node biopsy performed before delivery of neoadjuvant chemotherapy

Study	Sample size	Prechemotherapy sentinel lymph node (SLN) biopsy results		Postchemotherapy status	
		SLN ID rate	SLN-positive (%)	Management strategy	Postchemotherapy ALNDs negative for residual metastases (%)
Zirngibl, et al 2002 [77]	15	14/15 (93%)	6/14 (43%)	Completion ALND in SLN-positive patients only	6/6 (100%)
Sabel, et al 2003 [78]	24	24/24 (100%)	10/24 (42%)	Completion ALND in SLN-positive patients only	3/10 (30%)
Olilla, et al 2003 [79]	22	22/22 (100%)	10/22 (45%)	Completion ALND in all patients	12 SLN-negative patients: 12/12 (100%) 10 SLN-positive patients: 6/10 (60%)

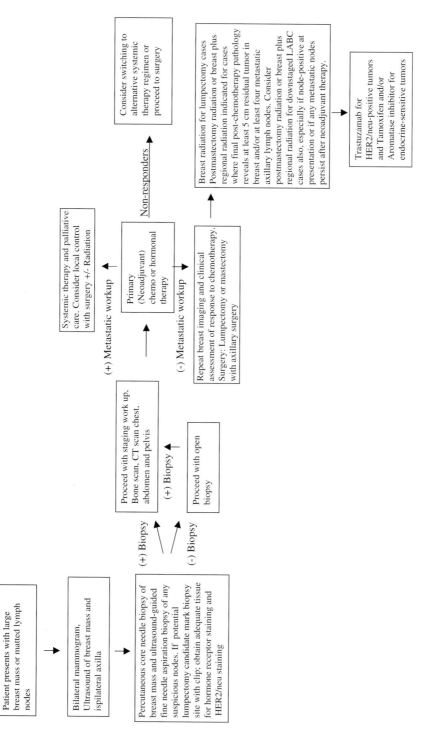

Fig. 1. Suggested diagnostic and treatment algorithm for locally advanced breast cancer. Individual programs should develop a consensus opinion from the multidisciplinary team regarding incorporation of sentinel lymph node biopsy into the neoadjuvant chemotherapy treatment sequence.

node-negative, and node-positive with chemo-resistant disease. Thus far, the final SLN biopsy appears to correlate well with the final axillary status, suggesting that lymphatic mapping is an accurate identifier of patients who have residual nodal metastases after induction chemotherapy [81]. In the future, we hope to avoid the completion ALND in the patients whose final (post-chemotherapy) sentinel lymph node biopsy indicates that their initial node-positive disease has been downstaged to node-negative status.

Postoperative systemic therapy

Patients with hormone receptor-positive breast cancer should receive at least 5 years of either tamoxifen or an aromatase inhibitor. Aromatase inhibitors should be given only to postmenopausal women, as these drugs do not block estrogen production from functioning ovaries. Any woman of unknown menstrual status can have ovarian function assessed by measurement of serum follicle-stimulating hormone (FSH), luteinizing hormone (LH), and estradiol levels. The role of ovarian ablation/suppression for premenopausal, hormone receptor-positive breast cancer patients is not yet defined. Tumors overexpressing HER2/neu also require treatment with adjuvant trastuzamab [82,83].

Management of locoregional recurrences

Chest wall recurrence following mastectomy, or any postlumpectomy recurrence requiring chest wall resection historically has been perceived as a grave event, indicating aggressive tumor biology. Downey and colleagues [84] and Chagpar and colleagues [85] recently reviewed the Memorial Sloan Kettering and Anderson experiences in managing this relapse pattern. These investigators reported that prolonged survival can be achieved when managed with aggressive resection. Five-year overall survival was 35% at Memorial and 47% at Anderson when chest wall recurrence was an isolated failure. Improved survival was associated with a disease-free interval of at least 2 years, node-negative disease, and a less than 4 cm recurrence focus. Resections sometimes included sternum and/or ribs, but surgical morbidity was low.

Summary

In summary, locally advanced breast cancer is defined as bulky T3 and T4 tumors of the breast, or breast cancer associated with matted axillary (N2) or supraclavicular (N3) adenopathy. Overall outcome and local control rates have improved markedly with multimodal therapy, including neoadjuvant chemotherapy plus surgery and locoregional radiation. Additional postoperative systemic treatments are determined by primary tumor molecular markers. BCT may be offered to selected patients after down-staging by neoadjuvant chemotherapy. Treatment with induction chemotherapy can stratify prognosis better based upon pathological response. Ongoing studies are underway to define the optimal induction chemotherapy regimen for maximizing response rates. Incorporation of lymphatic mapping into neoadjuvant chemotherapy protocols requires further study.

References

[1] Olivotto IA, Chua B, Allan SJ, et al. Long-term survival of patients with supraclavicular metastases at diagnosis of breast cancer. J Clin Oncol 2003;21:851–4.

[2] Brito RA, Valero V, Buzdar AU, et al. Long-term results of combined-modality therapy for locally advanced breast cancer with ipsilateral supraclavicular metastases: the University of Texas M.D. Anderson Cancer Center experience. J Clin Oncol 2001;19:628–33.

[3] Singletary SE, Allred C, Ashley P, et al. Revision of the American Joint Committee on Cancer staging system for breast cancer. J Clin Oncol 2002;20:3628–36.

[4] National Cancer Data Base, 1998–2004. Available at: http://web.facs.org/ncdbbmr/ncdbbenchmarks8.cfm. Accessed March 1, 2007.

[5] Haagensen C, Stout A. Carcinoma of the breast II. Criteria of operability. Ann Surg 1943; 118:859.

[6] Harris JR, Sawicka J, Gelman R, et al. Management of locally advanced carcinoma of the breast by primary radiation therapy. Int J Radiat Oncol Biol Phys 1983;9:345–9.

[7] Rao DV, Bedwinek J, Perez C, et al. Prognostic indicators in stage III and localized stage IV breast cancer. Cancer 1982;50:2037–43.

[8] Rubens RD, Armitage P, Winter PJ, et al. Prognosis in inoperable stage III carcinoma of the breast. Eur J Cancer 1977;13:805–11.

[9] Townsend CM Jr, Abston S, Fish JC. Surgical adjuvant treatment of locally advanced breast cancer. Ann Surg 1985;201:604–10.

[10] Arnold DJ, Lesnick GJ. Survival following mastectomy for stage III breast cancer. Am J Surg 1979;137:362–6.

[11] Montague ED, Fletcher GH. Local regional effectiveness of surgery and radiation therapy in the treatment of breast cancer. Cancer 1985;55:2266–72.

[12] Broadwater JR, Edwards MJ, Kuglen C, et al. Mastectomy following preoperative chemotherapy. Strict operative criteria control operative morbidity. Ann Surg 1991;213:126–9.

[13] Danforth DN Jr, Lippman ME, McDonald H, et al. Effect of preoperative chemotherapy on mastectomy for locally advanced breast cancer. Am Surg 1990;56:6–11.

[14] McCready DR, Hortobagyi GN, Kau SW, et al. The prognostic significance of lymph node metastases after preoperative chemotherapy for locally advanced breast cancer. Arch Surg 1989;124:21–5.

[15] De Lena M, Varini M, Zucali R, et al. Multimodal treatment for locally advanced breast cancer. Result of chemotherapy–radiotherapy versus chemotherapy–surgery. Cancer Clin Trials 1981;4:229–36.

[16] Perloff M, Lesnick GJ, Korzun A, et al. Combination chemotherapy with mastectomy or radiotherapy for stage III breast carcinoma: a Cancer and Leukemia Group B study. J Clin Oncol 1988;6:261–9.

[17] Papaioannou A, Lissaios B, Vasilaros S, et al. Pre- and postoperative chemoendocrine treatment with or without postoperative radiotherapy for locally advanced breast cancer. Cancer 1983;51:1284–90.

[18] Hortobagyi GN, Ames FC, Buzdar AU, et al. Management of stage III primary breast cancer with primary chemotherapy, surgery, and radiation therapy. Cancer 1988;62:2507–16.

[19] Lippman ME, Sorace RA, Bagley CS, et al. Treatment of locally advanced breast cancer using primary induction chemotherapy with hormonal synchronization followed by radiation therapy with or without debulking surgery. NCI Monogr 1986;153–9.

[20] Valagussa P, Zambetti M, Bignami P, et al. T3b-T4 breast cancer: factors affecting results in combined modality treatments. Clin Exp Metastasis 1983;1:191–202.

[21] Olson JE, Neuberg D, Pandya KJ, et al. The role of radiotherapy in the management of operable locally advanced breast carcinoma: results of a randomized trial by the Eastern Cooperative Oncology Group. Cancer 1997;79:1138–49.

[22] Cance WG, Carey LA, Calvo BF, et al. Long-term outcome of neoadjuvant therapy for locally advanced breast carcinoma: effective clinical downstaging allows breast preservation and predicts outstanding local control and survival. Ann Surg 2002;236:295–302 [discussion: 3].

[23] Mauriac L, Durand M, Avril A, et al. Effects of primary chemotherapy in conservative treatment of breast cancer patients with operable tumors larger than 3 cm. Results of a randomized trial in a single centre. Ann Oncol 1991;2:347–54.

[24] Mauriac L, MacGrogan G, Avril A, et al. Neoadjuvant chemotherapy for operable breast carcinoma larger than 3 cm: a unicentre randomized trial with a 124-month median follow-up. Institut Bergonie Bordeaux Groupe Sein (IBBGS). Ann Oncol 1999;10:47–52.

[25] Schwartz GF, Birchansky CA, Komarnicky LT, et al. Induction chemotherapy followed by breast conservation for locally advanced carcinoma of the breast. Cancer 1994;73:362–9.

[26] Schwartz GF, Lange AK, Topham AK. Breast conservation following induction chemotherapy for locally advanced carcinoma of the breast (stages IIB and III). A surgical perspective. Surg Oncol Clin N Am 1995;4:657–69.

[27] Powles TJ, Hickish TF, Makris A, et al. Randomized trial of chemoendocrine therapy started before or after surgery for treatment of primary breast cancer. J Clin Oncol 1995; 13:547–52.

[28] Makris A, Powles TJ, Ashley SE, et al. A reduction in the requirements for mastectomy in a randomized trial of neoadjuvant chemoendocrine therapy in primary breast cancer. Ann Oncol 1998;9:1179–84.

[29] Fisher B, Brown A, Mamounas E, et al. Effect of preoperative chemotherapy on local–regional disease in women with operable breast cancer: findings from National Surgical Adjuvant Breast and Bowel Project B-18. J Clin Oncol 1997;15:2483–93.

[30] Wolmark N, Wang J, Mamounas E, et al. Preoperative chemotherapy in patients with operable breast cancer: nine-year results from National Surgical Adjuvant Breast and Bowel Project B-18. J Natl Cancer Inst Monogr 2001;96–102.

[31] Newman LA, Buzdar AU, Singletary SE, et al. A prospective trial of preoperative chemotherapy in resectable breast cancer: predictors of breast conservation therapy feasibility. Ann Surg Oncol 2002;9:228–34.

[32] Bedrosian I, Bedi D, Kuerer HM, et al. Impact of clinicopathological factors on sensitivity of axillary ultrasonography in the detection of axillary nodal metastases in patients with breast cancer. Ann Surg Oncol 2003;10:1025–30.

[33] Krishnamurthy S, Sneige N, Bedi DG, et al. Role of ultrasound-guided fine-needle aspiration of indeterminate and suspicious axillary lymph nodes in the initial staging of breast carcinoma. Cancer 2002;95:982–8.

[34] Newman LA, Kuerer HM, Fornage B, et al. Adverse prognostic significance of infraclavicular lymph nodes detected by ultrasonography in patients with locally advanced breast cancer. Am J Surg 2001;181:313–8.

[35] Samant R, Ganguly P. Staging investigations in patients with breast cancer: the role of bone scans and liver imaging. Arch Surg 1999;134:551–3 [discussion: 4].

[36] Khan SA, Stewart AK, Morrow M. Does aggressive local therapy improve survival in metastatic breast cancer? Surgery 2002;132:620–7.

[37] Fisher B, Bryant J, Wolmark N, et al. Effect of preoperative chemotherapy on the outcome of women with operable breast cancer. J Clin Oncol 1998;16:2672–85.

[38] Kuerer HM, Newman LA, Smith TL, et al. Clinical course of breast cancer patients with complete pathologic primary tumor and axillary lymph node response to doxorubicin-based neoadjuvant chemotherapy. J Clin Oncol 1999;17:460–9.

[39] Singletary SE, McNeese MD, Hortobagyi GN. Feasibility of breast conservation surgery after induction chemotherapy for locally advanced breast carcinoma. Cancer 1992;69:2849–52.

[40] Scholl SM, Fourquet A, Asselain B, et al. Neoadjuvant versus adjuvant chemotherapy in premenopausal patients with tumours considered too large for breast-conserving surgery: preliminary results of a randomised trial: S6. Eur J Cancer 1994;30A:645–52.

[41] Scholl SM, Pierga JY, Asselain B, et al. Breast tumour response to primary chemotherapy predicts local and distant control as well as survival. Eur J Cancer 1995;31A:1969–75.

[42] Recht A, Edge SB, Solin LJ, et al. Postmastectomy radiotherapy: clinical practice guidelines of the American Society of Clinical Oncology. J Clin Oncol 2001;19:1539–69.

[43] Mamounas E. Preliminary results of the NSABP B-27 Trial. Presented at the San Antonio Breast Cancer Symposium 2001. San Antonio (TX), December 2001.

[44] Green M, Buzdar AU. Results from a prospective trial of neoadjuvant paclitaxel and doxorubicin for breast cancer. Presented at the American Society of Clinical Oncology 2002 Symposium. Orlando (FL), May 2002.

[45] Smith IC, Heys SD, Hutcheon AW, et al. Neoadjuvant chemotherapy in breast cancer: significantly enhanced response with docetaxel. J Clin Oncol 2002;20:1456–66.

[46] Heys SD, Hutcheon AW, Sarkar TK, et al. Neoadjuvant docetaxel in breast cancer: 3-year survival results from the Aberdeen trial. Clin Breast Cancer 2002;2(3 Suppl):S69–74.

[47] Dixon JM, Anderson TJ, Miller WR. Neoadjuvant endocrine therapy of breast cancer: a surgical perspective. Eur J Cancer 2002;38:2214–21.

[48] Ellis M, Coop A, Singh B. Letrozole is more effective neoadjuvant endocrine therapy than tamoxifen for ErbB-1 and/or ErbB-2-positive, estrogen receptor-positive primary breast cancer: evidence from a phase III randomized trial. J Clin Oncol 2001;19:3808–16.

[49] Pusztai L, Ayers M, Stec J, et al. Clinical application of cDNA microarrays in oncology. Oncologist 2003;8:252–8.

[50] Helvie MA, Joynt LK, Cody RL, et al. Locally advanced breast carcinoma: accuracy of mammography versus clinical examination in the prediction of residual disease after chemotherapy. Radiology 1996;198:327–32.

[51] Delille JP, Slanetz PJ, Yeh ED, et al. Invasive ductal breast carcinoma response to neoadjuvant chemotherapy: noninvasive monitoring with functional MR imaging pilot study. Radiology 2003;228:63–9.

[52] Abraham D, Jones R, Jones S, et al. Evaluation of neoadjuvant chemotherapeutic response of locally advanced breast cancer by magnetic resonance imaging. Cancer 1996;78:91–100.

[53] Wahl R, Zasadny K, Helvie M. Metabolic monitoring of breast cancer chemohormonal therapy using positron emission tomography: initial evaluation. J Clin Oncol 1993;11:2101–11.

[54] Mezi S, Primi F, Capoccetti F, et al. In vivo detection of resistance to anthracycline-based neoadjuvant chemotherapy in locally advanced and inflammatory breast cancer with technetium-99m sestamibi scintimammography. Int J Oncol 2003;22:1233–40.

[55] Wilczek B, von Schoultz E, Bergh J, et al. Early assessment of neoadjuvant chemotherapy by FEC courses of locally advanced breast cancer using 99mTc-MIBI. Acta Radiol 2003;44: 284–7.

[56] Newman LA, Kuerer HM, Hunt KK, et al. Feasibility of immediate breast reconstruction for locally advanced breast cancer. Ann Surg Oncol 1999;6:671–5.

[57] Styblo T, Lewis M, Carlson G, et al. Immediate breast reconstruction for stage III breast cancer using transverse rectus abdominis musculotaneous (TRAM) flap. Ann Surg Oncol 1996;3:375–80.

[58] Tran NV, Chang DW, Gupta A, et al. Comparison of immediate and delayed free TRAM flap breast reconstruction in patients receiving postmastectomy radiation therapy. Plast Reconstr Surg 2001;108:78–82.

[59] Mamounas E, Wang J, Bryant J, et al. Patterns of loco–regional failure in patients receiving neoadjuvant chemotherapy: results from NSABP B-18. Presented at the 26th Annual San Antonio Breast Cancer Symposium. San Antonio (TX), December 2003.

[60] Buchholz TA, Katz A, Strom EA, et al. Pathologic tumor size and lymph node status predict for different rates of locoregional recurrence after mastectomy for breast cancer patients treated with neoadjuvant versus adjuvant chemotherapy. Int J Radiat Oncol Biol Phys 2002; 53:880–8.

[61] Bedrosian I, Reynolds C, Mick R, et al. Accuracy of sentinel lymph node biopsy in patients with large primary breast tumors. Cancer 2000;88:2540–5.

[62] Chung M, Ye W, Giuliano A. Role for sentinel lymph node dissection in the management of large (> or + 5 cm) invasive breast cancer. Ann Surg Oncol 2001;8:688–92.

[63] Breslin TM, Cohen L, Sahin A, et al. Sentinel lymph node biopsy is accurate after neoadjuvant chemotherapy for breast cancer. J Clin Oncol 2000;18:3480–6.

[64] Nason KS, Anderson BO, Byrd DR, et al. Increased false-negative sentinel node biopsy rates after preoperative chemotherapy for invasive breast carcinoma. Cancer 2000;89:2187–94.

[65] Haid A, Tausch C, Lang A, et al. Is sentinel lymph node biopsy reliable and indicated after preoperative chemotherapy in patients with breast carcinoma? Cancer 2001;92:1080–4.

[66] Fernandez A, Cortes M, Benito E, et al. Gamma probe sentinel node localization and biopsy in breast cancer patients treated with a neoadjuvant chemotherapy scheme. Nucl Med Commun 2001;22:361–6.

[67] Tafra L, Verbanac K, Lannin D. Preoperative chemotherapy and sentinel lymphadenectomy for breast cancer. Am J Surg 2001;182:312–5.

[68] Stearns V, Ewing CA, Slack R, et al. Sentinel lymphadenectomy after neoadjuvant chemotherapy for breast cancer may reliably represent the axilla except for inflammatory breast cancer. Ann Surg Oncol 2002;9:235–42.

[69] Julian TB, Dusi D, Wolmark N. Sentinel node biopsy after neoadjuvant chemotherapy for breast cancer. Am J Surg 2002;184:315–7.

[70] Miller AR, Thomason VE, Yeh IT, et al. Analysis of sentinel lymph node mapping with immediate pathologic review in patients receiving preoperative chemotherapy for breast carcinoma. Ann Surg Oncol 2002;9:243–7.

[71] Brady E. Sentinel lymph node mapping following neoadjuvant chemotherapy for breast cancer. Breast J 2002;8:97–100.

[72] Piato J, Barros A, Pincerato K, et al. Sentinel lymph node biopsy in breast cancer after neoadjuvant chemotherapy. A pilot study. Eur J Surg Oncol 2002;29:118–20.

[73] Balch GC, Mithani SK, Richards KR, et al. Lymphatic mapping and sentinel lymphadenectomy after preoperative therapy for stage II and III breast cancer. Ann Surg Oncol 2003;10:616–21.

[74] Schwartz GF, Meltzer AJ. Accuracy of axillary sentinel lymph node biopsy following neoadjuvant (induction) chemotherapy for carcinoma of the breast. Breast J 2003;9: 374–9.

[75] Reitsamer R, Peintinger F, Rettenbacher L, et al. Sentinel lymph node biopsy in breast cancer patients after neoadjuvant chemotherapy. J Surg Oncol 2003;84:63–7.

[76] Mamounas EP, Brown A, Anderson S, et al. Sentinel node biopsy after neoadjuvant chemotherapy in breast cancer: results from National Surgical Adjuvant Breast and Bowel Project Protocol B-27. J Clin Oncol 2005;23:2694–702.

[77] Zirngibl C, Steinfeld-Birg D, Vogt H, et al. Sentinel lymph node biopsy before neoadjuvant chemotherapy- conservation of breast and axilla, abstract #516. San Antonio Breast Cancer Symposium. San Antonio, Texas; December 13, 2002.

[78] Sabel MS, Schott AF, Kleer CG, et al. Sentinel node biopsy prior to neoadjuvant chemotherapy. Am J Surg 2003;186:102–5.

[79] Ollila DW, Neuman HB, Sartor C, et al. Lymphatic mapping and sentinel lymphadenectomy prior to neoadjuvant chemotherapy in patients with large breast cancers. Am J Surg 2005; 190:371–5.

[80] Khan A, Sabel MS, Nees A, et al. Comprehensive axillary evaluation in neoadjuvant chemo-
     therapy patients with ultrasonography and sentinel lymph node biopsy. Ann Surg Oncol
     2005;12:697–704.
[81] Newman EA, Sabel M, Nees A, et al. Sentinel lymph node biopsy following neoadjuvant che-
     motherapy is Accurate in patients with documented nodal metastases at presentation. Ann
     Surg Onc, in press.
[82] Piccart-Gebhart MJ, Procter M, Leyland-Jones B, et al. Trastuzumab after adjuvant chemo-
     therapy in HER2-positive breast cancer. N Engl J Med 2005;353:1659–72.
[83] Romond EH, Perez EA, Bryant J, et al. Trastuzumab plus adjuvant chemotherapy for
     operable HER2-positive breast cancer. N Engl J Med 2005;353:1673–84.
[84] Downey R, Rusch V, Hsu F, et al. Chest wall resection for locally recurrent breast cancer: is it
     worthwhile? J Thorac Cardiovasc Surg 2000;119:420–8.
[85] Chagpar A, Meric-Bernstam F, Hunt K, et al. Chest wall recurrence after mastectomy does
     not always portend a dismal outcome. Ann Surg Oncol 2003;10:628–34.

ELSEVIER
SAUNDERS

SURGICAL
CLINICS OF
NORTH AMERICA

Surg Clin N Am 87 (2007) 399–415

Neoadjuvant Systemic Therapy and the Surgical Management of Breast Cancer

Jennifer F. Waljee, MD, MPH,
Lisa A. Newman, MD, MPH, FACS*

*Department of Surgery, Breast Care Center, University of Michigan,
1500 East Medical Center Drive, 3308 CGC, Ann Arbor, MI, USA*

Neoadjuvant systemic therapy (also called primary systemic therapy or induction therapy) has become a valuable strategy in the multidisciplinary treatment approach to breast cancer. Once reserved for women diagnosed with locally advanced or inflammatory breast cancer, the tumor downstaging benefits of the neoadjuvant therapy sequence are increasingly offered to women diagnosed with early-stage disease as well. Most of the neoadjuvant studies reported to date have involved delivery of chemotherapy as the induction therapy regimen.

Neoadjuvant chemotherapy offers several advantages compared with traditional postoperative regimens. Invasive breast cancer patients have a significant risk of harboring occult micrometastatic disease in distant organs. Neoadjuvant chemotherapy allows for earlier exposure of these micrometastases to chemotherapeutic agents, and an observed response to chemotherapy in the primary breast disease site indicates that the regimen has effective antitumor activity. Additionally, for women who experience significant regression of their tumor, neoadjuvant chemotherapy can allow for a more conservative surgical procedure. Neoadjuvant therapy clinical trials offer the promise of a rapid and less-costly means for evaluating the effectiveness of novel systemic therapy agents when compared to conventional adjuvant therapy trials. The latter format requires many thousands of participating patients followed over many years, and is extremely labor-intensive.

Several issues pertinent to the optimal utilization of neoadjuvant systemic therapy remain subject to extensive scrutiny and discussion. Some of these questions have been addressed through completed clinical trials, and others

---

* Corresponding author.
 E-mail address: lanewman@umich.edu (L.A. Newman).

0039-6109/07/$ - see front matter © 2007 Published by Elsevier Inc.
doi:10.1016/j.suc.2007.02.004

surgical.theclinics.com

continue to generate debate. First, can disease progression occur if the pre-operative regimen is ineffective? Does neoadjuvant therapy downstaging of the breast and axillary disease impair our ability to perform adequate tumor resections, or to make appropriate recommendations regarding adjuvant locoregional radiation? A final consideration is related to the fact that progress in the local and systemic treatment of breast cancer occur simultaneously. Although we would like for our patients to benefit from all of these advances, the oncologically-safest strategy for integrating these advances into a comprehensive management plan is not always clear. A perfect example of this dilemma is apparent in the controversy regarding integration of lymphatic mapping/sentinel lymph node (SLN) biopsy into neoadjuvant chemotherapy protocols. This article provides an overview of neoadjuvant chemotherapy, and its influence on current surgical management for breast cancer. An accompanying article on Locally Advanced Breast Cancer in this issue of *Surgical Clinics of North America* addresses several of these issues as well.

Indications for neoadjuvant chemotherapy

Neoadjuvant chemotherapy was initially explored several decades ago for management of locally advanced and inflammatory breast cancer, as a strategy for improving local control of these high-risk cases by transforming inoperable disease into tumors that were amenable to resection. The use of neoadjuvant chemotherapy has recently been extended to women who have early-stage breast cancer to improve eligibility for BCS among women presenting with tumors that are bulky in proportion to their breast size and to allow for an in vivo assessment of tumor chemosensitivity. Therefore, any patient expected to require postoperative chemotherapy may be an appropriate candidate for neoadjuvant chemotherapy, regardless of tumor size [1]. However, recommendations for neoadjuvant chemotherapy will also be influenced the hormone receptor status, tumor grade, primary tumor histopathology, axillary nodal status, and patient age.

Although neoadjuvant chemotherapy has been studied most extensively with invasive ductal carcinoma, data are now emerging regarding outcome for invasive lobular breast cancers treated with neoadjuvant chemotherapy. Cristofanilli and colleagues [2] studied 122 patients who had invasive lobular carcinoma. Although these patients were more likely to present with advanced disease, and less likely to have a pathologic response to neoadjuvant chemotherapy, women who had invasive lobular carcinoma had longer overall survival and recurrence-free survival compared with women who had invasive ductal tumors. Similarly, Newman and colleagues [3] reported on feasibility of breast-conserving surgery in 100 women treated on a prospective clinical trial of neoadjuvant chemotherapy and found that invasive lobular histology was associated with a significantly lower likelihood of successful downstaging to lumpectomy eligibility when compared with invasive ductal carcinoma. Thus, women who have lobular tumors can be considered for neoadjuvant chemotherapy protocols, although their response may differ from that of women who have other tumor biology.

Although the potential applications for neoadjuvant chemotherapy are broad, there are some patients in whom this approach is contraindicated. Patients who have large-volume or palpable ductal carcinoma in situ (DCIS) tumors or DCIS tumors with microinvasion are not candidates for neoadjuvant chemotherapy. It is therefore important to obtain multiple core biopsy specimens in patients with mass lesions of the breast; the biopsies must confirm that the bulk of the tumor is comprised of invasive cancer in order to proceed with consideration of neoadjuvant chemotherapy. Although patients who have multifocal disease, multicentric disease, or extensive calcifications on mammography can be treated with neoadjuvant chemotherapy (and may benefit from the resulting assessment of tumor chemosensitivity), these patients should be aware that neoadjuvant chemotherapy is unlikely to offer them the possibility of BCS [3].

Neoadjuvant chemotherapy regimens

Although the optimal regimen has not been explicitly defined, anthracycline-based regimens are the most extensively studied in clinical trials. The typical approach consists of at least four to six cycles of an anthracycline-based regimen, usually adriamycin and cyclophosphamide, with or without the addition of taxane-based agents. Several studies have reported higher pathologic clinical response rates and rates of BCS with the addition of preoperative docetaxel [4–6]. Other trials have explored the use of platinum agents, paclitaxel, and epirubicin in combination with anthracycline agents. Nonetheless, taxane and anthracycline regimens appear to be the most successful. Although a wide variety of timing schedules have been studied—sequential, concurrent, and dose-dense approaches—there is no consensus on the best timing for each chemotherapeutic agent [1,7].

Preoperative endocrine therapy has been studied primarily in postmenopausal women who have endocrine-responsive disease, but the optimal integration of endocrine therapy into neoadjuvant chemotherapy protocols remains unclear. Although there are limited data on the use of preoperative endocrine therapy in premenopausal patients, estrogen-receptor status, specifically an Allred score of 6 or higher, has been advocated as the best measure to identify patients appropriate for neoadjuvant endocrine therapy [8,9]. Current data suggest that aromatase inhibitors may offer significantly better clinical response rates compared with tamoxifen, with higher rates of local response and rates of BCS [10]. At least 3–4 months of neoadjuvant endocrine therapy is generally delivered in order to achieve a significant clinical response. Achievement of a complete pathologic response is rare, occurring in fewer than 10% of cases in most reported studies. However, there are limited data regarding the addition of these agents into chemotherapeutic regimens and the extent to which they can offer additional survival benefit [11,12]. An ongoing prospective clinical trial conducted by the American College of Surgeons Oncology Group [13] is randomizing postmenopausal Stage II/III, estrogen receptor-positive breast cancer patients to receive sixteen weeks of one of the three different commercially-available aromatase inhibitors for sixteen weeks preoperatively. This trial will provide valuable insights regarding the downstaging effectiveness of neoadjuvant endocrine therapy for individual agents in a direct, head-to-head comparison.

Neoadjuvant chemotherapy and outcomes

Tumor response and survival

To date, several clinical trials comparing neoadjuvant chemotherapy with postoperative therapy have demonstrated equivalent survival for the two different treatment sequences. These studies have also shown that patients achieving a complete pathologic response (no residual invasive cancer identified in post-chemotherapy surgical specimen) have significantly higher survival rates compared to women with less than a complete response. These findings confirm the oncologic safety of neoadjuvant chemotherapy: outcome is not compromised by delaying the surgery while chemotherapy is delivered. They also support the concept that assessment of pathologic response to the neoadjuvant regimen is a valid surrogate marker of disease chemosensitivity. Additionally, rapid assessment of tumor response to the selected chemotherapy regimen provides an opportunity to individualize treatment. If the primary neoadjuvant chemotherapy regimen fails to result in a significant clinical response (indicating chemoresistant disease), then the oncology team then has an opportunity to switch to an alternative regimen (or proceed to surgery) and thereby minimize exposing the patient to the toxicity of an ineffective regimen. In practice however, little data is available to document the results from "crossover" regimens following suboptimal initial response in the neoadjuvant setting. The potential advantages of early crossover to alternative chemotherapy regimens may be realized as advances are made with preoperative imaging modalities to assess tumor response.

The National Surgical Adjuvant Breast and Bowel Project (NSABP) B-18 trial compared outcomes between patients receiving adjuvant and neoadjuvant chemotherapy, using survival and breast-conserving surgery as endpoints. In this study, more than 1500 women who had operable breast cancer were randomized to four cycles of doxorubicin and cyclophosphamide either pre- or postoperatively, with 9 years of follow-up now reported. There were no significant differences in overall survival or disease-free survival between women who received neoadjuvant chemotherapy and women who received adjuvant chemotherapy, with an overall survival for both groups was 70% at 9 years of follow up. Disease-free survival for both groups ranged between 53% and 55% [14]. Among women receiving neoadjuvant chemotherapy, tumor size was reduced in 80%; 36% had a complete clinical response, and 13% had a complete pathologic response. Survival rates were significantly higher among the complete pathologic responders compared to other subsets [15].

Despite using a wide variety of chemotherapeutic agents, the majority of studies have shown that neoadjuvant chemotherapy offers similar overall survival and disease-free survival compared with adjuvant regimens. Several of these studies are summarized in Table 1. Both disease-free and overall survival from these studies range from 55% to 89%, but within studies the survival rates are equivalent for the neoadjuvant and adjuvant randomization arms. Variation in survival rates is observed between studies, this is likely related to study design and the stage distribution of trial participants.

A recent meta-analysis by Mauri and colleagues [16] summarized nine randomized controlled trials that randomized women to either neoadjuvant or adjuvant chemotherapy. These authors report no difference in mortality between patients who received neoadjuvant chemotherapy, and patients who received adjuvant chemotherapy (summary relative risk of death = 1.0, 95% CI, 0.9–1.12). Additionally, these authors did not find a significant increase in disease progression or distant recurrence among women who received neoadjuvant chemotherapy; however, the authors report a 22% higher rate of loco-regional recurrence among women who receive neoadjuvant chemotherapy (95% CI, 1.04–1.43).

Several studies have confirmed the NSABP B-18 trial evidence that the clinical and pathologic tumor response of the primary tumor to neoadjuvant chemotherapy is associated with improved long-term outcome. Kuerer and colleagues [17] retrospectively analyzed survival rates of 372 locally advanced breast cancer patients managed on two different prospective trials of neoadjuvant chemotherapy at the M.D. Anderson Cancer Center. A complete pathologic response occurred in 12%, and five year survival was 89% for these patients, compared to only 64% in patients with lesser degrees of response. Von Minckwitz and colleagues [18,19] reported in 2005 that early response to induction chemotherapy within the first one to two cycles can identify those patients who will have a high likelihood of achieving complete pathologic response. Feldman and colleagues [20] studied 90 patients who had inflammatory and locally advanced disease, and reported that patients who had a pronounced response following induction chemotherapy had a longer disease-free survival compared with patients who had lesser degrees of response. Thus, achievement of a mastectomy specimen free of residual macroscopic tumor after preoperative chemotherapy is an excellent prognostic factor for a prolonged disease-free and overall survival. Poor overall survival is associated with advanced nodal disease, failure to respond to preoperative chemotherapy, and an increased S phase fraction of the primary tumor. Additionally, increased metastatic recurrence is associated with age younger than 35 years, large clinical tumor size (>5 cm),

Table 1
Studies of neoadjuvant and adjuvant chemotherapy for breast cancer

Study	N	Stage	Regimen	Median follow-up	Rate of BCS (%) Preop CTX	Rate of BCS (%) Postop CTX	Local recurrence after BCS (%) Preop CTX	Local recurrence after BCS (%) Postop CTX	Overall survival at median follow-up (%) Preop CTX	Overall survival at median follow-up (%) Postop CTX	Disease-free survival (%) Preop CTX	Disease-free survival (%) Postop CTX
Institut Bergonie [22,23]	272	II–IIIa	E, Mth, V, Mt, Th, Vd	124 m	63.1	—	22.5	NA	55.0	55.0	NA	NA
Institut Curie [21,24,25]	414	IIa–IIIa	F, A, C	66 m	82.0	77.0	24	18	86.0	78.0	73.0	68.0
Royal Marsden [26–28]	309	I–IIIb	Mx, Mt, Mth, Tam	48 m	89.0	78.0	3	4	80.0	80.0	84.1	81.6
N.N. Petrov Research Institute of Oncology [29]	271	IIb–IIIa	Th, M, F	53 m	—	—	—	—	86.0	78.3	81.0	71.6
NSABP B-18 [14,15,68]	1523	I–IIIa	A, C	108 m	60.0	68.0	10.7	7.6	69.0	70.0	53.0	55.0
EORTC [32]	698	I–IIIa	F, E, C,	56 m	37.0	21.0	18.1	11.9	82.0	84.0	65.0	70.0
Gazet et al. 2001 [30]	210	T1–T4 No-N2	Mth, Mx, Mt + gosrelin, formestane	60 m	65.0	87.3	—	—	79.0	87.0	—	—
Danforth et al, 2003 [31]	53	II	F, L, A, C, G-CSF	9 years	42.3	40.7	—	—	88.5	77.8	65.4	59.3

Abbreviations: A, doxorubicin; C, cyclophosphamide; Doc, docataxel; E, epirubicin; EROTC, European Organization for the Research and Treatment of Cancer; F, flourouracil; G-CSF, granulocyte colony stimulating factors; L, leucovorin; Mt, mitomycin; Mth, methotrexate; Mx, mitoxantrone; P, prednisolone; Preop, preoperative; Postop, postoperative; Tam, tamoxifen; Th, thiopeta; V, vincristine; Vd, vindesine.

poor histological grade, and the failure to respond to preoperative chemotherapy [21].

Neoadjuvant chemotherapy and use of breast-conserving surgery

One of the most important benefits of neoadjuvant chemotherapy is that it offers tumor down-staging, expanding the number of women eligible for BCS. Typically, tumors 4 cm in size or less are best suited for BCS, but the cosmetic results improve with smaller tumors. Several large randomized controlled trials have reported the effect of neoadjuvant chemotherapy on rates of BCS; these are summarized in Table 1.

Investigators for the NSABP B-18 trial reported that women who received preoperative chemotherapy were significantly more likely to receive a lumpectomy compared with women who received adjuvant therapy (60% versus 67%, $P < .002$), with the greatest increase in lumpectomy rates among women who had tumors larger than 5 cm [15]. Other authors have studied BCS in the setting of neoadjuvant chemotherapy with comparable results. From these studies, detailed in Table 1 [22–31], the rates of BCS range from 37% to 89%, but in general are higher among women who received neoadjuvant chemotherapy. In fact, approximately one-quarter of women who are not initially eligible for BCS, but who receive neoadjuvant chemotherapy, may safely receive BCS following chemotherapy because of tumor shrinkage [32]. Singletary and colleagues [33] reviewed the post-mastectomy pathology records of women who received neoadjuvant chemotherapy, and reported that up to 23% of women became potential BCS candidates based on based on resolution of skin changes, shrinkage of the primary tumor to less than 5 cm, and the presence of unifocal disease; however, it remains challenging to accurately predict tumor size following neoadjuvant chemotherapy, with clinical examination and current imaging modalities such as mammography and ultrasound only moderately helpful in accurately predicting residual tumor size [34].

Nonetheless, BCS can be safely performed in women who receive neoadjuvant chemotherapy, with low rates of locoregional recurrence. Early studies documenting higher rates of breast tumor recurrence prompted skepticism in the ability of BCS to safely treat these women, with loco-regional recurrence rates ranging from 3–24% by ten years of follow-up (see Table 1) [35–37]. In general, reports of higher local recurrence rates were observed in women with inflammatory or locally advanced disease at presentation, and in patients where radiation-only was delivered as locoregional therapy (without surgery) after neoadjuvant chemotherapy.

Chen and colleagues [38] identified risk factors for loco-regional recurrence and developed selection criteria for women who will be best suited for BCS following neoadjuvant chemotherapy. In this study (a collective review of the M.D. Anderson Cancer Center experience with breast-conserving surgery after neoadjuvant chemotherapy), approximately 9% of women developed locoregional recurrence. Characteristics associated with increased likelihood of loco-regional recurrence included larger tumor sizes, advanced nodal disease, a multifocal pattern of residual disease following neoadjuvant chemotherapy, and the presence of lymphovascular invasion. The study authors propose the following contraindications for BCS following neoadjuvant chemotherapy: residual tumor size greater than 5 cm, residual skin edema or direct skin involvement, chest wall fixation, diffuse calcifications on post-chemotherapy mammography, multicentric disease, and contraindications to medical therapy. Notably, T3 or T4 tumors did not have an increased risk of locoregional recurrence if another contraindication was not present.

Diagnosis and management of axillary node metastases

Introduced over 10 years ago, lymphatic mapping with SLN biopsy is a well-established alternative to axillary lymph node dissection (ALND) to diagnose axillary node metastases in women who have clinically node-negative disease. Based on the concept that areas of the breast drain through different lymphatics to a "sentinel node," SLN biopsy uses either dye or a radioactive tracer to identify the axillary SLN, which can then be excised and examined for metastatic disease. Multiple studies have confirmed that the remainder of the axilla can be presumed to be disease-free if the sentinel node is free of disease, and full ALND is unnecessary. False-negative rates for SLN biopsy range from 1% to 10% [39–42]. Accurate and reliable assessment of the axillary lymph node basins is essential to identify axillary metastases in women who receive neoadjuvant chemotherapy, because most of these patients have locally advanced disease or large primary tumors, with a high likelihood of axillary metastases at diagnosis.

Both SLN biopsy and ultrasound- guided fine-needle aspiration (FNA) have been studied to detect axillary metastases before the initiation of preoperative chemotherapy. Ultrasound-guided FNA has been shown to be accurate and effective to detect and document axillary nodal disease, and aspiration of nonpalpable suspicious axillary lymph nodes is a reliable option for pre-chemotherapy staging of axillary disease [43]. Unfortunately, axillary ultrasound has a false-negative rate of 15–20%, because of limited sensitivity in detecting metastatic foci smaller than 5–10 mm. Many centers have therefore, opted to routinely perform a pre-neoadjuvant chemotherapy SLN biopsy. Not surprisingly, (given pre-existing experience with lymphatic mapping performed alongside primary breast surgery in early-stage breast cancer management) SLN biopsy before chemotherapy is both feasible and accurate to identify axillary metastases at time of disease presentation [44–46]. Results from these studies are detailed in Table 2. Identification of the SLN was performed without difficulty, and follow-up of those patients who were node-negative before chemotherapy has not revealed evidence of

Table 2
Studies assessing the use of SLN biopsy in the setting of neoadjuvant chemotherapy

Study	N	Pre/ postperative chemotherapy	Method of lymphatic mapping	SLN identified	Metastases in SLN only	False negative rate (%)
Schrenk et al, 2003 [45]	21	Pre	Dye alone, dye + tracer	100.0	NA	NA
Sabel et al, 2003 [44]	25	Pre	Dye + tracer	100.0	NA	NA
Olilla et al, 2005 [46]	21	Pre	Dye + tracer	100.0	NA	NA
Breslin et al, 2000 [49]	51	Post	Dye alone, dye + tracer	84.3	45.5	12.0
Nason et al, 2000 [50]	15	Post	Dye + tracer	86.7	Not Reported	33.0
Schwartz 2003 [51]	21	Post	Dye alone	100.0	63.6	9.0
Fernandez et al, 2001 [52]	40	Post	Tracer	85.0	25.0	22.0
Mamounas et al, 2005 [65]	428	Post	Dye alone, tracer, dye + tracer	84.8	56.0	10.7
Julian et al, 2002 [53]	34	Post	Dye alone, tracer, dye + tracer	91.2	38.7	0
Haid et al, 2001 [54]	33	Post	Dye + tracer	87.9	37.9	0
Reitsamer et al, 2003 [55]	30	Post	Dye + tracer	86.7	57.1	6.7
Aihara et al, 2004 [56]	36	Post	Dye alone	100	0.0	8.0
Kinoshita et al, 2006 [57]	77	Post	Dye + tracer	93.5	45.8	11.1
Khan et al, 2005 [47]	38	Post	Dye + tracer	97.0	33.0	4.5
Miller et al, 2002 [58]	35	Post	Dye alone, tracer, dye + tracer	86.0	22.2	0
Tafra et al, 2001 [59]	29	Post	Dye + tracer	93.0	—	0
Balch et al, 2003 [60]	32	Post	Dye + tracer	97.0	55	5
Brady et al, 2002 [61]	14	Post	Dye alone, tracer alone (1)	93.0	60.0	0
Stearns et al, 2002 [67]	34	Post	Dye alone	85.3	14.7	14.0
Piato et al, 2003 [62]	42	Post	Tracer	97.6	—	11.5
Shimazu et al, 2004 [63]	42	Post	Dye alone, Tracer, Dye + tracer	94.0	31.0	12.1
Jones et al, 2005 [64]	36	Post	—	80.6	16.7	11.0

Abbreviation: NA, not applicable.

recurrent disease. Furthermore, Ollila and colleagues [46] included routine completion ALND (after neoadjuvant chemotherapy) into the surgical management plan of all cases undergoing SLN biopsy prior to neoadjuvant therapy, regardless of whether or not this initial staging SLN was negative or positive. This study confirmed that patients staged as node-negative by pre-neoadjuvant chemotherapy SLN biopsy will remain node-negative, as the completion ALND revealed no metastatic disease in this subset of cases. Results from these pre-neoadjuvant chemotherapy SLN biopsy studies therefore suggest that patients who are node-negative by ultrasound-guided FNA or SLN biopsy may not require further axillary surgery [44–47]; however, future studies with long-term follow-up of these patients are needed to fully resolve this question.

An alternative approach involves performing the SLN biopsy after neoadjuvant chemotherapy, so that patients can avoid the additional operative procedure, and so that focus can be placed upon the final, post-neoadjuvant chemotherapy downstaged disease status. SLN biopsy following neoadjuvant chemotherapy has been met with controversy. Some postulate that SLN biopsy will only be accurate if the metastatic deposits within each axillary lymph node respond in the same way to preoperative chemotherapy. Additionally, tumor cells that necrose because of chemotherapy may block axillary lymphatics, causing impaired flow of the dye or tracer to the sentinel node, and shrinkage of the primary tumor may distort lymphatic drainage patterns. Furthermore, large primary tumors may drain to multiple lymph node basins, and it is not known if neoadjuvant chemotherapy would. Finally, neoadjuvant chemotherapy could potentially complicate subsequent ALND [39]. Neuman and colleagues [48] have reported that fewer lymph nodes are retrieved during ALND performed in patients who have received neoadjuvant chemotherapy, making it difficult to assess if a complete and therapeutic procedure has been performed.

Despite these concerns, SLN biopsy has been shown to be both accurate and feasible in women who receive neoadjuvant chemotherapy. These studies are detailed in Table 2 [49–64]. Early studies evaluating the use of SLN biopsy among women receiving neoadjuvant chemotherapy were limited by small sample size and single-center setting. Although estimates from these early studies vary widely, the collective data indicate that SLN biopsy among women receiving neoadjuvant chemotherapy has similar success in identifying the sentinel node, and similar false-negative rates as compared with SLN biopsy in women who receive adjuvant chemotherapy. SLN identification rates range from 80% to 100%, and false-negative rates range from 0% to 33%. The NSABP protocol B-27 is a clinical trial of neoadjuvant chemotherapy, however, it includes a large cohort of women that underwent SLN biopsy with completion ALND following delivery of the neoadjuvant therapy. In this study, false-negative rates were comparable to those reported in multicenter studies of women who have early-stage breast cancer treated with adjuvant chemotherapy. The NSABP authors report a SLN identification rate of 84.8%, and a false-negative rate of 10.7% [65]. Box 1 summarizes the advantages and disadvantages of performing a SLN biopsy before versus after delivery of neoadjuvant chemotherapy. Primary disadvantages of the pre-neoadjuvant chemotherapy strategy are related to the need for an additional operative procedure, and the concern that many women whose initial SLN reveals metastatic disease

---

Box 1. Advantages and disadvantages of sentinel lymph node biopsy performed before versus delivery of neoadjuvant chemotherapy

Sentinel lymph node (SLN) biopsy performed after delivery of neoadjuvant chemotherapy
Advantages
- Among neoadjuvant chemotherapy patients, there is more widespread experience with lymphatic mapping performed after chemotherapy, because breast and axillary surgery typically have been performed concomitantly upon completion of preoperative chemotherapy.
- Surgical sequence consistent with conventional neoadjuvant chemotherapy regimens

Disadvantages
- False-negative rates not yet optimized—range, 0% to 40%
- Significant learning curve

SLN biopsy performed before delivery of neoadjuvant chemotherapy
Advantages
- Significance of nodal status is understood better when axillary staging is performed at presentation.
- Preferred by many medical and radiation oncologists, who may modify their treatment recommendations on the basis of pretreatment nodal status
- Most surgeons already experienced with lymphatic mapping technology in the prechemotherapy setting

Disadvantages
- Commits some patients to unnecessary ALND (metastatic disease limited to the excised SLN in 30% to 50%; chemotherapy downstages 25% to 30% of patients to node negativity)
- Requires an additional surgical procedure

will then be subjected to an "unnecessary" ALND. The unnecessary ALNDs (completion ALNDs that are negative for residual axillary disease) might occur because the initial metastatic disease was limited to the resected SLN, or because the neoadjuvant chemotherapy sterilized all residual axillary metastases. Primary concerns regarding the post-neoadjuvant chemotherapy approach are related to skepticism regarding accuracy of lymphatic mapping in this setting. Also, many oncologists believe that definitive axillary staging information at presentation is just as important as knowing the definitive post-treatment stage. At the University of Michigan, we approach the axilla of neoadjuvant chemotherapy patients in a comprehensive fashion, allowing us to stratify patients into three different categories: node-negative cases at presentation; node-positive cases at presentation, that are downstaged to node-negative; and node-positive cases with resistent disease, that remains node-positive. We accomplish this stratification by performing pre-chemotherapy axillary ultrasound and ultrasound-guided FNA biopsy of any suspicious nodes. If the ultrasound is negative, then we proceed with definitive axillary staging by SLN biopsy. Definitively-node-negative cases do not undergo any additional axillary surgery after the neoadjuvant chemotherapy has been delivered. Node-positive cases undergo completion ALND after the neoadjuvant chemotherapy has been delivered, but we have been coupling this final ALND with a SLN biopsy, so that the accuracy of lymphatic mapping for identifying downstaged patients can be defined. The authors' results [47,66] thus far have been promising: our low false negative rate of 8% suggests that the SLN biopsy may be a reasonable strategy for assessing the final axillary stage and determining which of the initially node-positive cases have had their axillae sterilized and can therefore avoid the completion ALND.

SLN biopsy may not be appropriate for all patients receiving neoadjuvant chemotherapy, however. Stearns and colleagues [67] studied the use of SLN biopsy in women who received neoadjuvant chemotherapy in the setting of inflammatory breast cancer. These authors reports that the SLN was identified successfully in only 75% of women, compared with 89% in women who had locally advanced, but not inflammatory, disease. Although the study had a relatively small sample size, it does raise concern that SLN biopsy is excessively risky for patients who have inflammatory breast cancer.

In addition to offering complete pathologic response at the primary tumor, neoadjuvant chemotherapy can clear the axilla of nodal metastases before surgery in some patients [14,68,69]. Among women who have known axillary metastases, neoadjuvant chemotherapy has been shown to offer complete pathologic response in the axilla in up to 23% of these patients. These patients have a higher 5-year overall survival and disease-free survival compared with patients who do not achieve a complete pathologic response [70,71]. Unfortunately, for women who have persistent extensive nodal disease burden following neoadjuvant chemotherapy, the median survival is poor at 48 months, with a 10-year survival rate of 26% [72]. Predictors of complete conversion to node-negative disease are estrogen-receptor negative tumors, smaller primary tumors, and complete pathologic response in the primary tumor. These patients have significantly longer 5-year disease-free survival rates compared with patients who have residual disease (87% versus 51%) [70,73,74].

Summary

Neoadjuvant chemotherapy is standard management for women who have locally advanced or inflammatory breast cancer, but can also be considered for any case of early-stage breast cancer, if it is clear that postoperative would be administered. postoperative chemotherapy for early-stage breast cancer. Disease-free survival and overall survival are equivalent between patients treated with neoadjuvant chemotherapy and patients treated with the same regimen postoperatively. Preoperative chemotherapy can offer women less morbid surgical treatment by down-staging both the primary breast tumor and axillary metastases. Finally, response to chemotherapy can inform clinicians of the chemosensitivity of the tumor, and predict long-term outcome for women who have breast cancer. Use of neoadjuvant endocrine therapy and neoadjuvant therapy with targeted agents is currently being studied. The optimal strategy for incorporating lymphatic mapping into neoadjuvant therapy regimens has not yet been uniformly defined.

References

[1] Kaufmann M, Hortobagyi GN, Goldhirsch A, et al. Recommendations from an international expert panel on the use of neoadjuvant (primary) systemic treatment of operable breast cancer: an update. J Clin Oncol 2006;24(12):1940–9.

[2] Cristofanilli M, Gonzalez-Angulo A, Sneige N, et al. Invasive lobular carcinoma classic type: response to primary chemotherapy and survival outcomes. J Clin Oncol 2005;23(1):41–8.

[3] Newman LA, Buzdar AU, Singletary SE, et al. A prospective trial of preoperative chemotherapy in resectable breast cancer: predictors of breast-conservation therapy feasibility. Ann Surg Oncol 2002;9(3):228–34.

[4] Bear HD, Anderson S, Brown A, et al. The effect on tumor response of adding sequential preoperative docetaxel to preoperative doxorubicin and cyclophosphamide: preliminary results from National Surgical Adjuvant Breast and Bowel Project Protocol B-27. J Clin Oncol 2003;21(22):4165–74.

[5] Bear HD, Anderson S, Smith RE, et al. Sequential preoperative or postoperative docetaxel added to preoperative doxorubicin plus cyclophosphamide for operable breast cancer: National Surgical Adjuvant Breast and Bowel Project Protocol B-27. J Clin Oncol 2006;24(13): 2019–27.

[6] Smith IC, Heys SD, Hutcheon AW, et al. Neoadjuvant chemotherapy in breast cancer: significantly enhanced response with docetaxel. J Clin Oncol 2002;20(6):1456–66.

[7] Hamilton A, Hortobagyi G. Chemotherapy: what progress in the last 5 years? J Clin Oncol 2005;23(8):1760–75.

[8] Dixon JM, Jackson J, Renshaw L, et al. Neoadjuvant tamoxifen and aromatase inhibitors: comparisons and clinical outcomes. J Steroid Biochem Mol Biol 2003;86(3–5):295–9.

 [9] Ellis MJ, Coop A, Singh B, et al. Letrozole is more effective neoadjuvant endocrine therapy
     than tamoxifen for ErbB-1- and/or ErbB-2-positive, estrogen receptor-positive primary
     breast cancer: evidence from a Phase III randomized trial. J Clin Oncol 2001;19(18):3808–16.
[10] Eiermann W, Paepke S, Appfelstaedt J, et al. Preoperative treatment of postmenopausal
     breast cancer patients with letrozole: a randomized double-blind multicenter study. Ann On-
     col 2001;12(11):1527–32.
[11] von Minckwitz G, Costa SD, Raab G, et al. Dose-dense doxorubicin, docetaxel, and gran-
     ulocyte colony-stimulating factor support with or without tamoxifen as preoperative therapy
     in patients with operable carcinoma of the breast: a randomized, controlled, open Phase IIb
     study. J Clin Oncol 2001;19(15):3506–15.
[12] Abrial C, Mouret-Reynier MA, Cure H, et al. Neoadjuvant endocrine therapy in breast
     cancer. Breast 2006;15(1):9–19.
[13] American College of Surgeons Oncology Group Protocol Z1031. Available at: www.
     acosog.org. Accessed April 1, 2007.
[14] Wolmark N, Wang J, Mamounas E, et al. Preoperative chemotherapy in patients with
     operable breast cancer: nine-year results from National Surgical Adjuvant Breast and Bowel
     Project B-18. J Natl Cancer Inst Monogr 2001;(30):96–102.
[15] Fisher B, Brown A, Mamounas E, et al. Effect of preoperative chemotherapy on local-
     regional disease in women with operable breast cancer: findings from National Surgical
     Adjuvant Breast and Bowel Project B-18. J Clin Oncol 1997;15(7):2483–93.
[16] Mauri D, Pavlidis N, Ioannidis JP. Neoadjuvant versus adjuvant systemic treatment in
     breast cancer: a meta-analysis. J Natl Cancer Inst 2005;97(3):188–94.
[17] Kuerer HM, Newman LA, Smith TL, et al. Clinical course of breast cancer patients with
     complete pathologic primary tumor and axillary lymph node response to doxorubicin-based
     neoadjuvant chemotherapy. J Clin Oncol 1999;17:460–9.
[18] von Minckwitz G, Raab G, Caputo A, et al. Doxorubicin with cyclophosphamide followed
     by docetaxel every 21 days compared with doxorubicin and docetaxel every 14 days as pre-
     operative treatment in operable breast cancer: the GEPARDUO study of the German Breast
     Group. J Clin Oncol 2005;23(12):2676–85.
[19] von Minckwitz G, Blohmer JU, Raab G, et al. In vivo chemosensitivity-adapted preopera-
     tive chemotherapy in patients with early-stage breast cancer: the GEPARTRIO pilot study.
     Ann Oncol 2005;16(1):56–63.
[20] Feldman LD, Hortobagyi GN, Buzdar AU, et al. Pathological assessment of response to
     induction chemotherapy in breast cancer. Cancer Res 1986;46(5):2578–81.
[21] Scholl SM, Fourquet A, Asselain B, et al. Neoadjuvant versus adjuvant chemotherapy in
     premenopausal patients with tumours considered too large for breast conserving surgery:
     preliminary results of a randomised trial: S6. Eur J Cancer 1994;30(5):645–52.
[22] Mauriac L, MacGrogan G, Avril A, et al. Neoadjuvant chemotherapy for operable breast
     carcinoma larger than 3 cm: a unicentre randomized trial with a 124-month median fol-
     low-up. Institut Bergonie Bordeaux Groupe Sein (IBBGS). Ann Oncol 1999;10(1):47–52.
[23] Mauriac L, Durand M, Avril A, et al. Effects of primary chemotherapy in conservative treat-
     ment of breast cancer patients with operable tumors larger than 3 cm. Results of a random-
     ized trial in a single centre. Ann Oncol 1991;2(5):347–54.
[24] Scholl SM, Asselain B, Palangie T, et al. Neoadjuvant chemotherapy in operable breast
     cancer. Eur J Cancer 1991;27(12):1668–71.
[25] Scholl SM, Pierga JY, Asselain B, et al. Breast tumour response to primary chemotherapy
     predicts local and distant control as well as survival. Eur J Cancer 1995;31(12):1969–75.
[26] Powles TJ, Hickish TF, Makris A, et al. Randomized trial of chemoendocrine therapy
     started before or after surgery for treatment of primary breast cancer. J Clin Oncol 1995;
     13(3):547–52.
[27] Makris A, Powles TJ, Ashley SE, et al. A reduction in the requirements for mastectomy in
     a randomized trial of neoadjuvant chemoendocrine therapy in primary breast cancer. Ann
     Oncol 1998;9(11):1179–84.

[28] Makris A, Powles TJ, Dowsett M, et al. Prediction of response to neoadjuvant chemoendocrine therapy in primary breast carcinomas. Clin Cancer Res 1997;3(4):593–600.

[29] Semiglazov VF, Topuzov EE, Bavli JL, et al. Primary (neoadjuvant) chemotherapy and radiotherapy compared with primary radiotherapy alone in Stage IIb-IIIa breast cancer. Ann Oncol 1994;5(7):591–5.

[30] Gazet JC, Ford HT, Gray R, et al. Estrogen-receptor-directed neoadjuvant therapy for breast cancer: results of a randomised trial using formestane and methotrexate, mitozantrone and mitomycin C (MMM) chemotherapy. Ann Oncol 2001;12(5):685–91.

[31] Danforth DN Jr, Cowan K, Altemus R, et al. Preoperative FLAC/granulocyte-colony-stimulating factor chemotherapy for Stage II breast cancer: a prospective randomized trial. Ann Surg Oncol 2003;10(6):635–44.

[32] van der Hage JA, van de Velde CJ, Julien JP, et al. Preoperative chemotherapy in primary operable breast cancer: results from the European Organization for Research and Treatment of Cancer trial 10902. J Clin Oncol 2001;19(22):4224–37.

[33] Singletary SE, McNeese MD, Hortobagyi GN. Feasibility of breast-conservation surgery after induction chemotherapy for locally advanced breast carcinoma. Cancer 1992;69(11): 2849–52.

[34] Chagpar AB, Middleton LP, Sahin AA, et al. Accuracy of physical examination, ultrasonography, and mammography in predicting residual pathologic tumor size in patients treated with neoadjuvant chemotherapy. Ann Surg 2006;243(2):257–64.

[35] Touboul E, Lefranc JP, Blondon J, et al. Primary chemotherapy and preoperative irradiation for patients with Stage II larger than 3 cm or locally advanced non-inflammatory breast cancer. Radiother Oncol 1997;42(3):219–29.

[36] Rouzier R, Extra JM, Carton M, et al. Primary chemotherapy for operable breast cancer: incidence and prognostic significance of ipsilateral breast tumor recurrence after breast-conserving surgery. J Clin Oncol 2001;19(18):3828–35.

[37] Calais G, Berger C, Descamps P, et al. Conservative treatment feasibility with induction chemotherapy, surgery, and radiotherapy for patients with breast carcinoma larger than 3 cm. Cancer 1994;74(4):1283–8.

[38] Chen AM, Meric-Bernstam F, Hunt KK, et al. Breast conservation after neoadjuvant chemotherapy: the MD Anderson cancer center experience. J Clin Oncol 2004;22(12): 2303–12.

[39] Kuerer HM, Newman LA. Lymphatic mapping and sentinel lymph node biopsy for breast cancer: developments and resolving controversies. J Clin Oncol 2005;23(8): 1698–705.

[40] Krag DN, Weaver DL, Alex JC, et al. Surgical resection and radiolocalization of the sentinel lymph node in breast cancer using a gamma probe. Surg Oncol 1993;2(6):335–9 [discussion: 40].

[41] Schwartz GF. Clinical practice guidelines for the use of axillary sentinel lymph node biopsy in carcinoma of the breast: current update. Breast J 2004;10(2):85–8.

[42] Senn HJ, Thurlimann B, Goldhirsch A, et al. Comments on the St. Gallen Consensus 2003 on the primary therapy of early breast cancer. Breast 2003;12(6):569–82.

[43] Krishnamurthy S, Sneige N, Bedi DG, et al. Role of ultrasound-guided fine-needle aspiration of indeterminate and suspicious axillary lymph nodes in the initial staging of breast carcinoma. Cancer 2002;95(5):982–8.

[44] Sabel MS, Schott AF, Kleer CG, et al. Sentinel node biopsy prior to neoadjuvant chemotherapy. Am J Surg 2003;186(2):102–5.

[45] Schrenk P, Hochreiner G, Fridrik M, et al. Sentinel node biopsy performed before preoperative chemotherapy for axillary lymph node staging in breast cancer. Breast J 2003;9(4): 282–7.

[46] Ollila DW, Neuman HB, Sartor C, et al. Lymphatic mapping and sentinel lymphadenectomy prior to neoadjuvant chemotherapy in patients with large breast cancers. Am J Surg 2005; 190:371–5.

[47] Khan A, Sabel MS, Nees A, et al. Comprehensive axillary evaluation in neoadjuvant chemotherapy patients with ultrasonography and sentinel lymph node biopsy. Ann Surg Oncol 2005;12(9):697–704.

[48] Neuman H, Carey LA, Ollila DW, et al. Axillary lymph node count is lower after neoadjuvant chemotherapy. Am J Surg 2006;191(6):827–9.

[49] Breslin TM, Cohen L, Sahin A, et al. Sentinel lymph node biopsy is accurate after neoadjuvant chemotherapy for breast cancer. J Clin Oncol 2000;18(20):3480–6.

[50] Nason KS, Anderson BO, Byrd DR, et al. Increased false negative sentinel node biopsy rates after preoperative chemotherapy for invasive breast carcinoma. Cancer 2000;89(11): 2187–94.

[51] Schwartz GF, Meltzer AJ. Accuracy of axillary sentinel lymph node biopsy following neoadjuvant (induction) chemotherapy for carcinoma of the breast. Breast J 2003;9(5):374–9.

[52] Fernandez A, Cortes M, Benito E, et al. Gamma probe sentinel node localization and biopsy in breast cancer patients treated with a neoadjuvant chemotherapy scheme. Nucl Med Commun 2001;22(4):361–6.

[53] Julian TB, Dusi D, Wolmark N. Sentinel node biopsy after neoadjuvant chemotherapy for breast cancer. Am J Surg 2002;184(4):315–7.

[54] Haid A, Tausch C, Lang A, et al. Is sentinel lymph node biopsy reliable and indicated after preoperative chemotherapy in patients with breast carcinoma? Cancer 2001;92(5):1080–4.

[55] Reitsamer R, Peintinger F, Rettenbacher L, et al. Sentinel lymph node biopsy in breast cancer patients after neoadjuvant chemotherapy. J Surg Oncol 2003;84(2):63–7.

[56] Aihara T, Munakata S, Morino H, et al. Feasibility of sentinel node biopsy for breast cancer after neoadjuvant endocrine therapy: a pilot study. J Surg Oncol 2004;85(2):77–81.

[57] Kinoshita T, Takasugi M, Iwamoto E, et al. Sentinel lymph node biopsy examination for breast cancer patients with clinically negative axillary lymph nodes after neoadjuvant chemotherapy. Am J Surg 2006;191(2):225–9.

[58] Miller AR, Thomason VE, Yeh IT, et al. Analysis of sentinel lymph node mapping with immediate pathologic review in patients receiving preoperative chemotherapy for breast carcinoma. Ann Surg Oncol 2002;9(3):243–7.

[59] Tafra L, Verbanac KM, Lannin DR. Preoperative chemotherapy and sentinel lymphadenectomy for breast cancer. Am J Surg 2001;182(4):312–5.

[60] Balch GC, Mithani SK, Richards KR, et al. Lymphatic mapping and sentinel lymphadenectomy after preoperative therapy for Stage II and III breast cancer. Ann Surg Oncol 2003; 10(6):616–21.

[61] Brady EW. Sentinel lymph node mapping following neoadjuvant chemotherapy for breast cancer. Breast J 2002;8(2):97–100.

[62] Piato JR, Barros AC, Pincerato KM, et al. Sentinel lymph node biopsy in breast cancer after neoadjuvant chemotherapy. A pilot study. Eur J Surg Oncol 2003;29(2):118–20.

[63] Shimazu K, Tamaki Y, Taguchi T, et al. Sentinel lymph node biopsy using periareolar injection of radiocolloid for patients with neoadjuvant chemotherapy-treated breast carcinoma. Cancer 2004;100(12):2555–61.

[64] Jones JL, Zabicki K, Christian RL, et al. A comparison of sentinel node biopsy before and after neoadjuvant chemotherapy: timing is important. Am J Surg 2005;190(4):517–20.

[65] Mamounas EP, Brown A, Anderson S, et al. Sentinel node biopsy after neoadjuvant chemotherapy in breast cancer: results from National Surgical Adjuvant Breast and Bowel Project Protocol B-27. J Clin Oncol 2005;23(12):2694–702.

[66] Newman EA, Sabel M, Nees A, et al. Sentinel lymph node biopsy following neoadjuvant chemotherapy is Accurate in patients with documented nodal metastases at presentation. Ann Surg Onc, in press.

[67] Stearns V, Ewing CA, Slack R, et al. Sentinel lymphadenectomy after neoadjuvant chemotherapy for breast cancer may reliably represent the axilla except for inflammatory breast cancer. Ann Surg Oncol 2002;9(3):235–42.

[68] Singletary SE. Neoadjuvant chemotherapy in the treatment of Stage II and III breast cancer. Am J Surg 2001;182(4):341–6.

[69] Fisher B, Bryant J, Wolmark N, et al. Effect of preoperative chemotherapy on the outcome of women with operable breast cancer. J Clin Oncol 1998;16(8):2672–85.

[70] Kuerer HM, Sahin AA, Hunt KK, et al. Incidence and impact of documented eradication of breast cancer axillary lymph node metastases before surgery in patients treated with neoadjuvant chemotherapy. Ann Surg 1999;230(1):72–8.

[71] Hennessy BT, Hortobagyi GN, Rouzier R, et al. Outcome after pathologic complete eradication of cytologically proven breast cancer axillary node metastases following primary chemotherapy. J Clin Oncol 2005;23(36):9304–11.

[72] Pierga JY, Mouret E, Dieras V, et al. Prognostic value of persistent node involvement after neoadjuvant chemotherapy in patients with operable breast cancer. Br J Cancer 2000;83(11): 1480–7.

[73] Kuerer HM, Newman LA, Smith TL, et al. Clinical course of breast cancer patients with complete pathologic primary tumor and axillary lymph node response to doxorubicin-based neoadjuvant chemotherapy. J Clin Oncol 1999;17(2):460–9.

[74] Lenert JT, Vlastos G, Mirza NQ, et al. Primary tumor response to induction chemotherapy as a predictor of histological status of axillary nodes in operable breast cancer patients. Ann Surg Oncol 1999;6(8):762–7.

ELSEVIER
SAUNDERS

Surg Clin N Am 87 (2007) 417–430

SURGICAL
CLINICS OF
NORTH AMERICA

Pregnancy-Associated Breast Cancer:
A Literature Review

Dawn M. Barnes, MD*,
Lisa A. Newman, MD, MPH, FACS

Department of Surgery, University of Michigan Health System, 1500 East Medical Center Drive, B1-380 Taubman Center/Box 0305, Ann Arbor, MI 48109, USA

Breast cancer, along with cervical cancer, is one of the most commonly diagnosed cancers of pregnancy. Most would define gestational breast cancer as breast cancer that is diagnosed during pregnancy, lactation, and up to 12 months post-partum. The diagnostic and therapeutic implications in this clinical setting are special. These women typically present with a more advanced-stage disease that carries an associated poorer prognosis. Physicians thus are challenged to balance aggressive maternal care with appropriate modifications that will ensure fetal protection.

Epidemiology

Based on the National Cancer Institute's Surveillance, Epidemiology, and End Results Program Cancer Statistics Review and rates from 2001 to 2003, 12.67% of women will develop breast cancer during their lifetime. This lifetime risk translates into one in eight women. Additionally, this review notes that the mean age at diagnosis for breast cancer from 2000 to 2003 was 61 years, and only approximately 12.7% of women were between the ages of 20 and 44 [1]. Of women diagnosed with breast cancer younger than 40 years, only approximately 10% will be pregnant [2,3]. These data certainly suggest a low incidence of pregnancy-associated breast cancer. In fact, historically, the incidence is estimated at 1 in 3000 pregnancies [4–6]. Despite the overall low incidence, however, gestational breast cancer is one of the most common pregnancy-associated malignancies, second only to cervical cancer [4,6]. Notably, many have offered that this incidence will only increase as more women delay childbearing until later in life [4,7]. This concern is based on the fact that pregnancy-associated breast cancer is age-related, and women

---

* Corresponding author.
  E-mail address: dawnbarn@umich.edu (D.M. Barnes).

0039-6109/07/$ - see front matter © 2007 Elsevier Inc. All rights reserved.
doi:10.1016/j.suc.2007.01.008   *surgical.theclinics.com*

who have their first term pregnancy after the age of 30 years have a two to three times higher risk of developing breast carcinoma than women who have their first pregnancy before the age of 20 years [8]. Presently, most studies support a mean age at diagnosis of 32 to 34 years [8–11].

Prognosis

Clinical staging of these patients does not waver from the TNM staging system of the American Joint Committee on Cancer. Historically pregnancy-associated breast cancer was thought to be rapid in course, excessively malignant, and incurable [12,13]. More recently, the prognosis of gestational breast cancer has been shown to be similar to that of nonpregnant women when age and stage at presentation are accounted for (Table 1) [4,14,15]. Notably, both Anderson and colleagues [16] and Ishida and colleagues [9] document no difference in the prognosis of early cancers (when matched for age and stage), but a poorer prognosis is demonstrated for patients with more advanced disease. Numerous studies have documented that these women present with larger tumors and have a higher incidence of lymph node metastases (56% to 89% when compared with 38% to 54% in nonpregnant young women) that appears to translate into a more advanced stage [7–9,17–21]. Most women present with stage II or III disease (65% to 90% compared with 45% to 66% of nonpregnant controls) [8,9,17].

Table 2 references the 5- and 10-year survival for node-negative and node-positive disease for pregnancy-associated breast cancer as 60% to 100% and 31% to 52% respectively [7,22,23]. A delay in diagnosis, on the part of physician and patient alike, is thought to contribute to the advanced disease at presentation. This in part, is attributed to the engorgement and physiologic hypertrophy of the pregnant or lactating breast. It is no longer accepted that pregnancy is an independent risk factor for poor prognosis, and there is no clear evidence to support that the hyperestrogenic state of pregnancy contributes to development and rapid growth [24].

Pathology

Table 3 references the general pathology of pregnancy-associated breast cancer. Invasive ductal carcinoma predominates. As mentioned previously, these tumors are typically larger in size at presentation. Additionally, there is a higher frequency of lymphovascular invasion, high nuclear grade, and hormone independence. These histopathologic and immunohistochemical features are similar to those of nonpregnant young women with breast cancer, and they are felt to be determined by the age of diagnosis rather than pregnancy [4,25,26].

The degree of hormone receptor status negativity is consistently greater in the pregnant cohort of young women diagnosed with breast cancer. Several theories persist. The first is that the high circulating levels of

Table 1
Selected studies comparing prognosis of patients with gestational- and nongestational breast cancer controls

Author/date	Number of patients (GBC versus non-GBC)	Survival type	Subgroup	Survival rate (GBC) %	Survival rate (non-GBC) %
Nugent and O'Connell/ 1985 [2]	19 versus 157	5-year survival		57	56
Ishida et al/1992 [9]	192 versus 191	10-year survival	All	55	79
			Node-negative	85	93
			Node-positive	37	62
Zemlickis et al/1992 [14]	118 versus 269	10-year survival	All	40	48
Petrek/1994 [19]	22 versus 103	5-year survival	Node-negative	82	82
	47 versus 63		Node-positive	47	59
Anderson et al/1996 [16]	22 versus 205	10-year survival	Stage I-IIA	73	74
			Stage IIB-IIIA	17	47
Ezzat et al/1996 [15]	37 versus 84	7-year survival (overall)	All	57	61
		7-year survival (relapse-free)	All	37	33
Bonnier et al/1997 [27]	154 versus 308	5-year survival (metastases-free)	All	45	68
		5-year survival (recurrent-free)	Node-negative	63	77
			Node-positive	31	63
			All	69	81
		5-year overall survival	All	61	75

Abbreviation: GBC, gestational breast cancer.
Data from Loibl S, von Minckwitz G, Gwyn K, et al. Breast cancer during pregnancy—international recommendations from an expert meeting. Cancer 2005;106(2):237–46.

Table 2
Selected studies comparing 5-year survival rates, considering nodal status

Author/date	Node-negative (n)	Node-positive (n)
King et al/1985 [22]	82% (22)	36% (36)
Nugent and O'Connell/1985 [2]	100% (4)	50% (15)
Petrek et al/1991 [18]	82% (22)	47% (34)
Ishida et al/1992 [9]	90% (71)	52% (101)
Kuerer et al/1997 [23]	60% (14)	45% (12)
Bonnier et al/1997 [27]	63% (50)	31% (64)
Reed et al/2003 [17]	62% (31)	40% (69)

n = sample size.

estrogen and progesterone in pregnancy may occupy all of the hormone receptor binding sites; the second relates to receptor down-regulation during pregnancy [7,9,27,28].

Additionally, a retrospective and multi-institutional study from Bonnier and colleagues [27] found immunohistochemical assessment of hormone receptor status to be more reliable than a ligand-based assay. Ligand-based assays depend upon the availability of unbound hormone receptors, which may be less accurate during pregnancy secondary to interference by circulating steroid receptors. Finally, there is no consensus regarding the prevalence or implication of HER-2/neu overexpression in pregnancy-associated breast cancer.

Diagnostic evaluation

Most women diagnosed with pregnancy-associated breast cancer will present with a painless mass in the breast. A milk-rejection sign has been described rarely in case reports when a nursing infant refuses a lactating breast that harbors occult carcinoma [29,30]. The differential diagnosis of a pregnancy-associated breast mass is broad and includes:

Invasive carcinoma
Lactating adenoma
Fibroadenoma
Cystic disease
Lobular hyperplasia
Milk retention cyst (galactocele)
Abscess
Lipoma
Hamartoma and rarely leukemia
Lymphoma
Sarcoma
Neuroma
Tuberculosis [31]

Table 3
Selected studies examining pathologic features of pregnancy-associated breast cancer

Author/date	N	Histology	Histo–prognostic grade	ER (+) %	PR (+) %	Assay	Her-2/neu (+) %
Elledge et al/1993 [28]	15 (versus 411 NPCs)	N.E.	N.E.	33 (versus 52% in control group) 50 (n = 12)	47 (versus 43% in control group) 83 (n = 10)	LBA IHC	58 (versus 16 in control group)
Ishida et al/1992 [9]	192 (versus 411 NPCs)	92.1% IDC 1.6% in situ 1.6% mucinous 3.7% med	N.E.	44 (versus 57% in control group)	29 (versus 69 in control group)	LBA	N.E.
Bonnier et al/1997 [27]	154 (v. 308 NPCs)	88.2% IDC 8.2% ILC 2.7% med	12% I 48% II 40% III	45 (versus 63.7 in control group) 46.7 (versus 53.9 in control group)	46.2 (versus 75.7 in control group) 34.2 (versus 65.8)	LBA IHC	N.E.
Shousha/2000 [25]	14 (versus 13 NPCs)	71% IDC 7% ILC 7% in situ 14% mucinous	0% I 20% II 80% III	50 (versus 91 in control group)	30 (versus 64 in control group)	LBA	44 (versus 18 in control group)
Middleton/2003 [8]	39	100% IDC	84% poorly differentiated	28	24	IHC	28
Reed et al/2003 [17]	122	85% IDC 2.4% ILC 4% In Situ	4% I 37.7% II 48.3% III	31.5 (versus 44% in control group)	22.5 (versus 42% in control group)	IHC	40.5% (versus 28% in control group)
Gentilini et al/2005 [26]	38	95% IDC	N.E.	24 ER or PR+ 36.8 ER and PR+		IHC	21
Ives et al/2005 [10]	148	85% IDC 4.7% ILC 2.1% in situ	2.8% I 15.9% II 44.8% III	35.1	N.E.	Unknown	N.E.
Hahn et al/2006 [11]	57	85% IDC	16% II 82% III	31 (n = 36)	17 (n = 35)	IHC	29
Yang et al/2006 [33]	23	78% IDC	17% mod diff 63% poor diff	27 (n = 15)	13 (n = 15)	Unknown	36% (n = 14)

Abbreviations: diff, differentiated; IDC, invasive ductal carcinoma; IHC, immunohistochemical examination; ILC, invasive lobular carcinoma; LBA, ligand-based assay; med, medullary carcinoma; mod, moderately; N, number of subjects; N.E., not examined; NPCs, nonpregnant controls.

Although 80% of these masses are benign, further evaluation is warranted if findings persist more than 2 to 4 weeks [7,32]. Evaluation begins with a thorough clinical examination, and a baseline breast examination is recommended at the first prenatal visit [4].

Mammography in young nonpregnant and nonlactating women (<35 years) often reveals dense breast parenchyma, contributing to the recommendation that mammography should not be employed for routine screening purposes in this patient population. As breast size and parenchymal density increase during pregnancy and lactation secondary to hyperestrogenic proliferative changes, the corresponding efficacy of mammography historically has been questioned [7]. More recently, both the safety and efficacy of mammography during pregnancy have been supported, and mammographic sensitivity rates of 78% to 90% have been documented [33–36]. A retrospective review by Yang and colleagues [33] of 20 pregnant patients imaged during pregnancy preoperatively found mammography to be 90% sensitive in detecting suspicious features of malignancy. Importantly, 33% of these tumors exhibited secondary features of malignancy, considered to be more subtle (ie, increased breast density and architectural distortion) and felt to contribute to the false-negative rate associated with mammography during pregnancy [33]. Regarding the risk of fetal irradiation, with proper abdominal shielding, the estimated fetal dose of radiation from a standard two-view mammogram (200 to 400 mrad) is less than 0.004 Gy [7]. This is negligible and well below the threshold exposure of the 100 mGy that is associated with a 1% risk of fetal malformation and central nervous system problems as published by the International Commission of Radiological Protection [37].

Ultrasound offers an excellent adjuvant role in the early work-up of a breast mass with no risk of fetal irradiation. The same study by Yahg and colleagues noted ultrasound to be 100% sensitive in detecting a breast mass correlating with a palpable abnormality, supporting previously published data [33,35,36]. Additionally, ultrasound detected additional tumors in the breast in 20% of patients in this same series, and detected axillary metastases in 83% of those imaged (supported by US-guided fine needle aspiration [FNA]) [33]. It appears to be complimentary for staging and detecting mammographic false-negative disease, and it may aid in the assessment of response to neoadjuvant therapy [33].

Further acceptable imaging modalities for staging, as clinically indicated, include chest radiograph with abdominal shielding (fetal irradiation exposure <0.01 mGy), abdominal ultrasound or MRI and thoracic/lumbar MRI. As Gandolinium crosses the placenta and is associated with fetal abnormalities in rats (Category C), contrast-enhanced MRI is not recommended [4,7,37]. A routine bone scan results in 4.7 to 1.8 mGy of fetal exposure, which varies with gestational age; this is not recommended during pregnancy [4,37].

Despite negative findings on breast imaging, pathologic diagnosis with biopsy is recommended for persistent masses, as with breast cancer in general.

FNA, core needle biopsy, and excisional biopsy are all reasonable modalities. Historically pregnancy-related hyperplastic changes with atypia were thought to result in false-positive FNA results; however, several authors have demonstrated marked accuracy and a reduction in surgical biopsy rates when performed by a skilled pathologist made aware of the patient's pregnant or lactating state [38–41]. Core needle and excisional biopsy may be employed also. There are only case reports to support the frequency of milk fistula as a complication, and this may be reduced by emptying the breast of milk before biopsy with ice packs, breast binding, and bromocriptine [7,42].

Management

There is no longer a role for therapeutic abortion. The therapeutic approach to pregnancy-associated breast cancer is similar to that in nonpregnant women: to achieve local control of disease and prevent systemic metastases. Treatment guidelines for nonpregnant patients are followed, allowing for fetal-protective modifications. Each patient's approach must be individualized, taking into account gestational age at presentation, patient's stage of disease, and patient preference [4]. A multidisciplinary approach should be embraced, allowing for close coordination between medical oncology, surgical oncology, and high-risk obstetrics. Genetic counseling is recommended for all women. The need for psychological support is emphasized.

Surgery

The safety of surgical intervention during pregnancy is well supported, but it may be deferred until the 12th gestational week given that the risk of spontaneous abortion is greatest during the first trimester [7,11,24,43,44]. Historically, a modified radical mastectomy was considered the standard of care for all resectable disease during each trimester. This approach both eliminates the need for breast irradiation and definitively manages the axilla. Breast conservation therapy (BCT) increasingly is offered to these young women, although limited by the risks of fetal irradiation postoperatively. Although lumpectomy is considered safe during all trimesters, the required postoperative therapeutic irradiation necessary to complete BCT and obtain optimal local control is considered contraindicated during all trimesters. Appropriate candidates for BCT include women diagnosed late in the second trimester or third trimester so that radiation therapy may be deferred until after delivery, and those women with advanced-stage disease in which neoadjuvant therapy may acceptably delay definitive local resection [4].

Irradiation

Fetal radiation risks are most significant during the first trimester (before the completion of organogenesis) and least during the third trimester. Risks include teratogenicity, spontaneous abortion and childhood neoplasia, and hematologic disorders. During weeks 2 to 8, during organogenesis, fetal malformations may arise with exposure to a threshold dose greater than 100 to 200 mGy [37,45]. During weeks 8 to 25, the central nervous system is especially sensitive to radiation, and exposure to a threshold dose of 0.1 to 0.2 Gy may decrease the intelligent quotient (IQ), while fetal exposure to 1 Gy increases the probability of severe mental retardation [37,45]. Additionally, fetal exposure to 0.01 Gy increases the incidence of spontaneous childhood cancer and leukemia by 40% (over a background risk of three to four per 1000) [37,45].

The typical dose for therapeutic breast or chest wall irradiation is 50 Gy; this results in fetal exposure of 0.05 to 0.15 Gy and up to 2 Gy toward the end of gestation as the fetus lies closer to the irradiated field in position [45–47]. Notably, there have been case reports of normal infants born to irradiated mothers and successful radiation therapy for Hodgkin disease during pregnancy with appropriate supplemental shielding [32,45,47–49]. Additionally, the 2006 international recommendations from an expert meeting published by Loibl and colleagues [4] regarding therapeutic irradiation have recently been challenged by authors who feel the risks of fetal irradiation exposure have been overestimated [49]. These authors present that the fetal dose caused by leakage radiation from the tube head of the linear accelerator and scatter from collimator and blocks can be reduced with a factor two to four by proper shielding, thereby keeping the radiation dose below the threshold dose for deterministic effects in most cases [49].

Management of the axilla

Appropriate interrogation and management of the axilla are necessary to ensure correct staging at the time of presentation and to drive the appropriate definitive therapy. As mentioned previously, these women present with an increased frequency of nodal involvement. Notably, the early diagnosis of axillary metastases may increase patient stage such that she becomes an acceptable candidate for neoadjuvant chemotherapy, thereby allowing for BCT [4]. Certainly, axillary ultrasound with sonographic-guided FNA of suspicious nodes may be helpful in diagnosing metastatic disease [33]. Currently, axillary lymph node dissection remains the standard of care for these women.

Intraoperative lymph node mapping and sentinel lymph node biopsy remain controversial for two reasons. First, Isosulfan blue dye is classified as a pregnancy category C drug and subsequently is not recommended in these patients. The sensitivity of sentinel lymph node biopsy is reduced when using only the radiocolloid to guide mapping [4]. Second, there are justifiable concerns regarding the risk of fetal irradiation with the use of a radiocolloid in pregnancy, specifically ^{99m}Tc-Sulfur Colloid [50,51].

Nicklas and Baker suggested that sentinel lymph node biopsy might be safe during pregnancy with a minimal dose of 500 to 600 μCi using double-filtered ^{99m}Tc-Sulfur Colloid [7,51]. Several publications have followed to support that fetal radiation exposure from this procedure is actually quite minimal and that sentinel lymph node biopsy may serve more of a role during pregnancy. Using two nonpregnant patient exposures, Keleher and colleagues [52] in 2004 estimated the maximum absorbed dose to the fetus/embryo in pregnant women undergoing breast lymphoscintigraphy with 92.5MBq (2.5mCi) of ^{99m}Tc-Sulfur Colloid as 4.3 mGy using the Medical Internal Radiation Dosimetry (MIRD) program. The same year, Gentilini and colleagues [53] measured activity using thermoluminescent dosimeters combined with static and whole-body scintigraphic imaging in 26 nonpregnant patients exposed to lymphoscintigraphy and overestimated the fetal absorbed dose as 61 μGy. In 2006, Pandit-Taskar and colleagues [54] retrospectively assessed the absorbed doses to various organs and a modeled fetus using standard internal absorbed dose assessment methodologies and phantom models in 1021 nonpregnant women undergoing sentinel node mapping and biopsy and estimated the absorbed fetal dose as 14 μGy. Finally, also in 2006, Mondi and colleagues [50] reviewed one institution's experience with sentinel node mapping and biopsy during pregnancy for breast cancer and melanoma. Although limited (n = 9), the review noted no adverse reactions to the procedure itself; all pregnancies were delivered at term. Additionally, there have been no birth defects or discernable malformations.

It is unclear whether the lymphatic drainage of the breast is altered by pregnancy, but there is no evidence to support this [50,55]. Additionally, sentinel lymph node biopsy in pregnancy has not been evaluated systematically. The estimated fetal absorbed dose of radiation, however, is negligible, and recent recommendations from an international expert panel meeting in 2006 suggest that pregnant patient could be offered sentinel lymph node biopsy after extensive counseling regarding the amount of radiation involved, the overall safety, and efficacy [4].

Systemic therapy

Chemotherapy serves an important role in adjuvant and neoadjuvant therapy for patients who have pregnancy-associated breast cancer, especially as so many will present with advanced-stage disease. Although all chemotherapy agents used in the treatment of breast cancer in pregnancy are Category D (ie, teratogenic effects have occurred in people), a surprising safety profile has been demonstrated if administered outside of the first trimester [4,7,11,56–62]. Most frequently documented complications included preterm delivery, low birth weight, transient leukopenia of the newborn, and intrauterine growth restriction. Doll and colleagues [59] in 1989 note that the incidence of fetal malformations with first-trimester chemotherapy with various agents ranged from 14% to 19%. This value compared with the 1.3% incidence of fetal malformations associated with chemotherapy administered in the second and third trimesters.

The largest prospective series of pregnancy-associated breast cancer treated with cytotoxic chemotherapy in the second and third trimesters initially included 24 women and came from the University of Texas M.D. Anderson Cancer Center. In 1999 Berry and colleagues [56] evaluated the treatment of pregnancy-associated breast cancer with 5-Fluorouracil, Doxorubicin, and Cyclophosphamide (FAC: 500 mg/m^2 5-fluorouracil days 1 + 4; 50 mg/m^2 continuous 72-hour infusion of Doxorubicin days 1 through3; 500 mg/m^2 Cyclophosphamide day 1 of a 3-week cycle). This group reported no antepartum complications temporally attributed to systemic therapy and supported that Apgar scores, birth weights, and immediate postpartum health were normal for all children.

This data set expanded and was published recently by Hahn and colleagues [11] in September 2006. Fifty-seven women who had pregnancy-associated breast cancer were treated with FAC in the second and third trimesters, and parents/guardians were surveyed for longer-term follow-up (median follow-up duration 38.5 months). The authors reported no still-births, miscarriages, or perinatal deaths related to therapy. Only three patients delivered before 34 weeks gestational age, one being less than 29 weeks and associated with maternal preeclampsia. Only 6 children weighed less than 2500g. The most common documented neonatal complication was difficulty breathing, and 10% of neonates required mechanical ventilation. One child had a subarachnoid hemorrhage on postpartum day 2, coinciding with thrombocytopenia (platelet count 89 K/UL), and neutropenia. Finally, one child was born with Down syndrome. Only 2 of the 18 school-aged children required special attention at school, and the rest were thought to exhibit normal development [56].

There still remains a concern for anthracycline-associated fetal cardiotoxicity as children and adults reliably demonstrate a dose-dependent risk of cardiomyopathy with exposure. There have been several studies that support neonatal cardiac effects and in utero fetal death after exposure to idarubicin or epirubicin (among other agents) [62–64]. For this reason, Cardonick and colleagues endorse the use of doxorubicin rather than the aforementioned agents [60]. Meyer-Wittkopf and colleagues [65] performed fetal echocardiograms every 2 weeks in pregnant patients receiving doxorubicin and cyclophosphamide starting at 24 weeks. Using unexposed fetuses aged 20 to 40 weeks for comparison; the authors identified no notable difference in systolic function between the study and control groups. In fact, postnatal echocardiograms repeated until 2 years of age demonstrated no myocardial damage. Additionally, Peccatori and colleagues [66] support that epirubicin is preferable clinically in this setting given its better therapeutic index, fewer systemic and cardiac toxic effects, and shorter terminal half-life. These same authors relay their experience with epirubicin-based regimens for pregnancy-associated breast cancer and report no severe maternal or fetal complications, only one case of vesicoureteral reflux, mirroring other authors' experiences [66–68].

Methotrexate is a known abortifacient, and it should be avoided during pregnancy [7,58]. There are several case reports that support the safety of taxanes in treating pregnancy-associated breast cancer, but nothing to support the safety of dose dense anthracycline therapy with or without taxanes during pregnancy [69–73]. Finally, there are only case reports documenting the use of trastuzumab on pregnancy. Watson describes a case of reversible anhydramnios, while two other case reports report no immediate fetal or neonatal complications [74–76]. Tamoxifen therapy during pregnancy has been associated with ambiguous genitalia and Goldenhar's syndrome while other authors note no fetal/neonatal complication [77–82]. Tamoxifen is not recommended during gestation [4].

Present recommendations for chemotherapy dosing in pregnancy are weight-based. This dosing, however, may be complicated by increased plasma volume, increased hepatorenal function, decreased albumin concentration, decreased gastric motility, and the theoretical possibility of amniotic sac third-spacing [7]. Also, chemotherapy should be avoided 3 to 4 weeks before delivery (following the mother's nadir) to reduce the risk of infectious complications and hemorrhage from pancytopenia [7,60].

References

[1] Ries LAG, Harking D, Krapcho M, et al, editors. SEER cancer statistics review, 1975–2003. Bethesda (MD): National Cancer Institute. Available at: http://seer.cancer.gov/scr/1975_2003/. Accessed March 14, 2007.

[2] Nugent P, O'Connell T. Breast cancer and pregnancy. Arch Surg 1985;120:1221–4.

[3] Merkel D. Pregnancy and breast cancer. Semin Surg Oncol 1996;12:370–5.

[4] Loibl S, von Minckwitz G, Gwyn K, et al. Breast carcinoma during pregnancy. International recommendations from an expert meeting. Cancer 2006;106(2):237–46.

[5] White TT. Prognosis of breast cancer for pregnant and nursing women. Surg Gynecol Obstet 1955;100:661–6.

[6] Antonelli NM, Dotters DJ, Katz VL, et al. Cancer in pregnancy: a review of the literature. Part I. Obstet Gynecol Surv 1996;51:125–34.

[7] Woo JC, Taechin Y, Hurd T. Breast cancer in pregnancy—a literature review. Arch Surg 2003; 138:91–9.

[8] Middleton L, Amin M, Gwyn K, et al. Breast carcinoma in pregnant women—assessment of clinicopathologic and immunohistochemical features. Cancer 2003;98(5):1055–60.

[9] Ishida T, Yokoe T, Kasumi F, et al. Clinicopathologic characteristics and prognosis of breast cancer patients associated with pregnancy and lactation: analysis of case-control study in Japan. Jpn J Cancer Res 1992;83:1143–9.

[10] Ives A, Saunders C, Semmens J. The Western Australian Gestational Breast Cancer Project: a population-based study of the incidence, management, and outcomes. Breast 2005;14: 276–82.

[11] Hahn KME, Johnson PH, Gordon N, et al. Treatment of pregnant breast cancer patients and outcomes of children exposed to chemotherapy in utero. Cancer 2006;107(6):1219–26.

[12] Bernik SF, Bernik TR, Whooley BP, et al. Carcinoma of the breast during pregnancy: a review and update on treatment options. Surg Oncol 1999;7:45–9.

[13] Haagensen C, Stout A. Carcinoma of the breast. Ann Surg 1943;118:859–70.

[14] Zemlickis D, Lishner M, Degendorfer P, et al. Maternal and fetal outcome after breast cancer in pregnancy. Am J Obstet Gynecol 1992;166:781–7.

[15] Ezzat A, Raja MA, Berry J, et al. Impact of pregnancy of nonmetastatic breast cancer: a case control study. Clin Oncol 1996;8:367–70.

[16] Anderson BO, Petrek JA, Byrd D, et al. Pregnancy influences breast cancer stage at diagnosis in women 30 years of age and younger. Ann Surg Oncol 1996;3(2):204–11.

[17] Reed W, Hannisdal E, Skovlund E, et al. Pregnancy and breast cancer: a population-based study. Virchows Arch 2003;443:44–50.

[18] Petrek J, Dunkoff R, Rogatko A. Prognosis of pregnancy-associated breast cancer. Cancer 1991;67:869–72.

[19] Petrek J. Breast cancer during pregnancy. Cancer 1994;74(Suppl 1):518–27.

[20] Bunker M, Peters M. Breast cancer associated with pregnancy or lactation. Am J Obstet Gynecol 1963;85:312–21.

[21] Guinee VF, Olsson H, Moller T, et al. Effect of pregnancy on prognosis for young women with breast cancer. Lancet 1994;343:1587–9.

[22] King R, Welch J, Martin JJ, et al. Carcinoma of the breast associated with pregnancy. Surg Gynecol Obstet 1985;160:228–32.

[23] Kuerer HM, Cunningham JD, Brower ST, et al. Breast carcinoma associated with pregnancy and lactation. Surg Oncol 1997;6:93–8.

[24] Melnick DM, Wahl WL, Dalton V. Management of general surgical problems in the pregnant patient. Am J Surg 2004;187:170–80.

[25] Shousha S. Breast cancer presenting during or shortly after pregnancy and lactation. Arch Pathol 2000;124:1053–60.

[26] Gentilini O, Masullo M, Rotmensz N, et al. Breast cancer diagnosed during pregnancy and lactation: biological features and treatment options. Eur J Surg Oncol 2005;31:232–6.

[27] Bonnier P, Romain S, Dilhuydy JM, et al. Influence of pregnancy on the outcome of breast cancer: a case–control study. Int J Cancer 1997;72:720–7.

[28] Elledge R, Ciocca D, Langone G, et al. Estrogen receptor, progesterone receptor, and HER-2/neu protein in breast cancers from pregnant patients. Cancer 1993;71(8): 2499–506.

[29] Goldsmith HS. Milk rejection sign of breast cancer. Am J Surg 1974;127(3):280–1.

[30] Saber A, Dardik H, Ibrahim IM, et al. The milk rejection sign: a natural tumor marker. Am Surg 1996;62(12):998–9.

[31] Byrd BJ, Bayer D, Robertson J. Treatment of breast tumors associated with pregnancy and lactation. Ann Surg 1962;155:940–7.

[32] Ngu SL, Duval P, Collins C. Fetal radiation dose in radiotherapy for breast cancer. Australas Radiol 1992;36:321–2.

[33] Yang W, Dryden M, Gwyn K, et al. Imaging of breast cancer diagnosed and treated during pregnancy. Radiology 2006;239(1):52–60.

[34] Son E, Keun K, Kim EK. Pregnancy-associated breast disease: radiologic features and diagnostic dilemmas. Yonsei Med J 2006;47(1):34–42.

[35] Liberman L, Giess C, Dershaw DD, et al. Imaging of pregnancy-associated breast cancer. Radiology 1994;191:245–8.

[36] Ahn B, Kim HH, Moon WK, et al. Pregnancy- and lactation-associated breast cancer: mammographic and sonographic findings. J Ultrasound Med 2003;22:491–7.

[37] International Commission on Radiological Protection. Biological effects after prenatal irradiation (embryo and fetus). Ann ICRP 2003;33:205–6.

[38] Gupta RK, McHutchison AG, Dowle CS, et al. Fine-needle aspiration cytodiagnosis of breast masses in pregnant and lactating women and its impact on management. Diagn Cytopathol 1993;9(2):156–9.

[39] Mitre BK, Kanbour AI, Mauser N. Fine needle aspiration biopsy of breast carcinoma in pregnancy and lactation. Acta Cytol 1997;4(4):1121–30.

[40] Novotny DB, Maygarden SJ, Shermer RW, et al. Fine needle aspiration of benign and malignant breast masses associated with pregnancy. Acta Cytol 1991;35(6):676–86.

[41] Bottles K, Taylor RN. Diagnosis of breast masses in pregnant and lactating women by aspiration cytology. Obstet Gynecol 1985;66(Suppl 3):76S–8S.

[42] Schackmuth E, Harlow C, Norton L. Milk fistula: a complication after core breast biopsy. AJR Am J Roentgenol 1993;161:961–2.

[43] Duncan P, Pope W, Cohen M, et al. Fetal risk of anesthesia and surgery during pregnancy. Anesthesiology 1986;64:790–4.

[44] Mazze R, Kallen B. Reproductive outcome after anesthesia and operation during pregnancy: a registry study of 5405 cases. Am J Obstet Gynecol 1989;161:1178–85.

[45] Kal H, Struikmans H. Radiotherapy during pregnancy: fact and fiction. Lancet Oncol 2005; 6:328–33.

[46] Fenig E, Mishaeli M, Kalish Y, et al. Pregnancy and radiation. Cancer Treat Rev 2001;27: 1–7.

[47] Antypas C, Sandilos P, Kouvaris J, et al. Fetal dose evaluation during breast cancer radiotherapy. Int J Radiat Oncol Biol Phys 1998;40:995–9.

[48] Van der Giessen PH. Measurement of the peripheral dose for the tangential breast treatment technique with Co-60 gamma radiation and high energy x-rays. Radiother Oncol 1997;42: 257–64.

[49] Kal HB, Struikmans H. Breast carcinoma during pregnancy. International recommendations from an expert meeting. Cancer 2006;107(4):882–3; [discussion: author reply 883].

[50] Mondi MM, Cuenca RE, Ollilia DW, et al. Sentinel lymph node biopsy during pregnancy: initial clinical experience. Ann Surg Oncol 2007;14(1):218–21.

[51] Nicklas A, Baker M. Imaging strategies in pregnant cancer patients. Semin Oncol 2000;27: 623–32.

[52] Keleher A, Wendt R III, Delpassand E, et al. The safety of lymphatic mapping in pregnant breast cancer patients using Tc-99m sulfur colloid. Breast J 2004;10(6):492–5.

[53] Gentilini O, Cremonesi M, Trifirò G, et al. Safety of sentinel node biopsy in pregnant patients with breast cancer. Ann Oncol 2004;15:1348–51.

[54] Pandit-Taskar N, Dauer LT, Montgomery L, et al. Organ and fetal absorbed dose estimates from 99Tc-sulfur colloid lymphoscintigraphy and sentinel node localization in breast cancer patients. J Nucl Med 2006;47:1202–8.

[55] Krontiras H, Bland KI. When is sentinel node biopsy for breast cancer contraindicated? Surg Oncol 2003;12:207–10.

[56] Berry DL, Theriault RL, Holmes FA, et al. Management of breast cancer during pregnancy using a standardized protocol. J Clin Oncol 1999;17(3):855–61.

[57] Gwyn K. Children exposed to chemotherapy in utero. J Natl Cancer Inst Monogr 2005;34: 69–71.

[58] Ebert U, Loffler H, Kirch W. Cytotoxic therapy and pregnancy. Pharmacol Ther 1997;74: 207–20.

[59] Doll DC, Ringenberg QS, Yarbo JW. Antineoplastic agents and pregnancy. Semin Oncol 1989;16:337–46.

[60] Cardonick E, Iacobucci A. Use of chemotherapy during pregnancy. Lancet Oncol 2004;5: 283–91.

[61] Ring AE, Smith IE, Jones A, et al. Chemotherapy for breast cancer during pregnancy: an 18-year experience from five London teaching hospitals. J Clin Oncol 2005;23(18): 4192–7.

[62] Giacalone PL, Laffargue F, Benos P. Chemotherapy for breast carcinoma during pregnancy: a French National Survey. Cancer 1999;86:2266–72.

[63] Reynoso EE, Hueta F. Acute leukemia and pregnancy—fatal fetal outcome after exposure to idarubicin during the second trimester. Acta Oncol 1994;33:703–16.

[64] Karp GI, von Oeyen P, Valone F, et al. Doxorubicin in pregnancy: possible transplacental passage. Cancer Treat Rep 1983;67:773–7.

[65] Meyer-Wittkopf M, Barth H, Emons G, et al. Fetal cardiac effects of doxorubicin therapy for carcinoma of the breast during pregnancy: case report and review of the literature. Ultrasound Obstet Gynecol 2001;18:62–6.

[66] Peccatori F, Martinelli G, Gentillini O, et al. Chemotherapy during pregnancy: what is really safe? Lancet 2004;5:398.

[67] Germann N, Goffinet F, Goldwasser R. Anthracyclines during pregnancy: embryo–fetal outcome in 160 patients. Ann Oncol 2004;15:146–50.

[68] Andreadis C, Charalampidou M, Diamantopoulos N, et al. Combined chemotherapy and radiotherapy during conception and first two trimesters of gestation in a woman with metastatic breast cancer. Gynecol Oncol 2004;95:252–5.

[69] Potluri V, Lewis D, Burton GV. Chemotherapy with taxanes in breast cancer during pregnancy: case report and review of the literature. Clin Breast Cancer 2006;7(2):167–70.

[70] Nieto Y, Santisteban M, Aramendia JM, et al. Docetaxol administered during pregnancy for inflammatory breast carcinoma. Clin Breast Cancer 2006;6(6):533–4.

[71] Gonzalez-Angulo AM, Walters RS, Carpenter RJ, et al. Paclitaxel chemotherapy in a pregnant patient with bilateral breast cancer. Clin Breast Cancer 2004;5(4):317–9.

[72] Sood AK, Shahin MS, Sorosky JL. Paclitaxel and platinum chemotherapy for ovarian carcinoma during pregnancy. Gynecol Oncol 2001;83:599–600.

[73] De Santis M, Lucchese A, De Carolis S, et al. Metastatic breast cancer in pregnancy: first case of chemotherapy with docetaxel. Eur J Cancer Care 2000;9:235–7.

[74] Waterston AM, Graham J. Effect of adjuvant Trastuzumab on pregnancy. J Clin Oncol 2006;24(2):321–2.

[75] Watson WJ. Herceptin (Trastuzumab) therapy during pregnancy: association with reversible anhydramnios. Obstet Gynecol 2005;105:642–3.

[76] Fanale MA, Uyei AR, Theriault RL, et al. Treatment of metastatic breast cancer with Trastuzumab and vinorelbine during pregnancy. Clin Breast Cancer 2005;6(4):354–6.

[77] Barthelmes L, Gateley CA. Tamoxifen and pregnancy. Breast 2004;13:446–51.

[78] Tewari K, Bonebrake RG, Asrat T, et al. Ambiguous genitalia in infant exposed to tamoxifen in utero. Lancet 1997;350(9072):183.

[79] Cullins SL, Pridjian G, Sutherland CM. Goldenhar's syndrome associated with tamoxifen given to the mother during gestation. J Am Med Assoc 1994;271(24):1905–6.

[80] Oksuzoglu B, Guler N. An infertile patient with breast cancer who delivered a healthy child under adjuvant tamoxifen therapy. Eur J Obstet Gynecol Reprod Biol 2002;104(1):79.

[81] Koizumi K, Aono T. Pregnancy after combined treatment with bromocriptine and tamoxifen in two patients with pituitary prolactinomas. Fertil Steril 1986;46(2):312–4.

[82] Isaacs RJ, Hunter W, Clark K. Tamoxifen as systemic treatment of advanced breast cancer during pregnancy—case report and literature review. Gynecol Oncol 2001;80(3):405–8.

ELSEVIER
SAUNDERS

SURGICAL
CLINICS OF
NORTH AMERICA

Surg Clin N Am 87 (2007) 431–451

Complications in Breast Surgery

Angelique F. Vitug, MD,
Lisa A. Newman, MD, MPH, FACS*

*University of Michigan, Breast Care Center, 1500 East Medical Center Drive,
3308 CGC, Ann Arbor, MI 48167, USA*

The breast is a relatively clean organ comprised of skin, fatty tissue, and mammary glandular elements that have no direct connection to any major body cavity or visceral structures. In the absence of concurrent major reconstruction, breast surgery generally is not accompanied by large-scale fluid shifts, infectious complications, or hemorrhage. Thus, most breast operations are categorized as low-morbidity procedures. Because the breast is the site of the most common cancer afflicting American women, however, a variety of complications can occur in association with diagnostic and multidisciplinary management procedures. Some of these complications are related to the breast itself, and others are associated with axillary staging procedures. This article first addresses some general, nonspecific complications (wound infections, seroma formation, hematoma). It then discusses complications that are specific to particular breast-related procedures: lumpectomy (including both diagnostic open biopsy and breast-conservation therapy for cancer), mastectomy; axillary lymph node dissection (ALND), lymphatic mapping/sentinel lymph node biopsy, and reconstruction. Complications related to reconstruction are discussed in a separate article in this issue.

General wound complications related to breast and axillary surgery

Because it is a peripheral soft tissue organ, many wound complications related to breast procedures are relatively minor and frequently are managed on an outpatient basis. It therefore is difficult to establish accurate incidence rates for these events. As discussed later, however, reported studies

Support for this manuscript is via an Interdisciplinary Fellowship Grant from The Susan G. Komen Breast Cancer Foundation.

* Corresponding author.

E-mail address: lanewman@umich.edu (L.A. Newman).

document that surgical morbidity from breast and/or axillary wound infections, seromas, and hematomas occur in up to 30% of cases. Fewer than half of these cases require a prolongation of hospital stay or a readmission for inpatient care. A fourth complication, chronic incisional pain, also can occur in conjunction with various surgical breast procedures.

Rare complications that also can occur in conjunction with various breast procedures are not discussed in depth here. For example, pneumothorax can be related to either inadvertent pleural puncture during wire localization or to inadvertently deep dissection within an intercostal space. Also, patients can develop brachial plexopathy related to stretch injury caused by malpositioning in the operating room [1]. The American Society of Anesthesiology recommends upper extremity positioning such that maximal angle at the shoulder is 90°, with neutral forearm position, and use of padded armboards [2].

Mondor's disease, or thrombosis of the thoracoepigastric vein, can occur spontaneously, after any breast procedure such as lumpectomy, or even after percutaneous needle biopsy [3–7]. Although Mondor's disease is not an established risk factor in breast cancer, there are case reports of patients presenting with this condition at the time of the breast cancer diagnosis [4]. This condition typically presents as a palpable, sometimes tender cord running vertically from the mid-lower hemisphere of the breast toward the abdominal wall. It usually is self-limited; resolution can be expedited by soft tissue massage.

Wound infections

Rates of postoperative infections in breast and axillary incisions have ranged from less than 1% of cases to nearly 20%, as shown in Table 1 [8–21]. A meta-analysis by Platt and colleagues [22] from 1993 analyzed data from 2587 surgical breast procedures and found an overall wound infection rate of 3.8% of cases. Staphylococcal organisms introduced by means of skin flora usually are implicated in these infections [8,17]. Obesity, older age, and diabetes mellitus have been some of the most consistently identified risk factors for breast wound sepsis. Several investigators have found that patients undergoing definitive surgery for cancer had a lower risk for wound infection if the diagnosis had been established by prior needle biopsy rather than by an open surgical biopsy [11,14,21], but one investigator found the opposite effect [20]. Nicotine and other components of cigarettes have well-known adverse effects on small vessels of the skin, resulting in a nearly fourfold increase in the risk of wound infection after breast surgery [19]. As demonstrated by the various studies summarized in Table 1, there is no consistent correlation between the risk of wound infection and mastectomy versus lumpectomy as definitive breast cancer surgery.

Use of preoperative antibiotic coverage to minimize infection rates has been evaluated in multiple retrospective as trials and in prospective, randomized, controlled trials. These studies have yielded disparate results;

many have shown that a single dose of a preoperative antibiotic (usually a cephalosporin, administered approximately 30 minutes preoperatively) effectively reduces wound infection rates by 40% or more [8,13,21,22], and the meta-analysis by Platt and colleagues [22] revealed that antibiotic prophylaxis reduced wound infection rates by 38%, despite the selection bias of antibiotics being used predominantly in higher-risk cases. Furthermore, the lowest reported rates of breast wound infections occurred in a phase III study [16] of a long-acting versus a short-acting cephalosporin, revealing greater risk reduction with the former (0.45% versus 0.91%). In contrast, Wagman and colleagues [10] found no effect of perioperative cephalosporin in a placebo-controlled, phase III trial involving 118 patients who had breast cancer (5% versus 8%), however, in the antibiotic arm the infections were delayed in onset (17.7 days versus 9.6 days). Gupta and colleagues [17] reported similar rates of wound infection in a phase III study of prophylactic amoxicillin/clavulanic acid (17.7%) versus placebo (18.8%) and concluded that perioperative antibiotics are unnecessary in elective breast surgery. Because of these disparate results, and in an attempt to minimize cost, many clinicians limit antibiotic prophylaxis to high-risk patients and to cases involving foreign bodies, such as wire localization biopsies. Despite this common practice, it should be noted that wire localization procedures have not been identified specifically as a risk factor for wound infection [21].

Mild incisional cellulitis can be treated with oral antibiotics, but nonresponding or extensive soft tissue infection requires intravenous therapy. A minority of breast wound infections progress into a fully developed abscess. The pointing, fluctuant, and exquisitely tender mass of a breast abscess usually becomes apparent 1 to 2 weeks postoperatively and occurs at a lumpectomy, mastectomy, or axillary incision site. When there is uncertainty regarding the diagnosis (as may be the case with deep-seated abscesses after lumpectomy), ultrasound imaging is helpful occasionally, but the complex mass that is visualized can appear identical to a consolidating seroma or hematoma. Aspiration also may confirm the diagnosis, but sampling error can mislead the clinician. Definitive management of an abscess requires incision and drainage; curative aspiration of purulent material is rarely successful, and the abscess generally reaccumulates. Usually the incision and drainage can be accomplished by reopening the original surgical wound; the resulting cavity must be left open to heal by secondary intention. When recurrent cancer is a concern, biopsy of the abscess cavity wall is prudent.

Chronic recurrent periareolar abscess formation (also known as "Zuska's disease") does not necessarily develop as a consequence of primary breast surgical procedures, but this condition is notable for its high risk of complications after attempts at surgical treatment. This condition has been associated with cigarette smoking, and afflicted patients also should be checked for tuberculosis as a factor in their recurrent superficial soft tissue infections. Resection of the involved subareolar ductal system(s) frequently is offered in an attempt to break the cycle of repeated abscesses, but these procedures

Table 1
Selected studies evaluating wound infection rates following breast surgery

Study	Number of cases	Type of procedures analyzed	Type of study	Wound infection rate (%)	Study findings/risk factors for infection
Platt et al [8] 1990	606	Lumpectomy, mastectomy, ALND, reduction mammoplasty	Phase III study of preoperative antibiotics	9.4	Preoperative antibiotic coverage reduced wound infection rate (6.6% versus 12.2%)
Hoefer et al [9] 1990	101	Mastectomy	Retrospective review	8.9	Risk factor: cautery
Wagman et al [10] 1990	118	Mastectomy	Phase III study of preoperative antibiotics	6.8	Preoperative antibiotics had no effect on wound infection rates (5% versus 8%)
Chen et al [11] 1991	—	Mastectomy, lumpectomy	Retrospective review	2.6–11.1	Risk factors: older age; surgery performed in 1970s versus 1980s; prior open diagnostic biopsy versus ingle-stage surgery
Vinton et al [12] 1991	560	Mastectomy, lumpectomy, ALND	Retrospective review	15 (mastectomy) 13 (lumpectomy)	Risk factors: older age; mastectomy versus lumpectomy; tobacco smoking; obesity
Platt et al [13] 1992	1981	Mastectomy, lumpectomy, ALND, reduction mammoplasty	Retrospective review	3.4	Preoperative antibiotic coverage reduced wound infection rate (odds ratio 0.59; 95% confidence interval 0.35–0.99)
Lipshy et al [14] 1996	289	Mastectomy	Retrospective review	5.3	Risk factor: prior open diagnostic biopsy versus diagnostic needle biopsy (6.9% versus 1.6%)

Study	N	Procedure	Study type	Rate (%)	Comments
Bertin et al [15] 1998	18 cases 37 controls	Mastectomy, lumpectomy	Case control	NA	Preoperative antibiotic coverage reduced wound infection rate. *Risk factors*: obesity; older age
Thomas et al [16] 1999	1766	Mastectomy, lumpectomy, ALND	Phase III study of preoperative antibiotics	0.6	Short-acting versus long-acting preoperative cephalosporin (0.91% versus 0.45%)
Gupta et al [17] 2000	334	Mastectomy, lumpectomy, ALND	Phase III study of preoperative antibiotics	18.3	Preoperative antibiotics had no effect on wound infection rates (17.7% versus 18.8%)
Nieto et al [18] 2002	107	Mastectomy, lumpectomy, ALND	Prospective observational study	7 (mastectomy) 17 (lumpectomy)	*Risk factors*: lumpectomy versus mastectomy; older age; obesity
Sorensen et al [19] 2002	425	Mastectomy, lumpectomy, ALND	Retrospective review	10.5	*Risk factors*: tobacco smoking; diabetes mellitus; obesity; heavy ethanol consumption
Witt et al [20] 2003	326	Mastectomy, lumpectomy, ALND	Prospective observational study	15.3	*Risk factors*: older age; obesity; diabetes mellitus; prior diagnostic core needle biopsy versus open diagnostic biopsy
Tran et al [21] 2003	320	Mastectomy, lumpectomy	Retrospective review	6.1	Preoperative antibiotic coverage reduced wound infection rate. *Risk factors*: prior open diagnostic biopsy versus diagnostic needle biopsy (11.1% versus 9.7%)

Abbreviations: ALND, axillary lymph node dissection; NA, not applicable.

often are themselves complicated by wound infections and by chronically draining sinus tracts. Some patients suffering from the most refractory cases have resorted to complete resection of the entire nipple-areolar complex, but this strategy certainly should be reserved as a last-ditch effort.

Seroma

The rich lymphatic drainage of the breast from intramammary lymphatics to the axillary, supraclavicular, and internal mammary nodal basins establishes the tendency for seroma formation within any closed space that results from breast surgery. It has been proposed that the low fibrinogen levels and net fibrinolytic activity within lymphatic fluid collections account for seroma formation [23,24]. The closed spaces of lumpectomy cavities, axillary wounds, and the anterior chest wall cavity left under mastectomy skin flaps can all harbor seroma. After a lumpectomy, this seroma is advantageous to the patient, because it usually preserves the normal breast contour even after a large-volume resection, eventually being replaced by scar formation as the cavity consolidates. Occasionally the lumpectomy seroma is overly exuberant. If the patient experiences discomfort from a bulging fluid collection, simple aspiration of the excess is adequate management.

Seroma formation under the skin flaps of axillary or mastectomy wounds impairs the healing process; therefore drains are usually left in place to evacuate postoperative fluid collections. Most breast cancer surgery is performed in the outpatient setting, and patients must be instructed about proper drainage catheter care. After 1 to 3 weeks, the skin flaps heal and adhere to the chest wall, as evidenced by diminished drain output. Seroma collections that develop after drain removal can be managed by percutaneous aspiration. Aspiration usually is well tolerated because the mastectomy and axillary incisions tend to be insensate; these procedures can be repeated as frequently as necessary to ensure that the skin flaps are densely adherent to the chest wall. Seroma aspiration is necessary in 10% to 80% of ALND and mastectomy cases, according to reported series and as reviewed in detail by Pogson and colleagues [23]. Axillary surgery limited to the sentinel lymph node biopsy seems to confer a lower risk of seroma formation, but this procedure usually is performed without drain insertion; therefore occasional patients require subsequent seroma aspiration [25].

Several investigators have studied strategies that might minimize seroma formation to decrease the time that drainage catheters are needed or to obviate their need altogether. Talbot and Magarey [26] subjected 90 consecutive patients who had breast cancer undergoing ALND to (1) conventional, prolonged closed-suction drainage; (2) 2-day short-term drainage; or (3) no drainage. There were no differences in the rates of infectious wound complications in the three groups, and at a minimum follow-up of 1 year there were no differences in lymphedema risk. In group 1, the drain was removed at a median of nearly 10 days, with 73% of cases requiring subsequent seroma aspiration. As expected, the short-term and no-drain groups required more frequent seroma aspirations (86% and 97%, respectively). The mean duration of suction drainage and/or aspiration drainages was similar for all three groups (25–27 days). In all groups fluid accumulation had mostly resolved by 4 weeks, but in each group there were a few patients (approximately 16%) who had prolonged drainage lasting an additional 2 to 3 weeks. Similar findings have been reported in older studies [27,28]. The number of drains used and the use of low- versus high-vacuum suction do not seem to affect the results achieved with drainage catheters.

Shoulder immobilization with slings or special wraps to decrease seroma formation also has been proposed, but this approach carries the risk of possible long-term range-of-motion limitations and even may increase the risk of lymphedema [29]. A reasonable alternative approach endorsed by most breast surgeons is to recommend that patients simply limit motion at the shoulder to abduction no greater than 90° and that active upper extremity physiotherapy be delayed until drainage catheters have been removed. This strategy seems to decrease seroma formation more effectively than early physiotherapy programs and does not adversely affect long-term range-of-motion results [30,31].

The tissue effects of electrocautery are a well-recognized risk factor for increased seroma formation [23]. Two prospective clinical trials have randomly assigned patients who have breast cancer to undergo surgery with electrocautery or with scalpel only and have confirmed the lower incidence of seroma formation with the latter technique [32,33]. Few surgeons, however, are willing to relinquish the convenience and improved hemostasis associated with electrocautery dissection.

In a study from France, Classe and colleagues [34] reported successful use of axillary padding in lieu of catheter drains in 207 patients who had breast cancer undergoing ALND and found seroma formation in 22.2%. In contrast, the Memorial Sloan Kettering Cancer Center conducted a clinical trial that randomly assigned 135 patients undergoing ALND to receive a compression dressing for 4 days or standard wound coverage (all patients had conventional catheter drainage as well). This study found no benefit from compression dressings [35]. Both arms of this study had similar total drainage volumes and drainage catheter durations, and the compression arm furthermore had increased need for seroma aspiration (mean number of aspirations, 2.9 in the compression arm compared with 1.8 in the standard dressing arm; $P < .01$).

Chemical maneuvers to decrease seroma formation also have been investigated. Application of tetracycline as a sclerosing agent has been ineffective [36]. Bovine thrombin similarly has been unsuccessful in this regard [37]. Use of fibrin glues, patches, and/or sealants has seemed promising, but clinical studies in humans have yielded inconsistent results, and it therefore is unclear whether the added expense of these agents is justified [23,38–40].

Hematoma

Widespread use of electrocautery has reduced the incidence of hematoma formation in breast surgery dramatically, but this complication continues to occur in 2% to 10% of cases. Some cases of low-volume hematoma carry low morbidity, leaving the patient with a more extensive ecchymosis as the adjacent soft tissues absorb the hematoma. At the other end of the spectrum, large hematomas can be quite painful because of rapid expansion through the closed wound space and should be evacuated surgically, with aggressive wound irrigation and reclosure to optimize cosmesis.

An ongoing debate in breast surgery has revolved around defining the optimal technique for closure of a lumpectomy cavity. Leaving the cavity open to fill with seroma and closing the overlying skin with deep dermal sutures and a final subcuticular layer has become a conventional wound-closure strategy. This method allows prompt restoration of the breast contour through rapid filling of the lumpectomy cavity by seroma, but it requires meticulous attention to ensuring hemostasis along the lumpectomy cavity walls before skin closure. Many others therefore advocate the use of absorbable sutures to reapproximate the deeper lumpectomy tissues, and this maneuver has been reported to decrease the risk of hematoma complications [41]. The disadvantage of using the deep cavity sutures is the potential for compromising the final cosmetic result by altering the underlying breast architecture and causing focal areas of retraction.

The use of a support brassiere in the postoperative period will bolster efforts to sustain hemostasis and relieves tension on the skin closure imposed by the weight of the breast. This precaution can be especially important with large, pendulous breasts, in which blood vessels running alongside the cavity can be avulsed mechanically if the heavy breast is allowed to suspend unsupported. The patient should be encouraged to wear the support brassiere day and night for several days.

The use of particular medications in the perioperative period also has been implicated in the risk for bleeding complications. Aspirin-containing products and nonsteroidal anti-inflammatory drugs such as ibuprofen have well-known antiplatelet activity, and these medications should be avoided for 1 to 2 weeks before surgery (the lifespan of the affected platelets). Ketorolac has become a popular intravenous substitute for opiate analgesics during the postoperative period, but this agent also is characterized as a nonsteroidal anti-inflammatory drug and should be used cautiously to minimize risk of hematoma [42]. In addition, several widely used over-the-counter medications and herbal supplements have become recognized recently for contributing to a bleeding diathesis; these include ginseng, ginkgo biloba, and garlic [43,44].

Chronic pain

A minority of breast cancer patients experience chronic incisional pain that can be quite debilitating and refractory to standard analgesics, lasting for several months to years postoperatively. The exact etiology of this syndrome remains obscure, although it commonly is assumed to be neuropathic in nature. Frequently described as a "burning," "constricting," or "lancing-type" ache, it is reported among mastectomy as well as lumpectomy patients and often is accompanied by ipsilateral upper extremity symptoms. The incidence of this chronic pain syndrome is uncertain, but it has been reported to afflict 20% to 30% of patients who are specifically queried [45–49]. Surprisingly, it has been reported to occur more commonly after lumpectomy than after mastectomy [45,49]. Risk factors identified with this syndrome include younger age, larger tumors, radiation therapy, chemotherapy, depression, and poor coping mechanisms [46,49,50]. The occasionally intractable quality of this syndrome causes substantial frustration for both patients and surgeons. Fortunately, recent successful management has been reported with use of serotonin uptake inhibitors, such as the antidepressants amitriptyline and venlafaxine [51].

Venous thromboembolism

Cancer is an established risk factor for hypercoagulable states [52,53] and therefore is a risk factor for postoperative venous thromboembolic (VTE) complications. Breast surgical procedures (in the absence of immediate reconstruction) tend not to be prolonged cases, however, and many are performed on an ambulatory, outpatient basis. Therefore the usefulness of routinely prescribing systemic VTE prophylaxis for patients who have breast cancer (as has been advocated for patients undergoing surgery for other types of cancer) and who lack some other predisposition for VTE has been questioned. Furthermore, the risk of wound hematoma after breast and/or axillary surgery can be tripled by the practice of systemic anti-VTE prophylaxis [54]. Andtbacka and colleagues [55] studied this issue in 3898 patients undergoing surgery for breast cancer at the University of Texas M.D. Anderson Cancer Center (with anti-VTE management consisting of early ambulation and compression stockings only) and reported a VTE rate of 0.16%, detected at a median time of 2 weeks after surgery. The authors concluded that the risk of VTE after breast surgery is sufficiently low that systemic VTE prophylaxis is not indicated.

Complications specific to mastectomy procedures

Incisional dog-ears

Heavyset patients who have thick axillary fat pads are especially prone to being left with triangular or cone-shaped flaps of redundant skin and fatty tissue along the lateral aspect of the mastectomy incision, commonly known as "dog-ears." Frequently the incisional dog-ear is not readily apparent while the patient is lying supine on the operating room table, but when she sits or stands upright postoperatively, these unsightly protrusions of axillary fat become obvious. Because they are irritating to the ipsilateral upper extremity, these flaps create significant discomfort for the patient. Similar to the inframammary fold before mastectomy, these dog-ears sometimes can be sites for recurrent candidal/yeast infections.

Numerous surgical approaches have been recommended to prevent or eliminate the dog-ear problem. One option is to bring the redundant axillary tissue forward and create a "T" or "Y" configuration at the lateral aspect of the transverse mastectomy incision [56]. Alternatively, the redundant axillary skin and fatty tissue can be resected either by elongating the standard elliptical mastectomy wound or by using a broad tear-drop incision, with the point of the tear-drop oriented medially [57,58].

Complications specific to lumpectomy procedures

Breast fibrosis, breast lymphedema, and chronic/recurrent breast cellulitis

The presence of long-term adverse sequelae related to breast-conservation therapy for cancer is being acknowledged and reported increasingly [59,60]. These complications are secondary to the combined tissue effects of surgery and radiation therapy. The European Organization for Research and Treatment and the Radiation Therapy Oncology Group have proposed that late effects of breast-conservation therapy (including breast edema, fibrosis, and atrophy/retraction) be graded according to the Late Effects of Normal Tissue-Subjective, Objective, Management, and Analytic (LENT-SOMA) scales [61]. The LENT-SOMA system stratifies breast symptoms on the basis of pain magnitude as reported by the patient, measurable differences in breast appearance, need for intervention to control pain and/or lymphedema, and presence of image-documented breast sequelae (eg, photographs, mammography, CT/MRI, and other studies).

Using the LENT-SOMA four-point grading system, Fehlauer and colleagues [60] reported grade 3 to grade 4 toxicity in 4% to 18% of patients who had breast cancer treated between 1983 and 1984 (radiation therapy fractionation schedule, 2.5 Gy four times per week to 60 Gy; median follow-up duration, 171 months), and these rates declined to 2% or less for patients treated in 1994 and 1995 (radiation therapy fractionation schedule, 2.0 Gy five times per week to 55 Gy; median follow-up duration, 75 months). These findings suggest that extent of side effects is a function of both follow-up duration and radiation delivery technique. Similarly, Meric and colleagues [59] reported chronic breast symptoms in 9.9% of patients who had breast cancer treated by lumpectomy and radiation from 1990 to 1992 and followed for at least 1 year after treatment.

Recurrent episodes of breast cellulitis occurring several months to years after lumpectomy and/or breast radiation therapy is reported to afflict fewer than 5% of patients, but this unusual and delayed complication causes significant concern because of the need to rule out an inflammatory breast cancer recurrence [62–66]. This condition can present as a myriad of scenarios: acutely inflamed seroma formation, localized mastitis, or diffuse breast pain and swelling. Repeat breast imaging is indicated to look for parenchymal features suggesting recurrence, such as an underlying spiculated mass or calcifications; if such features are present, an image-guided biopsy should be pursued. Otherwise benign-appearing cases that are refractory to a standard course of antibiotics should undergo punch biopsy for further evaluation. Occasionally patients ultimately request mastectomy because of intractable pain and inflammation.

The cause of delayed breast edema and cellulitis is incompletely understood but is assumed to be related to lymphatic obstruction affecting intramammary drainage. Risk factors for this condition include a history of early postoperative complications such as hematoma and seroma; upper extremity lymphedema; and large-volume lumpectomies [63]. Most cases have followed resection of upper outer quadrant tumors. Rarely is a causative bacterial pathogen identified in these cases, but the conventional management nonetheless includes antibiotic coverage for skin flora. The development of this complication does not seem to carry any cancer-related prognostic significance.

Complications related to lumpectomy and brachytherapy

Several breast cancer programs are currently exploring strategies of partial breast irradiation that allow shortening of the conventional 5- to 6-week external beam program. One such strategy involves insertion of a balloon-type catheter (the MammoSite applicator; MammoSite Radiation Therapy System, MammoSite RTS, CYTYC, Palo Alto, California) into the lumpectomy cavity for delivery of brachytherapy. This device typically is inserted in the operating room at the time of lumpectomy, with the expectation that margin control will be achieved; if this is not the case, additional surgery and a second implantation is required. While investigations of the long-term efficacy of these accelerated breast-irradiation programs are being conducted, experience with catheter-related risks is accumulating. CT imaging is performed subsequently to ensure adequate balloon placement, as defined by a minimum applicator–skin distance of 5 mm, and appropriate conformance, with uniform contact between the balloon and lumpectomy walls. Optimal positioning can be challenging but is essential for delivery of therapy with minimal risk of local complications.

Results from a prospective, multicenter study of the MammoSite device revealed that of 70 patients enrolled, 21 (30%) could not complete the study because of lumpectomy-related issues (cavity size, skin spacing, or conformance) [67]. Of the 54 patients who had a balloon inserted, 57% experienced overlying skin erythema, and 2 patients developed wound infections, including one abscess.

Angiosarcoma related to breast-conservation therapy

Reviewed in detail by Monroe and colleagues [68], angiosarcomas of the breast following lumpectomy and radiation therapy for breast cancer are rare but are being reported with increasing infrequency. These secondary angiosarcomas are to be distinguished from primary breast angiosarcomas, which occur in relatively younger women and which have no well-defined risk factors. Secondary angiosarcomas occur 4 to 10 years after primary breast cancer treatment [68–70]. Lymphedema-related extremity angiosarcoma (Stewart-Treves syndrome, discussed later) has a longer latency period from time of breast cancer treatment. Furthermore, the occurrence of breast angiosarcomas in the irradiated field coupled with the implications for genetic predisposition to radiation-induced tumorigenesis (eg, ataxia-telangiectasia) has prompted speculation that these lesions have an etiology different from that of Stewart-Treves syndrome. Median survival, however, is similarly poor, at 1 to 3 years [68].

Complications specific to diagnostic open biopsy procedures

Sampling error

The primary potential risk specifically associated with a diagnostic open biopsy is related to missing a cancerous lesion and resecting adjacent fibrocystic tissue, thereby misdiagnosing the patient. This complication exists with palpable masses as well as with screen-detected nonpalpable lesions.

The risk of misdiagnosis with palpable breast masses can be minimized by complete preoperative breast imaging, including mammography and ultrasonography. Palpable lesions that have a suspicious-appearing imaging correlate should have an initial attempt at percutaneous core needle biopsy to establish a diagnosis. If malignancy is confirmed, cancer-directed management options can be addressed promptly. In eligible patients who have measurable disease, neoadjuvant chemotherapy is one option that offers the potential benefits of tumor downstaging to improve the success of breast-conservation therapy and of monitoring chemosensitivity [71]. If the percutaneous biopsy was performed freehand, and results are nondiagnostic, an image-guided needle biopsy (by either ultrasound or stereotactic/mammographic) can be attempted. Alternatively, if resources are available, the percutaneous biopsy may be performed with image guidance as the initial maneuver to improve the diagnostic accuracy.

If the palpable lesion does not have an imaging correlate, or if needle biopsy strategies are unavailable, a diagnostic open biopsy must be performed. Sampling errors with these procedures are uncommon, but sampling in patients who have extensive fibrocystic changes can be challenging, especially when the lesion is a self-detected mass that is less apparent on clinical examination. In these cases the breast should be assessed and marked just before surgery by the surgeon and patient together, but intraoperative surgical judgment remains critical, and any suspicious masses identified within the open breast wound should be biopsied and oriented appropriately.

The risk of sampling error with nonpalpable breast lesions is greater. Establishing a diagnosis for clinically occult lesions that are identified by mammogram or ultrasound necessarily depends on image guidance. As noted previously, there are advantages to proceeding with an image-guided percutaneous needle biopsy as the initial diagnostic strategy. Patients whose diagnosis pf cancer has been made by needle biopsy are more likely to have successful breast-conservation therapy and to require fewer re-excisions for margin control than patients who undergo an initial open biopsy for diagnostic purposes [72]. A core-needle biopsy is preferable to a fine-needle aspiration biopsy because he larger tissue yield can distinguish in situ from invasive architecture and also because the sampling error with a fine-needle aspiration biopsy can be as high as 30%, compared with only 5% to 10% with a core needle. If the targeted lesion is small and can be resected completely within the core specimens, a radiopaque clip should be left in place to facilitate subsequent localization in case surgery is required.

When high-risk lesions such as atypical hyperplasia, radial scar, or lobular carcinoma in situ are identified on core-needle biopsy, a follow-up open surgical biopsy should be performed. The sampling error rates associated with these findings are substantial, and 10% to 40% will be upstaged to cancer on subsequent open biopsy [73].

Open surgical biopsies of nonpalpable, image-detected breast lesions require image-guided wire localization. The localizing wire can be inserted under either ultrasound or mammographic guidance, depending on which modality best images the abnormal lesion. MRI-guided wire localization technology is available in some centers as well. Past strategies for localization have included external skin markings and preoperative injection of dye into the vicinity of the lesion, but these techniques have been largely abandoned because of higher sampling error rates. Insertion of a hooked wire, with two-view confirmatory mammography of the wire position in relation to the abnormal lesion, followed by mammographic (and/or ultrasonographic) imaging of the biopsy specimen to document inclusion of the suspicious target, is the most widely used technique in contemporary breast programs. With this algorithm, the target is likely to be missed in fewer than 5% of cases. Risk factors for a sampling error complication despite these precautions include suboptimal wire localization, migration of the localizing wire between the time of insertion and the time of surgical resection, and migration of a previously inserted clip that was intended to mark the site of a prior core-needle biopsy. When a sampling error is recognized intraoperatively, based on specimen imaging, it is quite difficult to reorient the breast anatomy intraoperatively without the localizing wire. In this circumstance it is prudent to resist multiple attempts at blind biopsies, because the likelihood of success is low, and the additional tissue resections will compromise cosmesis. The patient should be informed of the failed procedure, and repeat imaging should be repeated 2 to 4 weeks postoperatively, with plans for another wire localization made accordingly.

Complications related to axillary staging procedures

The axillary nodal status remains the most powerful prognostic feature in staging patients who have invasive breast cancer. Surgical staging of the axilla is necessary for most newly diagnosed patients, because currently available imaging modalities can easily miss small nodal metastases. The conventional level I/II ALND is the standard means of evaluating the axilla, but lymphatic mapping and sentinel lymph node biopsy has emerged recently as a viable alternative strategy for accurately determining the nodal status. Each of these staging procedures is associated with risks for various complications and is discussed separately.

Complications associated with auxiliary lymph node dissection

The level I/II ALND is the conventionally accepted staging procedure. Random axillary sampling procedures and ALND limited to level I can miss metastases in 20% to 25% of cases. On the other hand, a level III dissection generally is considered unnecessary (unless grossly apparent disease is present in the axillary apex), because skip metastases to level III only occur in 2% to 3% of cases. The presence of an axillary arch has been proposed as an anatomic variant that can increase the risk of sampling error when a standard level I and II ALND is performed [74]. The axillary arch is formed by an aberrant segment of latissimus dorsi muscle that extends toward the pectoralis. If the axillary dissection does not encompass the lymphatic tissue lateral to these fibers, significant nodal tissue can be missed. Failure to appreciate this anatomic variant has been implicated as a cause for subsequent axillary recurrence [75].

Upper extremity lymphedema is the complication that has generated the most concern after ALND, because it is a lifelong risk following the procedure and, when it occurs, is quite refractory to treatment. Lymphedema has been reported to develop in 13% to 27% of patients who have breast cancer [25,76–79], but detection rates vary based on how closely patients are followed and duration of follow-up. The risk of lymphedema is greater after a higher-level axillary dissection than after less extensive surgery but has been reported to occur even after axillary surgery limited to the sentinel lymph nodes [25]. Other risk factors include obesity and regional radiation therapy. Patients can minimize the risk of lymphedema by participating in an aggressive and regulated physical therapy program, and onset of this problem is aggravated by upper extremity trauma or infection.

One of the most feared long-term sequelae of chronic lymphedema is the development of upper extremity angiosarcoma [80,81]. This condition is also known as "Stewart-Treves syndrome" [82], named for the investigators who first reported a series of cases demonstrating the association between postmastectomy lymphedema and the onset of this malignancy. Stewart-Treves syndrome typically appears as bluish-reddish macular lesions or nodules on the skin of the ipsilateral upper extremity. This disease generally develops approximately 10 years after treatment for breast cancer, and it is usually (but not always) seen in patients whose risk of lymphedema has been amplified by regional irradiation in addition to ALND. Treatment strategies have included wide local excision, amputation, chemotherapy, and/or radiation, with disappointing results. Most patients succumb to hematogenously disseminated metastases to lung and visceral organs, with a median survival of approximately 2 years.

The axillary dissection surgical bed exposes the axillary vein, thoracodorsal, long thoracic ("nerve of Bell"), and intercostobrachial nerves, as well as the neurovascular bundle to the pectoralis musculature. The intercostobrachial nerves are sacrificed routinely during a conventional ALND because they course directly through the nodal tissue en route to the skin of the axilla and upper inner arm, leaving patients with sensory deficits in this distribution. Attempts to preserve these nerves can result in damage that leaves the patient with chronic neuropathic pain of the involved skin. The axillary vein is at risk for hemorrhagic complications as a consequence of direct injury or thrombosis secondary to traction and/or compression. The axillary artery and brachial plexus are relatively protected from intraoperative damage because of their deeper and more superior location. The thoracodorsal neurovascular bundle, which courses along the inner aspect of the latissimus dorsi muscle, should be exposed completely and preserved intact, unless there is gross encasement by nodal metastases. Sacrifice of these structures denervates the latissimus (leaving the patient with weakness of internal rotation and shoulder abduction) and renders the thoracodorsal vessels unavailable for possible future use in conjunction with microvascular anastomoses for free flap reconstructions. Disruption of the long thoracic nerve results in loss of serratus anterior function and a winged scapula deformity with an unsightly posterior shoulder bony protrusion. When the medial and lateral pectoral nerves are transected, denervation atrophy of the pectoral muscles eventually becomes apparent and can compromise the cosmetic result substantially.

Axillary webs are bands of scar tissue that develop after ALND in fewer than 10% of cases. They are readily apparent as cordlike structures coursing from the surgical bed toward the forearm and occasionally reaching the thumb [83]. They cause significant tightness and limitation of motion but in most cases resolve within a few months. Physical therapy and massage are frequently helpful in alleviating symptoms.

One final rare complication of the ALND is chyle leak, sometimes reputed to be secondary to thoracic duct injury [84]. Recently, octreotide has been recommended to control extensive lymphorrhea [85].

Complications associated with lymphatic mapping and sentinel lymph node biopsy

In 1993 and 1994 the initial reports of lymphatic mapping and sentinel lymph node biopsy for patients who had breast cancer appeared in the literature, by Krag and colleagues [86] using radiolabeled isotope, and by Giuliano and colleagues [87] using blue dye. The accuracy of the sentinel lymph node biopsy procedure is discussed elsewhere in this issue, but the procedure now is widely accepted for axillary staging in breast cancer.

Complications that have been reported after a sentinel lymph node biopsy are the same as those associated with ALND, including seroma, lymphedema, axillary web formation, and neurosensory disturbances, but the magnitude of risk is lower. Data on long-term follow-up of patients who have undergone sentinel lymph node biopsy alone are revealing adverse sequelae in fewer than 10% of cases [25,78,88,89]. Wilke and colleagues [89] reported on the outcomes of 5327 patients who had early-stage breast cancer participating in the American College of Surgeons Oncology Group prospective lymphatic mapping protocol and found axillary wound infections in 1%, axillary seroma in 7.1%, and axillary hematoma in 1.4%. Lymphedema was reported in 6.9% of cases.

Allergic reactions to the blue dye used for mapping procedures can occur with the use of isosulfan blue as well as patent blue dye. Within a few minutes to an hour after blue dye injection, up to 2% of patients may experience sudden hemodynamic instability and other sequelae of intraoperative anaphylaxis. Despite the dramatic presentation, these episodes usually respond readily to supportive care, which includes discontinuation of the gaseous anesthetics, 100% oxygen, aggressive fluid resuscitation, and pressor support. In most cases the anesthesia and surgical procedure have been resumed and completed uneventfully after the patient has been stabilized. Some surgeons, however, have elected to abort the surgical procedure and to reschedule the mapping without blue dye [90]. In one reported case, a planned lumpectomy was converted to a mastectomy so that the allergen focus would be resected completely [91]. Many other patients have proceeded to undergo successful lumpectomies, but they should be monitored closely for 24 hours because continued uptake of the blue dye from skin and soft tissue can result in protracted or delayed secondary (biphasic) reactions.

Blue urticaria, a less severe form of blue dye allergy characterized by blue-tinged hives, is another pattern that has been reported [92,93]. There is no correlation with past allergy history, and preoperative skin testing is unreliable in identifying highest-risk patients. One hypothesis is that many individuals have prior sensitization from exposure to industrial dyes in cosmetics, textiles, detergents, and other products. Routine premedication of all patients undergoing mapping with steroids, antihistamines, and/or histamine receptor blockade has been proposed, but the added expense and risks of this approach for a low-incidence allergic reaction have not been documented. Known allergy to triphenylmethane is a contraindication to blue dye use. Thus far, methylene blue seems to be less allergenic [94], but caution must be exercised to avoid skin necrosis from dermal injections of this agent.

Blue dyes also can cause a spurious decline in pulse oximetry measurements, related to intravascular uptake and interference with spectroscopy; in these circumstances arterial blood gases reveal normal oxygenation. Blue dyes are contraindicated during pregnancy, because the risk of teratogenicity is unknown.

References

[1] Grunwald Z, Moore JH, Schwartz GF. Bilateral brachial plexus palsy after a right-side modified radical mastectomy with immediate TRAM flap reconstruction. Breast J 2003;9(1):41–3.

[2] Warner M, Blitt C, Butterworth J, et al. Practice advisory for the prevention of perioperative peripheral neuropathies. A report by the American Society of Anesthesiologists' Task Force on the prevention of perioperative peripheral neuropathies. Anesthesiology 2000;92: 1168–82.

[3] Bejanga BI. Mondor's disease: analysis of 30 cases. J R Coll Surg Edinb 1992;37(5):322–4.

[4] Catania S, Zurrida S, Veronesi P, et al. Mondor's disease and breast cancer. Cancer 1992; 69(9):2267–70.

[5] Harris AT. Mondor's disease of the breast can also occur after a sonography-guided core biopsy. AJR Am J Roentgenol 2003;180(1):284–5.

[6] Hou MF, Huang CJ, Huang YS, et al. Mondor's disease in the breast. Kaohsiung J Med Sci 1999;15(11):632–9.

[7] Jaberi M, Willey SC, Brem RF. Stereotactic vacuum-assisted breast biopsy: an unusual cause of Mondor's disease. AJR Am J Roentgenol 2002;179(1):185–6.

[8] Platt R, Zaleznik DF, Hopkins CC, et al. Perioperative antibiotic prophylaxis for herniorrhaphy and breast surgery. N Engl J Med 1990;322(3):153–60.

[9] Hoefer R, DuBois J, Ostrow L, et al. Wound complications following modified radical mastectomy: an analysis of perioperative factors. J Am Osteopath Assoc 1990;90:47–53.

[10] Wagman LD, Tegtmeier B, Beatty JD, et al. A prospective, randomized double-blind study of the use of antibiotics at the time of mastectomy. Surg Gynecol Obstet 1990; 170(1):12–6.

[11] Chen J, Gutkin Z, Bawnik J. Postoperative infections in breast surgery. J Hosp Infect 1991; 17:61–5.

[12] Vinton AL, Traverso LW, Jolly PC. Wound complications after modified radical mastectomy compared with tylectomy with axillary lymph node dissection. Am J Surg 1991; 161(5):584–8.

[13] Platt R, Zucker JR, Zaleznik DF, et al. Prophylaxis against wound infection following herniorrhaphy or breast surgery. J Infect Dis 1992;166(3):556–60.

[14] Lipshy KA, Neifeld JP, Boyle RM, et al. Complications of mastectomy and their relationship to biopsy technique. Ann Surg Oncol 1996;3(3):290–4.

[15] Bertin M, Crowe J, Gordon S. Determinants of surgical site infection after breast surgery. Am J Infect Control 1998;26:61–5.

[16] Thomas R, Alvino P, Cortino GR, et al. Long-acting versus short-acting cephalosporins for preoperative prophylaxis in breast surgery: a randomized double-blind trial involving 1,766 patients. Chemotherapy 1999;45(3):217–23.

[17] Gupta R, Sinnett D, Carpenter R, et al. Antibiotic prophylaxis for post-operative wound infection in clean elective breast surgery. Eur J Surg Oncol 2000;26(4):363–6.

[18] Nieto A, Lozano M, Moro MT, et al. Determinants of wound infections after surgery for breast cancer. Zentralbl Gynakol 2002;124(8–9):429–33.

[19] Sorensen LT, Horby J, Friis E, et al. Smoking as a risk factor for wound healing and infection in breast cancer surgery. Eur J Surg Oncol 2002;28(8):815–20.

[20] Witt A, Yavuz D, Walchetseder C, et al. Preoperative core needle biopsy as an independent risk factor for wound infection after breast surgery. Obstet Gynecol 2003;101(4):745–50.

[21] Tran CL, Langer S, Broderick-Villa G, et al. Does reoperation predispose to postoperative wound infection in women undergoing operation for breast cancer? Am Surg 2003;69(10): 852–6.

[22] Platt R, Zucker JR, Zaleznik DF, et al. Perioperative antibiotic prophylaxis and wound infection following breast surgery. J Antimicrob Chemother 1993;31(Suppl B):43–8.

[23] Pogson CJ, Adwani A, Ebbs SR. Seroma following breast cancer surgery. Eur J Surg Oncol 2003;29(9):711–7.

[24] Bonnema J, Ligtensetein D, Wiggers T, et al. The composition of serous fluid after axillary dissection. Eur J Surg 1999;165:9–13.

[25] Giuliano AE, Haigh PI, Brennan MB, et al. Prospective observational study of sentinel lymphadenectomy without further axillary dissection in patients with sentinel node-negative breast cancer. J Clin Oncol 2000;18(13):2553–9.

[26] Talbot ML, Magarey CJ. Reduced use of drains following axillary lymphadenectomy for breast cancer. ANZ J Surg 2002;72(7):488–90.

[27] Cameron AE, Ebbs SR, Wylie F, et al. Suction drainage of the axilla: a prospective randomized trial. Br J Surg 1988;75(12):1211.

[28] Somers R, Jablon L, Kaplan M. The use of closed suction drainage after lumpectomy and axillary dissection for breast cancer: a prospective randomized trial. Ann Surg 1992;215: 146–9.

[29] Flew J. The effect of restriction of shoulder movement. Br J Surg 1979;66:302–5.

[30] Lotz M, Duncan M, Gerber L, et al. Early versus delayed shoulder motion following axillary dissection. Ann Surg 1981;193:288–95.

[31] Schultz I, Barrholm M, Grondal S. Delayed shoulder exercises in reducing seroma frequency after modified radical mastectomy: a prospective randomized study. Ann Surg Oncol 1997;4: 293–7.

[32] Porter KA, O'Connor S, Rimm E, et al. Electrocautery as a factor in seroma formation following mastectomy. Am J Surg 1998;176(1):8–11.

[33] Keogh G, Doughty J, McArdle C, et al. Seroma formation related to electrocautery in breast surgery—a prospective, randomized trial. Breast 1998;7:39–41.

[34] Classe J, Dupre P, Francois T, et al. Axillary padding as an alternative to closed suction drain for ambulatory axillary lymphadenectomy. Arch Surg 2002;137:169–73.

[35] O'Hea BJ, Ho MN, Petrek JA. External compression dressing versus standard dressing after axillary lymphadenectomy. Am J Surg 1999;177(6):450–3.

[36] Rice DC, Morris SM, Sarr MG, et al. Intraoperative topical tetracycline sclerotherapy following mastectomy: a prospective, randomized trial. J Surg Oncol 2000;73(4):224–7.

[37] Burak WE Jr, Goodman P, Young D. Seroma formation following axillary dissection for breast cancer: risk factors and lack of influence of bovine thrombin. J Surg Oncol 1997;64:27–31.

[38] Langer S, Guenther JM, DiFronzo LA. Does fibrin sealant reduce drain output and allow earlier removal of drainage catheters in women undergoing operation for breast cancer? Am Surg 2003;69(1):77–81.

[39] Berger A, Tempfer C, Hartmann B, et al. Sealing of postoperative axillary leakage after axillary lymphadenectomy using a fibrin glue coated collagen patch: a prospective randomised study. Breast Cancer Res Treat 2001;67(1):9–14.

[40] Moore M, Burak WE Jr, Nelson E, et al. Fibrin sealant reduces the duration and amount of fluid drainage after axillary dissection: a randomized prospective clinical trial. J Am Coll Surg 2001;192(5):591–9.

[41] Paterson ML, Nathanson SD, Havstad S. Hematomas following excisional breast biopsies for invasive breast carcinoma: the influence of deep suture approximation of breast parenchyma. Am Surg 1994;60(11):845–8.

[42] Sharma S, Chang DW, Koutz C, et al. Incidence of hematoma associated with ketorolac after TRAM flap breast reconstruction. Plast Reconstr Surg 2001;107(2):352–5.

[43] Hodges P, Kam P. The perioperative implications of herbal medicines. Anaesthesia 2002; 57(9):889–99.

[44] Ang-Lee M, Moss J, Yuan C. Herbal medicines and perioperative care. JAMA 2001;286(2): 208–16.

[45] Tasmuth T, von Smitten K, Kalso E. Pain and other symptoms during the first year after radical and conservative surgery for breast cancer. Br J Cancer 1996;74(12): 2024–31.

[46] Tasmuth T, Blomqvist C, Kalso E. Chronic post-treatment symptoms in patients with breast cancer operated in different surgical units. Eur J Surg Oncol 1999;25:38–43.

[47] Stevens P, Dibble S, Miastowski C. Prevalence, characteristics, and impact of postmastectomy pain syndrome: an investigation of women's experiences. Pain 1995;61:61–8.

[48] Carpenter J, Andrylkowski M, Sloan P, et al. Postmastectomy/postlumpectomy pain in breast cancer survivors. J Clin Epidemiol 1998;51:1285–92.

[49] Tasmuth T, von Smitten K, Hietanen P, et al. Pain and other symptoms after different treatment modalities of breast cancer. Ann Oncol 1995;6:453–9.

[50] Bishop SR, Warr D. Coping, catastrophizing and chronic pain in breast cancer. J Behav Med 2003;26(3):265–81.

[51] Tasmuth T, Hartel B, Kalso E. Venlafaxine in neuropathic pain following treatment of breast cancer. Eur J Pain 2002;6(1):17–24.

[52] Rickles FR, Edwards RL. Activation of blood coagulation in cancer: Trousseau's syndrome revisited. Blood 1983;62(1):14–31.

[53] Duggan C, Marriott K, Edwards R, et al. Inherited and acquired risk factors for venous thromboembolic disease among women taking tamoxifen to prevent breast cancer. J Clin Oncol 2003;21(19):3588–93.

[54] Friis E, Horby J, Sorensen LT, et al. Thromboembolic prophylaxis as a risk factor for postoperative complications after breast cancer surgery. World J Surg 2004;28(6): 540–3.

[55] Andtbacka RH, Babiera G, Singletary SE, et al. Incidence and prevention of venous thromboembolism in patients undergoing breast cancer surgery and treated according to clinical pathways. Ann Surg 2006;243(1):96–101.

[56] Farrar WB, Fanning WJ. Eliminating the dog-ear in modified radical mastectomy. Am J Surg 1988;156(5):401–2.

[57] Chretien-Marquet B, Bennaceur S. Dog ear: true and false. A simple surgical management. Dermatol Surg 1997;23(7):547–50 [discussion: 551].

[58] Mirza M, Sinha KS, Fortes-Mayer K. Tear-drop incision for mastectomy to avoid dog-ear deformity. Ann R Coll Surg Engl 2003;85(2):131.

[59] Meric F, Buchholz TA, Mirza NQ, et al. Long-term complications associated with breast-conservation surgery and radiotherapy. Ann Surg Oncol 2002;9(6):543–9.

[60] Fehlauer F, Tribius S, Holler U, et al. Long-term radiation sequelae after breast-conserving therapy in women with early-stage breast cancer: an observational study using the LENT-SOMA scoring system. Int J Radiat Oncol Biol Phys 2003;55(3):651–8.

[61] LENT-SOMA scales for all anatomic sites. Int J Radiat Oncol Biol Phys 1995;31: 1049–91.

[62] Zippel D, Siegelmann-Danieli N, Ayalon S, et al. Delayed breast cellulitis following breast conserving operation. Eur J Surg Oncol 2003;29(4):327–30.

[63] Brewer VH, Hahn KA, Rohrbach BW, et al. Risk factor analysis for breast cellulitis complicating breast conservation therapy. Clin Infect Dis 2000;31(3):654–9.

[64] Staren ED, Klepac S, Smith AP, et al. The dilemma of delayed cellulitis after breast conservation therapy. Arch Surg 1996;131(6):651–4.

[65] Rescigno J, McCormick B, Brown AE, et al. Breast cellulitis after conservative surgery and radiotherapy. Int J Radiat Oncol Biol Phys 1994;29(1):163–8.

[66] Miller SR, Mondry T, Reed JS, et al. Delayed cellulitis associated with conservative therapy for breast cancer. J Surg Oncol 1998;67(4):242–5.

[67] Keisch M, Vicini F, Kuske RR, et al. Initial clinical experience with the MammoSite breast brachytherapy applicator in women with early-stage breast cancer treated with breast-conserving therapy. Int J Radiat Oncol Biol Phys 2003;55(2):289–93.

[68] Monroe AT, Feigenberg SJ, Mendenhall NP. Angiosarcoma after breast-conserving therapy. Cancer 2003;97(8):1832–40.

[69] Edeiken S, Russo DP, Knecht J, et al. Angiosarcoma after tylectomy and radiation therapy for carcinoma of the breast. Cancer 1992;70(3):644–7.

[70] Feigenberg SJ, Mendenhall NP, Reith JD, et al. Angiosarcoma after breast-conserving therapy: experience with hyperfractionated radiotherapy. Int J Radiat Oncol Biol Phys 2002; 52(3):620–6.

[71] Fisher B, Brown A, Mamounas E, et al. Effect of preoperative chemotherapy on local-regional disease in women with operable breast cancer: findings from National Surgical Adjuvant Breast and Bowel Project B-18. J Clin Oncol 1997;15(7):2483–93.

[72] Liberman L, Goodstone S, Dershaw D. One operation after percutaneous diagnosis of non-palpable breast cancer: frequency and associated factors. AJR Am J Roentgenol 2002;178: 673–9.

[73] Newman L. Surgical management of high-risk breast lesions. Curr Probl Surg 2004.

[74] Petrasek AJ, Semple JL, McCready DR. The surgical and oncologic significance of the axillary arch during axillary lymphadenectomy. Can J Surg 1997;40(1):44–7.

[75] Wright FC, Walker J, Law CH, et al. Outcomes after localized axillary node recurrence in breast cancer. Ann Surg Oncol 2003;10(9):1054–8.

[76] Erickson VS, Pearson ML, Ganz PA, et al. Arm edema in breast cancer patients. J Natl Cancer Inst 2001;93(2):96–111.

[77] Beaulac SM, McNair LA, Scott TE, et al. Lymphedema and quality of life in survivors of early-stage breast cancer. Arch Surg 2002;137(11):1253–7.

[78] Sener SF, Winchester DJ, Martz CH, et al. Lymphedema after sentinel lymphadenectomy for breast carcinoma. Cancer 2001;92(4):748–52.

[79] Roses DF, Brooks AD, Harris MN, et al. Complications of level I and II axillary dissection in the treatment of carcinoma of the breast. Ann Surg 1999;230(2):194–201.

[80] Grobmyer SR, Daly JM, Glotzbach RE, et al. Role of surgery in the management of post-mastectomy extremity angiosarcoma (Stewart-Treves syndrome). J Surg Oncol 2000;73(3): 182–8.

[81] Janse AJ, van Coevorden F, Peterse H, et al. Lymphedema-induced lymphangiosarcoma. Eur J Surg Oncol 1995;21(2):155–8.

[82] Stewart FW, Treves N. Classics in oncology: lymphangiosarcoma in postmastectomy lymphedema: a report of six cases in elephantiasis chirurgica. CA Cancer J Clin 1981;31(5):284–99.

[83] Moskovitz AH, Anderson BO, Yeung RS, et al. Axillary web syndrome after axillary dissection. Am J Surg 2001;181(5):434–9.

[84] Caluwe GL, Christiaens MR. Chylous leak: a rare complication after axillary lymph node dissection. Acta Chir Belg 2003;103(2):217–8.

[85] Carcoforo P, Soliani G, Maestroni U, et al. Octreotide in the treatment of lymphorrhea after axillary node dissection: a prospective randomized controlled trial. J Am Coll Surg 2003; 196(3):365–9.

[86] Krag DN, Weaver DL, Alex JC, et al. Surgical resection and radiolocalization of the sentinel lymph node in breast cancer using a gamma probe. Surg Oncol 1993;2(6):335–9 [discussion: 340].

[87] Giuliano AE, Kirgan DM, Guenther JM, et al. Lymphatic mapping and sentinel lymphadenectomy for breast cancer. Ann Surg 1994;220(3):391–8 [discussion: 398–401].

[88] Leidenius M, Leppanen E, Krogerus L, et al. Motion restriction and axillary web syndrome after sentinel node biopsy and axillary clearance in breast cancer. Am J Surg 2003;185(2): 127–30.

[89] Wilke LG, McCall LM, Posther KE, et al. Surgical complications associated with sentinel lymph node biopsy: results from a prospective international cooperative group trial. Ann Surg Oncol 2006;13(4):491–500.

[90] Laurie SA, Khan DA, Gruchalla RS, et al. Anaphylaxis to isosulfan blue. Ann Allergy Asthma Immunol 2002;88(1):64–6.

[91] Efron P, Knudsen E, Hirshorn S, et al. Anaphylactic reaction to isosulfan blue used for sentinel node biopsy: case report and literature review. Breast J 2002;8(6):396–9.

[92] Sadiq TS, Burns WW 3rd, Taber DJ, et al. Blue urticaria: a previously unreported adverse event associated with isosulfan blue. Arch Surg 2001;136(12):1433–5.

[93] Cimmino VM, Brown AC, Szocik JF, et al. Allergic reactions to isosulfan blue during sentinel node biopsy—a common event. Surgery 2001;130(3):439–42.

[94] Mostafa A, Carpenter R. Anaphylaxis to patent blue dye during sentinel lymph node biopsy for breast cancer. Eur J Surg Oncol 2001;27:610.

ELSEVIER
SAUNDERS

SURGICAL
CLINICS OF
NORTH AMERICA

Surg Clin N Am 87 (2007) 453–467

Breast Reconstruction

Emily Hu, MD[a], Amy K. Alderman, MD, MPH[a,b,*]

[a]Section of Plastic Surgery, Department of Surgery, The University of Michigan
Medical Center, Ann Arbor, MI 48109, USA
[b]VA Center for Practice Management and Outcomes Research, Ann Arbor
VA Health Care System, Ann Arbor, MI 48109, USA

During the last century, breast reconstruction after mastectomy has become an important part of comprehensive treatment for patients who have breast cancer. Breast reconstruction initially was created to reduce complications of mastectomy and to diminish chest wall deformities. Now, however, it is known that reconstruction also can improve the psychosocial well-being and quality of life of patients who have breast cancer [1]. The primary goal of breast reconstruction is to recreate form and symmetry by correcting the anatomic defect while preserving patient safety and health. The primary reconstructive options involve the use an implant (usually with an expander first), the patient's own tissue (autogenous tissue reconstruction), or both. The reconstructive process can start at the time of the mastectomy (immediate reconstruction) or any time afterwards (delayed reconstruction).

Historical background

Silicone breast implants were introduced in the early 1960s [2], but in 1992, the Food and Drug Administration (FDA) placed a moratorium on silicone implants due to concern regarding its safety of use in patients. Since then saline implants had been exclusively used in the United States, until recently. In November 2006, after an extensive scientific review revealed no significant risks, the FDA approved the use of silicone implants for breast reconstruction in women of all ages. Now that the silicone implant has been deemed safe, the FDA is requiring a 10 year follow-up to continue to monitor these implants as part of a post-approval study [3]. The initial implant reconstructions were placed under the thin mastectomy skin flaps

---

* Corresponding author.
E-mail addresses: aalder@umich.edu (A.K. Alderman); ehu@umich.edu (E. Hu).

without prior expansion of the tissue, a practice that led to frequent complications such as skin loss. The introduction of the latissimus dorsi myocutaneous flap provided better soft tissue coverage over the implant and
decreased postoperative complications [4]. In 1982, Radovan [5] introduced
tissue expansion with placement of an uninflated implant under the residual
skin and muscle, followed by intermittent filling of the implant. This process
resulted in a gradual expansion of the overlying tissue. As the final stage of
breast reconstruction, permanent implants replaced the expander implant.
This technique, however, remained plagued by complications such as capsular
contracture (scarring around the implant). Breast reconstruction advanced
further with the popularization of the transverse rectus myocutaneous
(TRAM) flap by Hartrampf and colleagues [6] in 1982, followed by the
microsurgical free TRAM flap. The latest technical advances in breast
reconstruction, perforator flaps, were introduced by Allen and colleagues in
1994 and 1995 [7,8].

The other major advance that has occurred in breast reconstruction has
been on the health policy front. In 1998, the federal government passed the
Women's Health and Cancer Rights Act (WHCRA), which mandated insurance coverage of reconstruction if the insurance plan provided mastectomy
coverage. The law also mandated coverage of breast symmetry procedures
and the treatment of surgical complications at all stages of the mastectomy
and reconstruction [9].

Goals

In keeping with the Hippocratic oath, one of the goals of breast reconstruction is to "first do no harm." Reconstruction after mastectomy should
not impede the patient's oncologic treatment (ie, delay administration of
chemotherapy or radiation therapy), should not delay the diagnosis of a recurrence, and should not add an unacceptable increase in operative morbidity or mortality. Current data indicate that reconstruction is safe and does
not delay adjuvant therapy or the detection of cancer recurrence [10–12].
In addition, although the most frequent site of recurrent breast cancer is
in the remaining chest wall skin, immediate reconstruction has not been
shown to increase the rate of local recurrence in the long term [10].

The specific surgical goals of the plastic surgeon are to optimize the aesthetic result while keeping in mind the patient's preferences and surgical limitations. For instance, some women may be happy with recreation of just
a breast mound, whereas other women may desire supple soft tissue and
complete nipple reconstruction.

Preoperative counseling

After appropriate discussion between the oncologic team and the patient,
if the woman desires reconstruction, a consultation with a plastic surgeon

should be offered at the time of initial surgical decision making. This preoperative consultation should cover several areas, such as the type and timing of reconstruction. Reconstructive options are based on the patient's overall goals, physical examination, and clinical factors. For example, autogenous tissue reconstructions are best in women who value the creation of the most natural-looking and -feeling breast. Other women may place more value on limiting potential morbidity to other body areas, such as the abdomen, and therefore prefer an expander/implant reconstruction. Clinical contraindications or significant risk factors to reconstruction, such as obesity, nicotine use, chronic obstructive pulmonary disease, diabetes, and other chronic conditions, should be assessed. (Such contraindications are discussed in further detail later in this article.) Although patient preference certainly is important, the highest priority is providing appropriate treatment of the breast cancer. Thus, input from a multidisciplinary team consisting of oncologic surgeons, medical and radiation oncologists, as well as reconstructive surgeons is necessary to provide the most comprehensive and appropriate treatment.

Timing of reconstruction

Immediate reconstruction

"Immediate" reconstruction is defined as reconstruction that starts at the same time as the mastectomy. This option can be an excellent one for women who have ductal carcinoma in situ and stage 1 or stage 2 disease. The advantages of immediate breast reconstruction are multiple. Women who have immediate reconstruction have less distress and better body image, self-esteem, and satisfaction, in general, than women who have delayed reconstruction [13]. From an aesthetic standpoint, autogenous tissue reconstructions performed at the time of the mastectomy generally have produced a better aesthetic result than delayed procedures because the skin envelope is preserved [14,15]. The overall cost is less because fewer major operations are needed, the patient is anesthetized already, the defect does not have to be recreated, and the patient can recover from the mastectomy and the reconstruction simultaneously [16].

Disadvantages of immediate reconstruction include the potential delay of adjuvant therapy should a postoperative complication such as delayed wound healing occur. Most studies, however, have not shown reconstruction to delay therapy [12]. Another potential pitfall of immediate reconstruction is the partial loss of the mastectomy skin flaps, especially if the oncologic surgeon needs to create thin skin flaps. In addition, residual disease or close surgical margins may necessitate the use of postoperative radiation therapy, which can adversely affect the reconstruction.

Relative contraindications to immediate reconstruction include advanced disease (stage 3 or higher), need for postoperative radiation (although this contraindication is controversial and varies by center), and medical comorbidities such as use of nicotine, morbid obesity, or cardiopulmonary disease. In addition, use of implants is a relative contraindication in women who have rheumatologic disorders.

Delayed reconstruction

Delayed reconstruction, defined as a reconstructive procedure that starts after the mastectomy, can be started any time after the wound has healed and adjuvant therapy has been administered. Postradiation skin changes should have stabilized, and the hematologic effects of chemotherapy should have normalized before reconstruction is begun. Delayed reconstruction has its own advantages. First, all guess work regarding whether radiation therapy will be required is eliminated, so surgeons and patients can appraise to their reconstructive options more accurately. Second, studies have shown that delayed reconstructions have overall fewer complications than immediate reconstruction [10]. Disadvantages of delayed reconstruction include prolonging the overall treatment of the patient, a poorer cosmetic result with autogenous tissue reconstruction because the skin envelope is not preserved, and potentially higher costs to the health care system.

Reconstructive techniques

Implant without tissue expansion

The simplest reconstruction for a mastectomy defect involves the placement of an implant, without prior expansion of the remaining tissue envelope. This simple technique requires that the skin flaps remaining after the mastectomy to be sufficient to cover the implant. Often, the remaining flaps are not sufficient. If an implant is placed without prior expansion, there is a greatly increased risk of skin necrosis secondary to tension. In addition, implants placed under nonexpanded mastectomy skin flaps often have poor cosmetic results because of constricted skin envelopes. For these reasons, this technique is generally discouraged.

Tissue expansion followed by permanent implant placement

Indications/contraindications

Tissue expansion followed by permanent implant placement is a frequently used technique in breast reconstruction. The most appropriate patients for this type of reconstruction are patients who do not qualify for autogenous reconstruction, patients who do not want additional scars from other donor sites, patients who prefer a typically quicker postoperative recovery period, and patients who have relatively small breasts. A contraindication for this type of reconstruction is mastectomy flaps that are too thin for adequate implant coverage. In these cases, one should consider using a latissimus dorsi muscle flap for additional coverage. Another relative contraindication is the completed or planned use of adjuvant radiation therapy because of higher implant complication rates [17].

Technique

The most common technique used for expander/implant placement is placing the expander in a subpectoral pocket (Fig. 1). For immediate tissue expander reconstructions, the goal is to obtain total submuscular coverage that protects the implant from becoming exposed if a minimal amount of skin necrosis occurs. To achieve this coverage, a portion of the serratus muscle is raised laterally and is plicated to the pectoralis major muscle. Occasionally, the superior aspect of the rectus abdominis muscle must be elevated also. Overall, the pocket size should match the size of the expander (as determined preoperatively based on measurements of the patient's chest wall). It is critical to not alter or undermine the inframammary fold, because this important landmark is difficult to reconstruct and is crucial to the long-term cosmetic result. If there is concern that the mastectomy flaps have compromised vascular supply, the expander placement should be delayed. Typically, the expansion is done weekly, and the volume instilled depends on patient comfort and skin quality (eg, tightness, erythema). The expander typically is overexpanded by 25% to improve the skin drape over the implant, to allow for the skin recoil that occurs after expansion, and to allow for differences in the profile of the expander versus the implant.

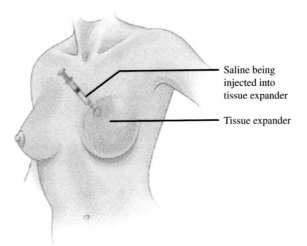

Saline being injected into tissue expander

Tissue expander

Fig. 1. Tissue expander technique. (*From* Wilkins E. The University of Michigan Breast Reconstruction Handbook. p. 3. Available at: http://www.med.umich.edu/surgery/plastic/clinical/breast/index.shtml. Accessed September 20, 2006; with permission.)

Advantages/disadvantages

Advantages of this technique include the avoidance of donor site morbidity and the low overall functional impairments for the patient. Expander and subsequent implant placement often requires less operative time than autogenous reconstruction, and the recovery period is shorter (typically patients are discharged on postoperative day one). One major disadvantage of this technique is the overall time required. Typically, tissue expansion is started 2 to 3 weeks postoperatively (if the wounds are healed), followed by weekly expansions in the clinic that can last several months before the tissue envelope is sufficiently expanded. Once expansion is complete, an additional 2 to 4 months are allowed for tissue equilibrium to occur before the skin envelope is ready for the expander to be exchanged for a permanent implant. The exchange of the expander for the implant also requires an additional, albeit relatively short, surgery. In addition, implants lack natural ptosis (or droop) and usually feel unnatural (especially saline implants).

Complications

Complications associated with expander/implant reconstructions can occur in the acute and long-term settings. Acute complications that often require removal of the expander or implant include exposure of the device, infection, malposition, or deflation. In addition, a hematoma or seroma may occur. Long-term complications include capsular contracture (scar tissue around the implant causing visible deformity and/or discomfort), visible wrinkling of the implant (especially with saline implants in thin women), and implant deflation (the devices typically last 10–15 years). The rate of reported complications with tissue expander/implant reconstructions in the setting of radiation approaches 50% [17–19].

Pedicled transverse rectus myocutaneous flap

Indications/contraindications

Many surgeons prefer to use autogenous tissue (ie, TRAM flap), in part because of greater patient satisfaction with these techniques [20,21]. Patient indications for the TRAM flap include patients in whom non-TRAM reconstruction was unsuccessful, who have mastectomy defects requiring a large amount of tissue for reconstruction, or who have a history of chest wall irradiation. TRAM reconstructions are also useful in women who have a ptotic contralateral breast that will be hard to match using an implant. For TRAM reconstructions, women must have adequate soft tissue in the lower abdomen and, preferably, have a body mass index less than 30. Contraindications to this procedure include prior abdominal surgery that may have divided the pedicle or blood supply, such as an open cholecystectomy, coronary artery bypass graft using the internal mammary artery or an abdominoplasty that transects the perforator blood vessels to the skin. Obesity also is a contraindication: it is well documented that complications are directly associated with a higher body mass index [10,22]. With increased abdominal fat, the blood supply to the skin and subcutaneous fat becomes unreliable, leading to partial flap loss or fat necrosis. Other relative contraindications include severe comorbidities (eg, vascular disease, chronic obstructive pulmonary disease) or active use of nicotine.

Technique

The blood supply to the TRAM flap is considered bipedicled (double), from the superior and inferior epigastric arteries, with the most direct supply from the inferior epigastric artery. In a pedicled TRAM flap, the inferior epigastric artery is severed, and the rectus muscle and overlying skin and subcutaneous tissue are rotated into the mastectomy defect based on the superior epigastric artery and the periumbilical perforators (Fig. 2). When this superior pedicle is used, the blood flows through the choke vessels (vessels that dilate based on need, Fig. 3) between the two pedicles before reaching the skin through perforating arteries. When the blood supply may be more tenuous (as in obese patients and patients who use nicotine), or when a large amount of tissue is needed for the reconstruction, the surgeon can dilate the choke vessels by severing the inferior epigastric artery 2 to 3 weeks before the actual reconstruction. This surgical-delay procedure is thought to improve the blood flow through these choke vessels and can be done at the time of the general surgeon's sentinel lymph node biopsy. Another way to improve the arterial inflow and venous outflow to the pedicled TRAM flap is to take the inferior epigastric vessels and anastomose it

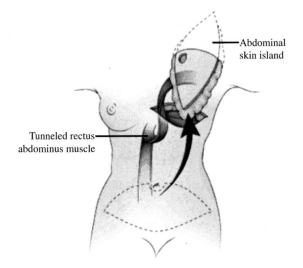

Fig. 2. Pedicled transverse rectus myocutaneous flap technique. (*From* Wilkins E. The University of Michigan Breast Reconstruction Handbook. p. 9. Available at: http://www.med.umich.edu/surgery/plastic/clinical/breast/index.shtml. Accessed September 20, 2006; with permission.)

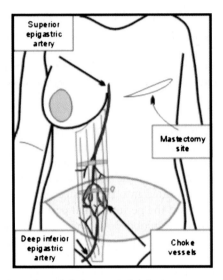

Fig. 3. Buntic R. Blood supply and choke vessels for the transverse rectus myocutaneous flap technique. (*From* Buntic R. Available at: www.microsurgery.net; with permission.)

microsurgically to the thoracodorsal or internal mammary vessels, a procedure termed "supercharging."

Advantages/disadvantages

Advantages of the TRAM flap include a natural-appearing and -feeling reconstruction that will have an aging process similar to an unreconstructed breast. Disadvantages of this type of reconstruction include a long operative time (4–6 hours), relatively long hospitalization (3–5 days), and long postoperative recovery. It takes most women 2 to 4 months to return to their preoperative physical functioning.

Complications

Complications in the acute period include infection (12%), hematoma or seroma of the breast or abdomen (4%), umbilical necrosis, and partial (16%) or total flap loss (1%) [10]. In the long term, potential complications include abdominal wall laxity or hernia (8%) [10].

Microsurgical transverse rectus myocutaneous flap

Another option with the TRAM flap is to perform a microsurgical or "free" transfer of the abdominal tissue to the mastectomy defect (Fig. 4). In this procedure, the blood supply is the deep inferior epigastric artery and its venae comitantes, which are severed at their origin. These vessels are anastomosed microsurgically to the thoracodorsal or internal mammary vessels. Relative indications for this procedure are similar to those for the pedicled TRAM flap. Unlike the pedicled TRAM flap, however, this

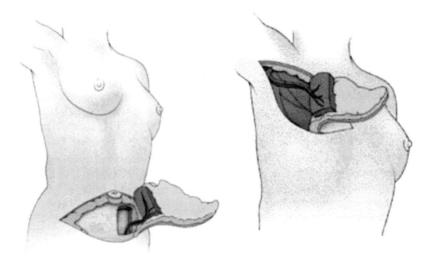

Fig. 4. Free transverse rectus myocutaneous flap technique. (*From* Wilkins E. The University of Michigan Breast Reconstruction Handbook. p. 12. Available at: http://www.med.umich.edu/surgery/plastic/clinical/breast/index.shtml. Accessed September 20, 2006; with permission.)

technique can be used when the superior epigastric artery has been divided (eg, in a patient who has had a previous open cholecystectomy). Some surgeons also believe that this procedure provides a more robust blood supply than obtained with a pedicled technique. Disadvantages of this technique include a potentially longer operating time and the need for microsurgical expertise. Complications in the acute period include infection (18%), hematoma or seroma of the breast or abdomen (4.5%–9%), umbilical necrosis, and partial (15%) or total flap loss (1.5%) [10]. In the long term, potential complications include abdominal wall laxity or hernia (12%) [10]. Although the microsurgical technique often is considered in obese patients, these patients still have a significantly higher risk of certain complications (total flap loss, flap hematoma, flap seroma, mastectomy skin flap necrosis, donor-site infection, donor-site seroma, and hernia) than normal-weight patients [23].

Perforator flaps

Deep inferior epigastric perforator

A more recently described technique, the deep inferior epigastric perforator (DIEP) flap, is similar to the free TRAM flap, but the blood supply to this flap is based on only one or two of the perforator arteries off of the deep inferior epigastric artery. This procedure does not require harvest of the rectus abdominis muscle, resulting in less abdominal wall morbidity. Specifically, the incidence of abdominal wall laxity or hernia is less than with techniques that remove abdominal wall fascia with the rectus muscle. A recent study also has reported a shorter hospitalization and faster recovery because there is less abdominal wall pain with perforator flaps than with traditional TRAM flap reconstructions [24]. This technique still has disadvantages. Significant microsurgical expertise is required, operative times are longer, and the incidence of partial or total flap loss is higher than with traditional TRAM procedures [25]. Earlier studies showed that the DIEP flap had a less robust blood supply, leading to an increased risk for fat necrosis [25]. More recent studies, however, suggest that the rates of fat necrosis or partial flap loss are no higher with perforator flaps than with pedicle TRAM procedures [15]. Nevertheless, the choice between the free TRAM and the DIEP flap should be based on the patient's weight, the breast volume required, the amount of abdominal fat available, and on the number, caliber, and location of the perforating vessels [26]. For the properly selected patient, some microsurgeons now prefer the DIEP flap to the free TRAM flap.

Superficial inferior epigastric artery flap

Another option that is used less frequently is the superficial inferior epigastric artery (SIEA) flap. This flap option was presented by Allen [27] in 1990 but was dismissed at that time because of a high flap failure rate (in three of seven clinical cases). A more recent prospective study comparing the SIEA flap with the DIEP and free TRAM flaps found a 2% flap loss with the SIEA [28]. Advantages of the SIEA flap include minimal donor-site morbidity because the rectus abdominis fascia and muscle are not violated and less postoperative pain [28].

Gluteal artery perforator flap

For patients who do not have sufficient abdominal tissue for breast reconstruction but still prefer the use of autologous tissue, an option is the use of the buttock as donor tissue. This donor site can also be used for unilateral or bilateral breast reconstructions. There are two options for blood supply to the flap. When the superior gluteal artery is used, the flap is called a "superior gluteal artery perforator" (SGAP) flap, and the upper buttock tissue is used. The scar lies in the upper buttock region and is hidden easily with underwear. When the inferior gluteal artery is used, the flap is called an "inferior gluteal artery perforator" (IGAP) flap, and the lower buttock tissue is used. The scar lies within the lower buttock crease.

The advantage of these flaps is the readily available donor tissue in most patients. Disadvantages include the technical challenge of raising this flap, the potential risk of injury to the sciatic nerve or postoperative pain from an insufficiently padded sciatic nerve, and a potentially disfiguring donor site. Although the selection of the donor site depends on preference and the patient's anatomy, Allen and colleagues [29] recently reported his preference for using the IGAP, rather than the SGAP, as the primary alternative to the DIEP flap because of its better aesthetic outcome.

Latissimus dorsi flap

Indications/contraindications

Another reliable workhorse for breast reconstruction is the latissimus dorsi muscle or myocutaneous (muscle and skin) flap. Indications for this flap include previous implant or TRAM flap failure, need to reconstruct a partial mastectomy or lumpectomy defect, abdominal obesity, or extreme thinness resulting in inadequate infraumbilical soft tissue. Contraindications to this technique include prior surgery that may have interrupted the blood supply (eg, posterior thoracotomy), the inability of the patient to be positioned on her side, severe comorbidities, and the patient not desiring implant placement.

Technique

The dominant blood supply to this flap is the thoracodorsal artery (off the subscapular artery), with segmental blood supply from the posterior intercostals and lumbar vessels (Fig. 5). If the thoracodorsal artery is damaged more proximally during the mastectomy, this flap also may survive on retrograde blood flow from the serratus branch off the thoracodorsal artery. This flap can be transferred either on its pedicle or as a free tissue microsurgical transfer.

Advantages/disadvantages

The advantages of this technique include the ability to provide single-stage implant reconstruction (the latissimus muscle is excellent soft tissue coverage of the implant) and its reliability. Most plastic surgeons, however, believe that a better aesthetic result is obtained by first using a tissue expander under the flap and then replacing the expander with a permanent implant. Disadvantages of this flap include a significant donor-site scar

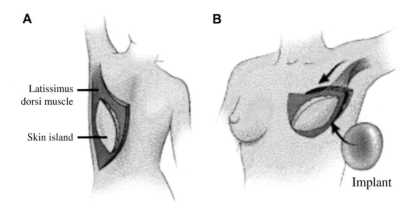

Fig. 5. Latissimus flap. (*From* Wilkins E. The University of Michigan Breast Reconstruction Handbook. p. 16. Available at: http://www.med.umich.edu/surgery/plastic/clinical/breast/index. shtml. Accessed September 20, 2006; with permission.)

(especially if skin is also harvested) and the frequent need for implant and/or tissue expander placement because of insufficient tissue.

Complications

Most complications related to this procedure are related either to the implant or the donor site. Implants have a risk of rupture, displacement, contracture, or infection. The donor site is at risk of hematoma, seroma, infection, and hypertrophic scarring. There also is a risk of flap necrosis at the recipient site.

Treatment of the contralateral breast

Once the mastectomy site has been reconstructed, often the next challenge for the plastic surgeon is to create symmetry with the contralateral breast. Ideally, the contralateral breast should be evaluated preoperatively (at the same time as consultation for reconstruction), and discussion with the patient should elicit her preferences and explain her realistic options. Surgery to achieve contralateral symmetry can be performed at the time of the initial reconstruction or later. In addition, surgery to create contralateral symmetry can be considered in patients who undergo breast-conservation treatment. The 1998 WHCRA mandates that alteration of the contralateral breast in cases of breast cancer reconstruction be covered by insurance.

Options for symmetry procedures include breast reduction, breast augmentation, mastopexy (breast lift), or a combination of the procedures [30]. For example, in a woman who has very large breasts and undergoes a mastectomy with reconstruction, a contralateral breast reduction would improve symmetry and patient comfort. A woman who has small breasts may require an augmentation on the contralateral side for symmetry. Although autogenous reconstruction often provides a better overall outcome when contralateral surgery is not performed, breast reconstruction rarely produces a breast that is symmetrical to the contralateral breast.

Nipple and areolar reconstruction

The final stage of total breast reconstruction is nipple and areolar reconstruction. Typically, this reconstruction is performed as a separate procedure and can be done any time after the reconstructed breast form has stabilized (at least 6–8 weeks after reconstruction). This procedure can be performed either in the operating room or under local anesthesia in an office setting. The goal of nipple and areolar reconstruction is to achieve symmetry of position of the nipple-areolar complex in the bilateral breasts with comparable appearance and color, because even small discrepancies are obvious.

Areolar reconstruction may be achieved by using a full-thickness skin graft or by tattooing alone [31]. Possible donor sites for the skin graft include the contralateral areola (if large), remnant excess abdominal tissue at the incision after a TRAM is performed, the medial thigh, or the mastectomy scar. A favorable aesthetic outcome also can be achieved with medical tattooing alone.

The type of papule reconstruction often is based on surgeon preference and the patient's size preference. Typically, local tissue is raised to create flaps for papule projection. Nipple projection decreases postoperatively, requiring a 50% overcorrection at the time of surgery. Another option includes a nipple-sharing technique that uses a papule graft from the contralateral nipple. There is, however, a risk of complications at the site of the contralateral nipple, including scarring and loss of nipple sensation, and thus use of local skin flaps is often the procedure of choice.

Nonsurgical options

Some women may choose not to have breast reconstruction or are poor surgical candidates for reconstruction. For these women, a breast prosthesis is an option. The advantages of not wearing a breast prosthesis include simplicity, comfort, and convenience [32]. The disadvantages include a feeling of imbalance and difficulty wearing certain clothes [32]. Prostheses can be purchased at surgical supply stores, pharmacies, custom lingerie shops, or through a private home shopping service [32]. Some stores have trained fitters who can help the woman find the appropriate prosthesis that fits her chest and matches the contralateral breast. Specialty clothing is available with pockets to hold the prosthesis in place, and some prostheses come with adhesive Velcro patches to keep the prosthesis in place on the chest. Most insurances cover a new prosthesis every 2 years and two brassieres with a prosthesis pocket each year [31].

References

[1] Wilkins E, Cederna P, Lowery J, et al. Prospective analysis of psychosocial outcomes in breast reconstruction: one year postoperative results from the Michigan Breast Reconstruction Outcome Study. Plast Reconstr Surg 2000;106(6):1014–125.
[2] Cronin TD, Gerow FJ. Augmentation mammaplasty: a new "natural feel" prosthesis. Excerpta Medica International Congress Series 1963;66:41.
[3] Food and Drug Administration. Available at: http://www.fda.gov/bbs/topics/NEWS/2006/NEW01512.htm. Accessed February 20, 2006.
[4] Hollos P. Breast augmentation with autologous tissue: an alternative to implants. Plast Reconstr Surg 1995;96:381–4.
[5] Radovan C. Breast reconstruction after mastectomy using the temporary expander. Plast Reconstr Surg 1982;69(2):195–208.
[6] Hartrampf CR, Scheflan M, Black PW. Breast reconstruction with a transverse abdominal island flap. Plast Reconstr Surg 1982;69(2):216–25.
[7] Allen RJ, Treece P. Deep inferior epigastric perforator-flap for breast reconstruction. Ann Plast Surg 1994;32:32–8.

[8] Allen RJ, Tucker C Jr. Superior gluteal artery perforator free flap for breast reconstruction. Plast Reconstr Surg 1995;95:1207–12.

[9] US Department of Labor. Your rights after a mastectomy… Women's Health & Cancer Rights Act of 1998. Available at: http://www.dol.gov/ebsa/publications/whcra. Accessed September 14, 2006.

[10] Alderman AK, Wilkins E, Kim M, et al. Complications in post-mastectomy breast reconstruction: two year results of the Michigan breast reconstruction outcome study. Plast Reconstr Surg 2002;109:2265–74.

[11] Wilson CR, Brown IM, Weiller-Mithoff E, et al. Immediate breast reconstruction does not lead to a delay in the delivery of adjuvant chemotherapy. Eur J Surg Oncol 2004;30(6):624–7.

[12] Newman LA, Kuerer HM, Hunt KK, et al. Presentation, treatment, and outcome of local recurrence after skin-sparing mastectomy and immediate breast reconstruction. Ann Surg Oncol 1998;5(7):620–6.

[13] Al-Ghazal SK, Sully L, Fallowfield L, et al. The psychological impact of immediate rather than delayed breast reconstruction. Eur J Surg Oncol 2000;26:17–9.

[14] Slavin SA, Schnitt SJ, Duda RB, et al. Skin-sparing mastectomy and immediate reconstruction: oncologic risks and aesthetic results in patients with early-stage breast cancer. Plast Reconstr Surg 1998;102(1):49–62.

[15] Ramon Y, Ullman Y, Moscona R, et al. Aesthetic results and patient satisfaction with immediate breast reconstruction using tissue expansion: a follow-up study. Plast Reconstr Surg 1997;99(3):686–91.

[16] Khoo A, Kroll SS, Reece GP, et al. A comparison of resource costs of immediate and delayed breast reconstruction. Plast Reconstr Surg 1998;101(4):964–8.

[17] Chawla A, Kachnic L, Taghian A, et al. Radiotherapy and breast reconstruction: complications and cosmesis with TRAM versus tissue expander/implant. Int J Radiat Oncol Biol Phys 2002;54(2):520–6.

[18] Spear SL, Onyewu C. Staged breast reconstruction with saline-filled implants in the irradiated breast: recent trends and therapeutic implications. Plast Reconstr Surg 2000;105(3): 930–42.

[19] Tallet AV, Salem N, Moutardier V, et al. Radiotherapy and immediate two-stage breast reconstruction with a tissue expander and implant: complications and esthetic results. Int J Radiat Oncol Biol Phys 2003;57(1):136–42.

[20] Alderman AK, Wilkins E, Lowery J, et al. Determinants of patient satisfaction in post-mastectomy breast reconstruction. Plast Reconstr Surg 2000;106:769–76.

[21] Cederna PS, Yates WR, Chang P, et al. Postmastectomy reconstruction: comparative analysis of the psychosocial, functional, and cosmetic effects of transverse rectus abdominis musculocutaneous versus breast implant reconstruction. Ann Plast Surg 1995;35:458–68.

[22] Kroll SS, Netscher DT. Complications of TRAM flap breast reconstruction in obese patients. Plast Reconstr Surg 1989;84:886–92.

[23] Chang DW, Wang B, Robb GL, et al. Effect of obesity on flap and donor-site complications in free transverse rectus abdominis myocutaneous flap breast reconstruction. Plast Reconstr Surg 2000;105(5):1640–8.

[24] Garvey PB, Buchel EW, Pockaj BA, et al. DIEP and pedicled TRAM flaps: a comparison of outcomes. Plast Reconstr Surg 2006;117(6):1711–9.

[25] Kroll SS. Fat necrosis in free transverse rectus abdominis myocutaneous and deep inferior epigastric perforator flaps. Plast Reconstr Surg 2000;106(3):576–83.

[26] Nahabedian MY, Momen B, Galdino G, et al. Breast reconstruction with the free TRAM or DIEP flap: patient selection, choice of flap, and outcome. Plast Reconstr Surg 2002;110(2): 466–75.

[27] Allen R. The superficial inferior epigastric artery free flap: an anatomic and clinical study for the use in reconstruction of the breast. Presented at the 33rd Annual Meeting of the Southeastern Society of Plastic and Reconstructive Surgeons. Kiawah (SC), June 3–7, 1990.

[28] Chevray PM. Breast reconstruction with superficial inferior epigastric artery flaps: a prospective comparison with TRAM and DIEP flaps. Plast Reconstr Surg 2004;114(5):1077–83.

[29] Allen RJ, Levine JL, Granzow JW. The in-the-crease inferior gluteal artery perforator flap for breast reconstruction. Plast Reconstr Surg 2006;118(2):333–9.

[30] Kroll SS. Options for the contralateral breast in breast reconstruction. In: Spear SL, editor. Surgery of the breast: principles and art. Philadelphia: Lippincott-Raven; 1998.

[31] Bhatty MA, Berry RB. Nipple-areola reconstruction by tattooing and nipple sharing. Br J Plast Surg 1997;50(5):331–4.

[32] Wilkins E. University of Michigan Breast Reconstruction Handbook. Available at: http://www.med.umich.edu/surgery/plastic/clinical/breast/index.shtml. Accessed September 20, 2006.

ELSEVIER
SAUNDERS

SURGICAL
CLINICS OF
NORTH AMERICA

Surg Clin N Am 87 (2007) 469–484

Use of Ultrasound in Breast Surgery

Margaret Thompson, MD[a],
V. Suzanne Klimberg, MD[a,b,*]

[a]Division of Breast Surgical Oncology, Department of Surgery,
University of Arkansas for Medical Sciences, 4301 West Markham,
Slot 725, Little Rock, AR 72205-7199, USA
[b]Department of Pathology, University of Arkansas for Medical Sciences,
4301 West Markham Street, Little Rock, AR 72205-7199, USA

The use of ultrasound (US) first was described in 1951 when Wild and Neal [1] demonstrated that high-frequency ultrasonic waves detect texture changes in living tissues. Twenty years later, US use in breast surgery increased as more breast-specialized equipment developed. Presently, breast sonogram is performed with a hand-held, 7.5 to 10 MHz linear array US that has a penetration depth of 4 to 6 cm.

There are over 1 million breast biopsies performed each year in the United States [2]. Studies have shown that blinded open excisional breast biopsy (EBB), when compared with those with a known diagnosis by prior percutaneous breast biopsy, increases the need for repeated surgery, costs, and the time to complete treatment [3]. Breast US should be considered an extension of the physical examination, and it will improve the care available to patients and subsequently improve outcomes. US can expedite diagnosis and treatment.

The advantages of using US in a breast practice include accurate surgical planning when the preoperative diagnosis is known, ability to remove benign lesions, and the fact that it does not require radiation and contrast and is readily available and easy to repeat to allow comparison with previous findings.

Supported by the Susan G. Komen Breast Cancer Clinical Fellowship and the Arkansas Breast Cancer Act.

* Corresponding author.
E-mail address: klimbergsuzanne@uams.edu (V.S. Klimberg).

Characteristics of ultrasound lesions

When describing lesions on US, the following characteristics should be included: margins, echogenicity, internal echo pattern, retrotumoral pattern, lateral/anterior–posterior (AP) pattern, and compressibility. Benign lesions often are characterized by the following characteristics:

- Smooth, well-defined margin
- Anechoic or hypoechoic echogenicity
- Homogenous or no internal echo pattern; posterior or no enhancement, regular bilateral shadowing
- A lateral AP pattern greater than one
- Compressibility (Fig. 1)

Malignant lesions can be characterized by any one of the following:

- Irregular, ill-defined, jagged margins
- Heterogenous internal echo pattern
- Retrotumoral pattern that has an irregular posterior shadowing related to is heterogenous internal nature
- A lateral AP less than one (malignant lesions grow into the plane of tissues, whereas benign lesions grow along the plane of tissues)
  No compressibility due to their solid nature (Fig. 2)

For lesions to be considered benign, all US characteristics need to be benign. Even if just one US finding is suspicious, the lesion is considered

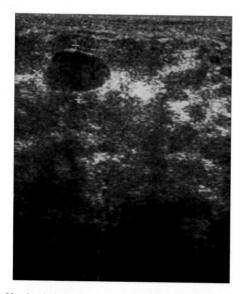

Fig. 1. Ultrasound of benign lesion with smooth margins, homogenous internal echoes, no retrotumoral pattern, wider than taller.

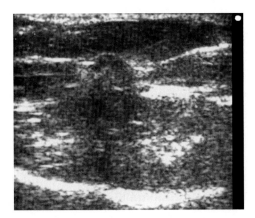

Fig. 2. Ultrasound findings of malignant lesion with jagged margins, irregular shadowing, heterogenous internal echoes, taller than wider.

suspicious and requires biopsy. For those breast complaints where there is a benign physical examination, benign imaging, and negative biopsy, this is considered a triple-negative test, and the benign lesion does not require excisional biopsy. Patients can be followed safely. The classification of US lesions includes simple cysts, fatty or glandular nodules, fibroadenoma, indeterminate (complex cyst, or solid versus cystic nature that is indeterminate), and suspicious.

Clinical indications for breast ultrasound

Abnormal physical examination

Mass

Breast US can clarify abnormalities found on physical examination. US imaging can help to determine if the abnormality is solid or fluid-filled, and also identify additional features of the abnormal area. It can be an additive benefit during the physical examination in young high-risk women who have a dense breast, where mammography is difficult, and also in pregnant women, thus avoiding the exposure to radiation. During examination of the axillary lymph nodes, US can identify the likelihood of regional metastasis and/or recurrence. In a patient who has an equivocal examination, US often will delineate a peak of glandular tissue.

Nipple discharge

US also may be used to evaluate the cause of nipple discharge and direct surgery. US can identify dilated, fluid-filled ducts by scanning in a radial manner parallel to its axis. Occasionally, a solid papillary lesion may be identified within this dilated duct (Fig. 3).

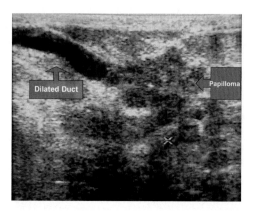

Fig. 3. Dilated duct with papilloma.

Abscess

US is very useful in accurately demonstrating the presence or absence of a fluid collection in the acutely inflamed breast. Although it is often difficult to tell a seroma, an abscess usually presents as a hypoechoic lesion with multiple internal echoes. Debris within the abscess may layer out in a dependent fashion, forming a fluid/debris level (Fig. 4). US can be used to direct surgical drainage.

Mammographic abnormalities

Currently, mammography is the only imaging modality with proven effectiveness for breast cancer screening. Mammography has reduced mortality by 17% in women ages 40 to 49 and approximately 44% in women older 50 [4]. Some benign-appearing lesions on mammogram need further investigation, however. For cases where the mammographic abnormality is nonpalpable, US is an extremely useful diagnostic adjunct in localizing

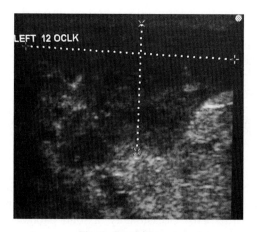

Fig. 4. Breast abscess.

and characterizing the lesion, and it allows for an easier method of biopsy than stereotactic biopsy.

Breast implants

MRI has a sensitivity of 78% and specificity of 91% for evaluating implant rupture, and it has the ability to detect intracapsular and extracapsular ruptures [5]. MRI is expensive and time-consuming, however. It also is contraindicated in women who have pacemakers, an aneurysm clip, or other metallic foreign objects, and it is untenable for women who have claustrophobia. Many insurers are no longer paying for MRI to evaluate breast implants, because, US is a quick, reliable, inexpensive, and safe method for assessing implant rupture [6].

US is also useful for women who have undergone reconstruction with breast implants and re-present with recurrent chest wall lesions. US can visualize the distance between the lesion and implant, and guide biopsy, thus avoiding injury to the implant (Fig. 5).

Screening

US is not used for primary breast cancer screening, because it does not consistently identify microcalcifications, and it is not recommended as a routine screening test of an asymptomatic breast. For value as a sole screening modality, US would need to detect all cancers that would be visible on mammogram and a substantial number of nonpalpable cancers that are not mammographically visible. US does not satisfy either of these requirements. Although its usefulness as a screening examination of the breast is limited, it may be useful in women who have very dense breasts in whom lesions may be missed using mammography, and particularly useful when such women have difficult physical examinations and/or strong individual or family histories for breast cancer. The role of US in the screening of these specific groups of patients is being investigated [7].

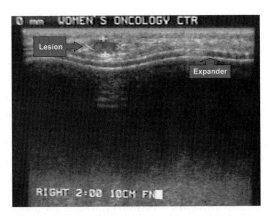

Fig. 5. Ultrasound identification of recurrent chest wall tumor over tissue expander.

Postoperative—MammoSite insertion

US can be used postoperatively in the clinic for insertion of a breast brachytherapy balloon catheter. US allows visualization of the lumpectomy cavity and measurement of the balloon-to-skin distance. After the administration of local anesthetic, the manufacturer-supplied trocar is inserted under US guidance either through a lateral 1-cm skin incision or through a lateral site of the scar. Once the balloon is in place and inflated, US is used to confirm balloon symmetry and balloon-to-skin distance [8].

Postoperative—fluid collection

Frequently, fluid collection occurs at the surgical site postoperatively. US can be used to localize and assess this fluid collection and guide drainage. This is especially true in expanders or implants that have been placed.

Learning curve and limitations

Breast surgeons have to be experienced with US, and there is a learning curve. Experience of the user and variability of equipment can affect interpretation of findings. It is recommended to begin US-guided biopsies on palpable masses and then expand to nonpalpable ones. Also start with superficial lesions instead of ones close to the chest wall.

Although US provides an effective and painless way to identify many breast abnormalities, it does have its limitations. Unlike a mammogram, an US does not have good spatial resolution, and therefore it does not provide as much detail for deeply located breast abnormalities. As stated before, US is also unable to reliably detect microcalcifications.

Outpatient ultrasound-guided interventions

General technique for percutaneous biopsy

Breast US is performed with a high-frequency (7.5 to 10 MHz) linear array transducer with the patient supine and the ipsilateral arm behind the head. For lesions located on the lateral aspect of the breast, visualization can be enhanced by positioning the patient at a 45-degree turn of the ipsilateral side up. A focused US examination is performed with attention to the appropriate quadrant/area. The transducer is moved in a radial, skiing, or back-and-forth pattern. By maintaining the long axis of transducer parallel to normal ductal architecture, ductal echography is another US technique that can be performed. In addition to using high-quality US equipment, it is essential to have an accurate knowledge of normal and abnormal breast US anatomy.

After preparing and draping in sterile fashion, the lesion is localized on US and positioned to allow for the shortest needle pathway. Local anesthesia then is obtained at the skin, the anticipated needle tract, deep, superior, and on both sides of the lesion. An 11-blade scalpel is used to make a stab incision into the skin. The biopsy needle is inserted while maintaining the needle parallel to long axis of transducer so as to visualize the entire pathway of needle to the lesion. Needle guides can be used or the free-hand technique. Needle guides are advantageous to the inexperienced US user. The disadvantages of this technique are that the user is unable to reposition the needle, unable to perform fan-like sampling, and the technique requires specialized equipment [9–11].

Ultrasound fine needle aspiration

Once the diagnosis of a simple cyst is made, it can be aspirated with US guidance. Fine needle aspiration (FNA) is performed with a 22-gauge needle, but a 20-guage needle can be used to aspirate thicker fluid. Complete aspiration can be confirmed on US, and excision will be required if there is incomplete aspiration. There is no need for cytologic examination if the fluid is clear. The shape, size, and location must be correlated on physical examination, mammogram, and US. US-guided FNA can be done for other fluid collections of the breast, such as lymphoceles, abscesses, seromas, and hematomas.

FNA of solid masses also can be performed with US-guidance. This technique yields cytological information, not histological, and can result in insufficient data for diagnosis and high false-negative rates for malignant lesions [12].

Ultrasound core needle biopsy

US-guided core needle biopsy (CNB) is the preferred biopsy technique for palpable and nonpalpable abnormalities. It is more comfortable for patients, because they are supine instead of prone as with stereotactic technique. US CNB is more advantageous, because it avoids radiation. Additionally, it is more rapid and provides more tissue for histologic examination.

The biopsy guns typically used for US CNB range from 12-gauge up to 14-gauge with a throw of 1 to 2.3 cm. The needle is inserted under US guidance, while holding the transducer in one hand and the biopsy gun in the other. This allows visualization of the needle tip arriving at the edge of the lesion. Once the needle is deployed, obtain documentation of the needle traversing the lesion. Five to 10 cores are obtained to ensure adequate tissue sampling. Lesions in close proximity to the chest wall can be problematic, because the risk of pneumothorax is increased. To decrease this problem, several methods can be employed:

- Approach the lesion more parallel to the chest wall
- Infiltrate the local anesthetic between the lesion and chest wall to increase distance
- Use the needle tip to elevate the lesion away from the chest wall

If the pathological diagnosis and US features are benign, the lesion can be followed with a 6-month mammogram and US. For those lesions where there is discordance between pathology and US, open excisional biopsy will be necessary. Patients who also have atypical hyperplasia or radial scar should have open excisional biopsy because of the increased risk of breast cancer [13].

Ultrasound vacuum-assisted breast biopsy

Vacuum-assisted core biopsy is based on the same general principle as the core needle biopsy but represents a significant advance in technology [13–15]. Vacuum is used to pull tissue into a sampling chamber, where it is removed with high-speed internal rotating knives. The specimen then is suctioned to a chamber outside the breast, where it can be retrieved. Multiple samples can be removed through this single-insertion technology, which has been approved for complete removal of benign imaged abnormalities under US or stereotactic guidance.

Vacuum-assisted core biopsy offers the ability of obtaining larger (2 to 3 mm × 19 mm) contiguous samples from the same area by rotating the device rather than by withdrawing and reinserting, as is necessary with the core biopsy needle. Theoretically, this minimizes seeding of the core tract and affords more accurate diagnosis [16,17]. Patients diagnosed by vacuum-assisted or standard core needle biopsy have shown no difference in recurrence rates compared with patients diagnosed by excisional breast biopsy, suggesting that limited seeding of the needle tract does not affect outcome [18].

Ultrasound vacuum-assisted excisional breast biopsy

A multi-institutional study demonstrated that the hand-held device can be used for diagnostic purposes and therapeutic management, facilitating the complete removal of benign-appearing lesions under US guidance with minimal complications and better cosmesis [19,20]. Patients enrolled in this study underwent an US-guided minimally invasive excisional breast biopsy through a 3 mm incision (Fig. 6). Complete removal of the imaged abnormality was accomplished with a hand-held 8- or 11-gauge image-guided vacuum device (Mammotome, Ethicon Endo-Surgery, Cincinnati, Ohio), which uses a high-speed rotating cutter to remove intact cores of breast tissue. Cores measuring 2 to 5 mm × 19 mm were removed until the visualized abnormality was excised completely. The gauge of the device was determined by lesion size. Lesions greater than or equal to 1.5 cm were excised with the 8-gauge device. If smaller lesions were removed, the 11-gauge mammotome was used. Complete removal of the US-visualized abnormality was achieved in 100% of patients. In patients older than 40 years, a 6-month follow-up with mammography documented total resolution of the mammographic lesion, demonstrating that vacuum-assisted excisional breast biopsy under US guidance is an effective technique for therapeutic management of benign lesions, with minimal morbidity and optimal

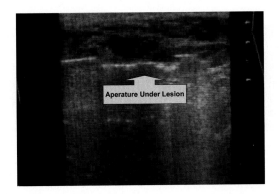

Fig. 6. Ultrasound-guided vacuum-assisted excisional breast biopsy.

cosmesis. The disadvantage of using this technique for both obtaining a diagnosis and completely excising a lesion is the inability to reconstruct the margin status of a malignant tumor. Thus, after an ultrasound excisional breast biopsy procedure for diagnostic purposes, a malignant diagnosis requires lumpectomy for margins. At present, the authors routinely remove benign-appearing lesions in this fashion [20].

Radiofrequency cutting devices

Alternative image-guided excisional techniques may remove the tumor intact. Present available systems include Rubicor (Redwood City, California) (Fig. 7) and the Intact (Natick, Massachusetts) Breast Lesion Excision System (BLES) (Fig. 8). Using a radiofrequency cutting loop attached to a retrieval bag, the Rubicor device is able to remove entire lesions up to 25 × 30 mm while preserving the architecture. A single Rubicor device can be used for up to seven passes. US with this device is viewed transversely to the axis of the device to view the loop enveloping the mass. Another similar single-use device, Intact (see Fig. 8), uses a radiofrequency basket to remove the entire lesion, and it is viewed in the standard long axis of the

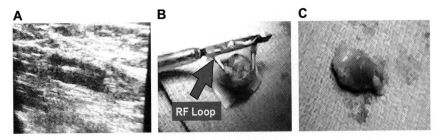

Fig. 7. Rubicor device. (*A*) Ultrasound localization of lymph node. (*B*) Rubicor device with radiofrequency ablation (RF) loop and bag capturing the lymph node. (*C*) Excised lymph node in its entirety.

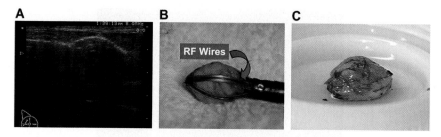

Fig. 8. Intact device. (*A*) Ultrasound localization of intact (BLES) device capturing the lesion. (*B*) Five small RF-enabled wires deploy from the wand to circumscribe the lesion. (*C*) Excised lesion in its entirety. (*Courtesy of* Pat Whitworth, MD, Nashville Breast Center, Nashville, Tennessee.)

device. Studies are needed on cautery distortion of diagnosis and tract seeding. These devices can remove up to 30 mm lesions in one pass and are US Food and Drug Administration (FDA)-approved for benign and breast cancer biopsy but not complete breast cancer removal.

Ultrasound injection for tumor or peri-tumoral injection for sentinel lymph node

For those surgeons who inject peri-tumorally for sentinel lymph node (SLN) biopsy, there may be difficulty injecting around the tumor or concern that injection into the tumor will not drain. US can be used to localize the non-palpable tumors for injection. This technique has been demonstrated to be more accurate for tracer injection when performing an SLN biopsy [21].

Ultrasound needle localization

If intraoperative US is not available, US can be used to localize the lesion preoperatively, and a wire can be placed for needle localization breast excision. This can be done in the preoperative holding area or in the clinic adjacent to the hospital operating room (OR), thus avoiding delays and scheduling difficulties with the radiology department.

Ultrasound central line/port insertions

Some cancer patients may require insertion of long-term subcutaneous central venous access devices (ports) for chemotherapy. Insertion of these central lines traditionally has been performed in the OR using fluoroscopic guidance. At the Arkansas Cancer Research Center, ports are placed using local anesthesia, without fluoroscopy, and with US to localize the veins (Fig. 9). Postprocedural chest radiographs confirm catheter position and rule out pneumothorax. Ports can be inserted safely and successfully in a dedicated central venous line clinic, where it eliminates the need for OR time and staff, fluoroscopy, and thus is more cost-effective and prevents scheduling-generated delays for the patient [22].

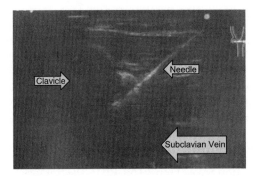

Fig. 9. Ultrasound to localize subclavian vein for central line insertion.

Intraoperative ultrasound

Ultrasound-guided excision of nonpalpable masses

Traditionally, surgeons have relied on palpation of masses or the needle localization of nonpalpable masses to guide surgical resection. Intraoperative US can assess correctly size in T1 lesions [23] and more accurately guide excision and improve first-time margin negativity in palpable and nonpalpable breast masses [24–26]. Intraoperative US excision of nonpalpable lesions avoids the additional delay and cost of radiology. Other benefits of include the avoidance of discomfort or radiation to the patient. A consistent finding of intraoperative US has been the ability to obtain better margin clearance (Table 1) [22–35].

Table 1
Studies on the use of intraoperative use of ultrasound in breast surgery

Author/Year	# Cases	Procedure	Margins (+)
DiGiorgio, et al 1996 [28]	35	Inoperative use of ultrasound (IOUS)	—
Harlow, et al 1999 [25]	65	IOUS	3%
Snider, et al 1999 [29]	29 versus 22	IOUS versus needle localization breast biopsy (NLBB)	18% versus 18%
Paramo, et al 1999 [30]	15 versus 15	IOUS versus NLBB	—
Smith, et al 2000 [24]	81	IOUS	4%
Moore, et al 2001 [26]	27 versus 24	IOUS versus no ultrasound	3% versus 29%
Feld, et al 2001 [31]	113	IOUS	—
Rahusen, et al 2002 [32]	26 versus 23	IOUS versus NLBB	11% versus 45%
Bumen and Clark 2005 [33]	130	IOUS	15%
Bennett, et al 2005 [34]	115	IOUS	7%
Thompson, et al 2007 [35]	123 versus 63	IOUS versus NLBB	22% versus 73%

Needle localization breast biopsy

For those lesions not visible by US and require needle localization breast biopsy (NLBB), intraoperative US can be used to localize the needle while it is in the breast and further guide the excision. US gives a better perception of the lesion by keeping it image-guided as opposed to just palpating the needle. This technique better directs the location for the incision and avoids unnecessary dissection.

Hematoma ultrasound guided (HUG) breast excision

Needle localization breast biopsy (NLBB) is the primary means of localizing nonpalpable lesions for excision. The disadvantages of NLBB include vasovagal episodes, patient discomfort, scheduling problems, and miss rates possibly because of localizing clip movement. Because hematomas naturally fill the cavity after vacuum-assisted breast biopsies (VABB), the authors have used US consistently to find and more accurately excise the actual biopsy site of nonpalpable breast lesions (HUG) without a needle [35,36]. HUG involves localizing the hematoma with a sterile US probe and using the line-of-sight technique straight down toward the chest wall to a depth seen on lateral US. A block of tissue encompassing the hematoma then is excised visualizing a 1 cm margin. *Ex vivo* specimen US then confirms excision of the hematoma (Fig. 10). Thompson and colleagues [35] were able to demonstrate that HUG was more accurate in localizing nonpalpable lesions than NLBB and that margin positivity was significantly higher for NLBB than HUG. Because it eliminated the additional procedure needed for NLBB and all other localizing methods, HUG was easier on the patient and also more time- and cost-efficient.

Ultrasound localization of nonpalpable lesions by iatrogenically induced hematomas

US also can be used to identify iatrogenically induced hematomas and guide the excision of nonpalpable lesions. Smith and colleagues [37]

A   **B**   **C**

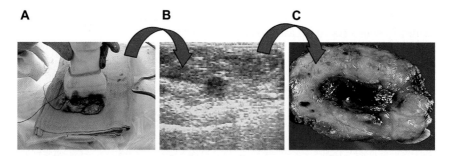

Fig. 10. Specimen ultrasound (US). (*A*) Specimen US is performed after excising from breast and before passing off to the back table. (*B*) Specimen US image confirms hematoma in the specimen and also shows wide margins. (*C*) Bivalved specimen on the back table confirms hematoma grossly.

demonstrated this technique by injecting a hematoma, which consisted of 2 to 5 cc of the patient's own blood, in the breast under MRI-guidance to target the nonpalpable lesion. Intraoperative US of the hematoma was used to direct the excisional biopsy. All of the hematomas (19/19) used to recognize targeted lesions were identified successfully at surgery by US and removed without complication.

Margin assessment/specimen ultrasound

Before the excision of the lesion, US can be used to assure the appropriate margin size is taken (see Table 1). This is done by placing the probe on one edge of the lesion and marking the skin, then moving the probe to the other edge of the lesion and marking the skin. Next, rotate the probe 90 degrees and repeat the maneuver (Fig. 11).

After excision of tumor from the breast and before it is passed off for pathology, specimen US is performed to confirm that the tumor/hematoma is in the specimen (see Fig. 10). Specimen US also will reveal the closest margin, allowing new margins to be taken. Postexcision US of the lumpectomy cavity also can performed to confirm no missed lesions.

Ablative ultrasound-guided procedures

Cryosurgery involves the use of argon gas to create an ice ball around the lesion. Real-time US is used to visualize the growth of the ice ball and the distance to the skin or underlying pectoralis major muscle. Fibroadenomas are the only FDA-approved indication for the cryoablation as treatment. This technique also can be done in an office-based setting with local anesthesia [38–41].

Radiofrequency ablation (RFA) involves coagulative necrosis from frictional heat that is produced by alternating high-frequency current; this current agitates tissue ions between the prongs of the RFA probe. After the lesion is localized by US, the RFA probe is inserted under US guidance and deployed. The lesion ablated at 100 degrees for 15 minutes [42]. The ablated area is visualized continuously on Doppler US, assuring appropriate distance from skin to ablation zone (Fig. 12).

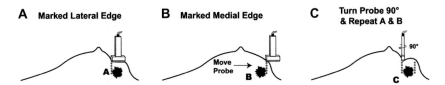

Fig. 11. Tumor/margin assessment. (*A*) Place the probe on one edge of the lesion and mark the skin. (*B*) Move the probe to the other edge of the lesion and mark the skin. (*C*) Rotate the probe 90 degrees and repeat the maneuver.

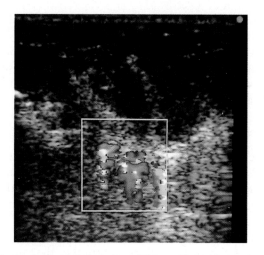

Fig. 12. Doppler Image during radiofrequency ablation of breast lesion demonstrating the effective ablation zone at the site of a tumor.

Laser ablation involves tissue coagulation from heat generated from infrared low-power laser light. Laser requires precise targeting to ablate a specific limited area, done thru MRI-guided laser or stereotactic mammography. During therapy, color Doppler US is used to verify thermal sensor needle and laser needle. Follow-up US can be used to visualize ablation zone and guide needle biopsy and/or surgical excision [43].

Summary

The use of US by the breast surgeon has gained a tremendous momentum, because it allows immediate assessment, diagnosis, and treatment of breast masses, often during the same clinic visit. To become quickly facile with US, scan all breasts so as to readily appreciate normal versus abnormal breast tissue. For US-guided procedures, start simply with palpable lesions and progress to nonpalpable lesions. Documentation is very important and should include patient demographics, date, location (clinic, operating room), machine, probe, and frequency. Also include findings (site-specific) and outcome (correlate with mammogram or operative findings). Print several copies of any ultrasounds. Back-up on a computer is necessary for various clinical documents, use in the operating room, and insurance documentation.

Breast US certification is offered by several surgical societies and is also available online (http://www.breastsurgeons.org). The goal is to improve the quality of care for patients who have breast disease by encouraging education and training to advance expertise and clinical competency for surgeons who use US and US-guided procedures in their practices [44].

References

[1] Wild JJ, Neal D. The use of high-frequency ultrasonic waves for detecting changes of texture in the living tissue. Lancet 1951;1:655–7.

[2] Burns RP. Image-guided breast biopsy. Am J Surg 1997;173:9–11.

[3] Edge SB, Ottesen RA, Lepisto EM, et al. Surgical biopsy to diagnose breast cancer adversely affects outcomes of breast cancer care: finding from the National Comprehensive Cancer Network. Presented at the San Antonio Breast Cancer Symposium; San Antonio, TX: December, 2005.

[4] Tabar L, Fagerberg CJ, Gad A, et al. Reduction in mortality from breast cancer after mass screening with mammography. Randomised trial from the Breast Cancer Screening Working Group of the Swedish National Board of Health and Welfare. Lancet 1985;1(8433): 829–32.

[5] Cher DJ, Conwell JA, Mandel JS. MRI for detecting silicone breast implant rupture: meta-analysis and implications. Ann Plast Surg 2001;47(4):367–80.

[6] Park AJ, Walsh J, Reddy PS, et al. The detection of breast implant rupture using ultrasound. Br J Plast Surg 1996;49(5):299–301.

[7] Parikh JR, Porter B. Understanding breast ultrasound. Available at: http://www.imagingeconomics.com/. Accessed August 1, 2006.

[8] Zannis V, Beitsch P, Vicini F, et al. Descriptions and outcomes of insertion techniques of a breast brachytherapy balloon catheter in 1403 patients enrolled in the American Society of Breast Surgeons MammoSite breast brachytherapy registry trial. Am J Surg 2005; 190(4):530–8.

[9] Staren ED. Ultrasound-guided biopsy of nonpalpable breast masses by surgeons. Ann Surg Oncol 1996;3:476–82.

[10] Fornage BD, Coan JD, David CL. Ultrasound-guided needle biopsy of the breast and other interventional procedures. Radiol Clin North Am 1992;30(1):167–85.

[11] Parker SH, Burbank F, Jackman RJ, et al. Percutaneous large-core breast biopsy: a multi-institutional study. Radiology 1994;193:359–64.

[12] Kopans DB. Fine-needle aspiration of clinically occult breast lesions. Radiology 1989;170: 313–4.

[13] Bassett LW, Caplan RB, Dershaw DD, et al. Stereotactic core needle biopsy of the breast. A report of the Joint Task Force of the American College of Radiology, American College of Surgeons, College of American Pathologists. Cancer J Clin 1997;47:171–90.

[14] Liberman L, LaTrenta LR, Van Zee KJ, et al. Stereotactic core biopsy of calcifications highly suggestive of malignancy. Radiology 1997;203:673–7.

[15] Velanovich V, Lewis F, Nathanson D, et al. Comparison of mammographically guided breast biopsy techniques. Ann Surg 1999;229(5):625–33.

[16] Youngson BJ, Liberman L, Rosen PP. Displacement of carcinomatous epithelium in surgical breast specimens following stereotaxic core biopsy. Am J Clin Pathol 1995;103: 598–602.

[17] Diaz LK, Wiley EL, Venta LA. Are malignant cells displaced by large-gauge needle core biopsy of the breast? Am J Roentgenol 1999;173:1303–13.

[18] King TA, Hayes DH, Cederbom GJ, et al. Biopsy technique has no impact on local recurrence after breast-conserving therapy. Breast J 2001;7:1–6.

[19] Fine RE, Whitworth PW, Kim JA, et al. Low-risk palpable breast masses removed using a vacuum-assisted hand-held device. Am J Surg 2003;186(4):362–7.

[20] Johnson AT, Henry-Tillman R, Smith L, et al. Percutaneous excisional breast biopsy. Presented at the Southwestern Surgical Congress; Coronado, CA: April 17, 2002. Am J Surg 2002;184(6):550–4.

[21] Miner TJ, Shriver CD, Jaques DP, et al. Ultrasonographically guided injection improves localization of the radiolabeled sentinel lymph node in breast cancer. Ann Surg Oncol 1998;5(4):315–21.

[22] Thompson M, Rowe M, Henry-Tillman R, et al. Insertion of ports in the clinic should replace operating room placement. Presented at the Association of Vascular Access; Indianapolis IN: September, 2006.

[23] Hieken TJ, Harrison J, Herreros J, et al. Correlating sonography, mammography, and pathology in the assessment of breast cancer size. Am J Surg 2001;182(4):351–4.

[24] Smith LF, Rubio IT, Henry-Tillman RS, et al. Intraoperative ultrasound-guided breast biopsy. Am J Surg 2000;180(6):419–23.

[25] Harlow SP, Krag DN, Ames SE, et al. Intraoperative ultrasound localization to guide surgical excision of nonpalpable breast carcinoma. J Am Coll Surg 1999;189(3):241–6.

[26] Moore MM, Whitney LA, Cerilli L, et al. Intraoperative ultrasound is associated with clear lumpectomy margins for palpable infiltrating ductal breast cancer. Ann Surg 2001;233(6): 761–8.

[27] Henry-Tillman R, Johnson AT, Smith LF, et al. Intraoperative ultrasound and other techniques to achieve negative margins. Semin Surg Oncol 2001;20(3):206–13.

[28] Di Giogio A, Meli C, Canavese A, et al. Nonpalpable lesions of the breast. A new technique of ultrasound-guided excision biopsy. Minerva Chir 1996;51(12):1139–43.

[29] Snider HC Jr, Morrison DG. Intraoperative ultrasound localization of nonpalpable breast lesions. Ann Surg Oncol 1999;6(3):308–14.

[30] Paramo JC, Landeros M, McPhee MD, et al. Intraoperative ultrasound-guided excision of nonpalpable breast lesions. Breast J 1999;5(6):389–94.

[31] Feld RI, Rosenberg AL, Nazarian LN, et al. Intraoperative sonographic localization of breast masses: success with specimen sonography and surgical bed sonography to confirm excision. J Ultrasound Med 2001;20(9):959–66.

[32] Rahusen FD, Bremers AJ, Fabry HF, et al. Ultrasound-guided lumpectomy of nonpalpable breast cancer versus wire-guided resection: a randomized clinical trial. Ann Surg Oncol 2002; 9(10):994–8.

[33] Buman SJ, Clark DA. Breast intraoperative ultrasound: prospective study in 112 patients with impalpable lesions. ANZ J Surg 2005;75(3):124–7.

[34] Bennett IC, Greenslade J, Chiam H. Intraoperative ultrasound-guided excision of nonpalpable breast lesions. World J Surg 2005;29(3):369–74.

[35] Thompson M, Henry-Tillman R, Margulies A, et al. Hematoma-directed ultrasound-guided (HUG) breast lumpectomy. Ann Surg Oncol 2007;14(1):148–56 [Epub 2006 Oct 22].

[36] Smith LF, Henry-Tillman R, Rubio IT, et al. Intraoperative localization after stereotactic breast biopsy without a needle. Am J Surg 2001;182(6):584–9.

[37] Smith LF, Henry-Tillman R, Harms S, et al. Hematoma-directed ultrasound-guided breast biopsy. Ann Surg 2001;233(5):669–75.

[38] Staren ED, Sabel MS, Gianakakis LM, et al. Cryosurgery of breast cancer. Arch Surg 1997; 132(1):28–33 [discussion: 34].

[39] Edwards MJ, Broadwater R, Tafra L, et al. Progressive adoption of cryoablative therapy for breast fibroadenoma in community practice. Am J Surg 2004;188(3):221–4.

[40] Tafra L, Smith SJ, Woodward JE, et al. Pilot trial of cryoprobe-assisted breast-conserving surgery for small ultrasound-visible cancers. Ann Surg Oncol 2003;10(9):1018–24.

[41] Nurko J, Mabry CD, Whitworth P, et al. Interim results from the fibroadenoma cryoablation treatment registry. Am J Surg 2005;190(4):647–51 [discussion: 651–2].

[42] Singletary SE. Radiofrequency ablation of breast cancer. Am Surg 2003;69(1):37–40.

[43] Huston TL, Simmons RM. Ablative therapies for the treatment of malignant diseases of the breast. Am J Surg 2005;189(6):694–701.

[44] American Society of Breast Surgeons. Available at: http://www.breastsurgeons.org.

ELSEVIER
SAUNDERS

Surg Clin N Am 87 (2007) 485–498

SURGICAL
CLINICS OF
NORTH AMERICA

Integrating Partial Breast Irradiation into Surgical Practice and Clinical Trials

Regina M. Fearmonti, MD[a], Frank A. Vicini, MD[b],
Timothy M. Pawlik, MD[c],
Henry M. Kuerer, MD, PhD[a],*

[a]The University of Texas M.D. Anderson Cancer Center,
Department of Surgical Oncology–Unit#444, 1400 Holcombe Boulevard,
#FC.12.3000, Houston, TX 77030, USA
[b]Beaumont Cancer Institute, William Beaumont Hospital, 3601 W. 13 Mile Road,
Royal Oak, MI 48072, USA
[c]Department of Surgery, Johns Hopkins School of Medicine, Johns Hopkins Hospital,
600 North Wolfe Street, Halsted 614, Baltimore, MD 21287, USA

The use of accelerated partial breast irradiation (APBI) in place of whole-breast irradiation (WBI) for breast-conservation therapy (BCT) is an area of intensive clinical investigation. With WBI, the entire breast is irradiated, and radiation therapy is delivered over a period of several weeks. With APBI, in contrast, radiation is focused on the area at greatest risk for tumor recurrence—the area of the lumpectomy cavity—and the entire course of radiation therapy is completed in a matter of days.

APBI can be delivered using brachytherapy or three-dimensional conformal radiation therapy (3D-CRT). Brachytherapy initially was used in the treatment of breast cancer as a means of providing a boost dose to the lumpectomy cavity following breast-conserving surgery and standard WBI [1]. Since that time, brachytherapy has evolved into a technique for APBI that is the subject of numerous clinical trials. Two different brachytherapy techniques can be used to deliver APBI. Brachytherapy can be delivered by means of interstitially implanted catheters placed intraoperatively or postoperatively in the portion of the breast centered around the lumpectomy cavity, or brachytherapy can be delivered using the MammoSite® Radiation Therapy System, a modification of the standard interstitial catheter technique that involves insertion of a single balloon-tipped catheter. With

* Corresponding author.
E-mail address: hkuerer@mdanderson.org (H.M. Kuerer).

0039-6109/07/$ - see front matter © 2007 Elsevier Inc. All rights reserved.
doi:10.1016/j.suc.2007.02.001   *surgical.theclinics.com*

3D-CRT, the radiation dose to the lumpectomy cavity is delivered externally by means of custom-configured beams in the postoperative period.

A large randomized clinical trial is evaluating interstitial catheter-based brachytherapy, balloon-based intracavitary brachytherapy, and 3D-CRT compared with WBI. Although only preliminary results with APBI are available, physician and patient interest in these new modes of radiation therapy underscore the need for a review of the techniques of APBI, the basis for the ongoing clinical trials of APBI, and the relevance of APBI to surgical practice.

Importance of radiation therapy as a component of breast-conservation therapy

At least seven prospective randomized trials have demonstrated that the combination of segmental mastectomy, level I and II axillary lymph node dissection, and WBI is equivalent to modified radical mastectomy in patients who have stage I or II breast cancer [2–4]. The National Surgical Adjuvant Breast and Bowel Project (NSABP) trial B-06 demonstrated no significant difference in disease-free or overall survival in patients who had primary tumors up to 4 cm in diameter treated with modified radical mastectomy, segmental mastectomy with axillary lymph node dissection, or segmental mastectomy with axillary lymph node dissection and WBI [5]. Twenty-year follow-up of that study, however, revealed a decrease in the local recurrence rate from 39.2% to 14.3% with the addition of WBI and established not only that BCT is equivalent to modified radical mastectomy for patients with stage I or II breast cancer, but that radiation delivery to the remaining breast is an essential component of BCT [6].

Studies of breast cancer recurrence following BCT have demonstrated that most recurrences are at or close to the tumor bed; an update of the NSABP B-06 trial demonstrated this to be the case in 75% of locoregional recurrences [7,8]. Studies that have distinguished true local recurrences from new primary tumors have demonstrated lower survival rates and increased rates of metastases in patients with true local recurrences [9]. Radiation therapy after breast-conserving surgery is essential to prevent local recurrence and, in doing so, to maximize survival.

Theoretical advantages of accelerated partial breast irradiation

Conventional WBI commences after segmental mastectomy and involves administering radiation to the whole breast by means of paired tangential fields 5 days per week for 5 to 7 weeks followed by 1 to 2 weeks of radiation to the tumor bed. The targeted radiation field is defined superiorly by the base of the clavicular head, inferiorly as 1 cm beyond the inframammary fold, laterally by the midaxillary line, and medially by the sternum. There is no consensus on which radiation therapy schedule should be used for WBI.

In fact, different radiation therapy schedules were used in the very prospective randomized trials that established the efficacy of WBI for reducing local recurrence risk following segmental mastectomy [10–12]. A schedule commonly used in clinical practice and employed in all the NSABP trials, however, is 50 Gy administered in 25 fractions of 2 Gy to the whole breast, delivered daily Monday through Friday over 35 days [8,9]. Studies that have evaluated the efficacy of different dosing schedules have not found differences between them in terms of disease-free or overall survival rates [13].

Studies have demonstrated that only about one fourth of women in the United States who are potential candidates for BCT on the basis of cancer stage actually undergo BCT, and among potential candidates, there are notable differences in BCT rates by age and geographic variation [14–17]. Misapplication of patient exclusion criteria by physicians and patient preference for mastectomy are possible explanations for the observed underutilization of BCT. Unwillingness or inability to undergo 5 to 7 weeks of outpatient WBI owing to transportation difficulties and employment status also may be contributing factors. The well-documented adverse effects of radiation therapy—ranging from lymphedema of the ipsilateral extremity and first-degree burns to the skin to fatigue and neutropenia—may also dissuade potential candidates from undergoing BCT.

APBI shortens the duration of treatment to about 5 days, offers greater patient convenience and cost-effectiveness than WBI, and delivers less radiation to vital structures (mediastinum, ipsilateral lung, great vessels) and the surrounding skin. All of these factors could make BCT more attractive to potential candidates. APBI also makes biologic sense, because it targets the region of the breast at greatest risk for recurrence. These potential benefits of APBI have led to the development of several modes of APBI delivery, each undergoing testing in the setting of a clinical trial.

Techniques of accelerated partial breast irradiation

Techniques of APBI are outlined in Table 1 [18] and discussed in the following paragraphs.

Interstitial catheter-based brachytherapy

Interstitial catheter-based brachytherapy begins with placement of 10 to 20 Silastic implants, or catheters, into the tumor bed under ultrasound guidance (Fig. 1A). At the beginning of each treatment session, the catheters are connected to a high-dose brachytherapy delivery system, and technologists insert pellets containing the radiation source through the catheters.

Interstitial catheter-based brachytherapy can be delivered with either low-dose-rate or high-dose-rate radiation sources. With low-dose-rate delivery, 45 Gy is delivered to the target volume over a course of 5 days on an inpatient basis. This method requires radiation-shielded inpatient facilities

Table 1

Comparison of whole-breast irradiation and three modes of accelerated partial breast irradiation

Feature	Whole-breast irradiation	Interstitial catheter-based brachytherapy	Balloon-based intracavitary brachytherapy	Three-dimensional conformal radiation therapy
Dose of radiation and duration of therapy	50 Gy in 25 fractions, monday through friday, over 35 days	45 Gy to target over 5 days (continuous low-dose-rate therapy) or 3.4 Gy, 2 times a day, for 5 days (high-dose-rate therapy)	34 Gy in 10 fractions over 5 days [18]	30 Gy in 5 fractions over 10 days
Complications and problems	■ Lymphedema of ipsilateral extremity ■ First-degree burn to chest wall ■ Fatigue ■ Neutropenia	■ Difficult catheter placement ■ Infection risk associated with indwelling catheters ■ Dose-related skin injury (erythema, moist desquamation, pain, fibrosis, fat necrosis)	■ Only two balloon inflation volumes (70 and 125 cm^3) ■ Difficult to achieve adequate skin spacing	■ Larger target volume needed to overcome motion artifact

and entails leaving the catheters in place for a longer duration. Alternatively, treatment can be delivered via a high-dose-rate source. This approach allows the patient to receive treatment on an outpatient basis: twice-daily, 3.4 Gy fractions delivered in 30-minute sessions over 5 days [19]. As with WBI, the different treatment schedules have not been shown to result in significant differences with regard to local recurrence or survival [20].

Catheter implantation can be performed by open or closed (percutaneous) techniques, either at the time of the lumpectomy or during a separate procedure. The catheters are placed by a radiation oncologist after careful calculation of dose and homogeneity patterns (Fig. 1B) [19]. Proper placement requires technical expertise and has served as a barrier to widespread implementation of interstitial catheter-based brachytherapy. Likewise, the indwelling catheters pose an infection risk, which is more pronounced after open placement, and a significant dose-related risk of poor cosmetic outcomes. Reported grade 1 to 2 adverse effects have included skin erythema, moist desquamation, pain, and fibrosis, and reported grade 3 adverse effects,

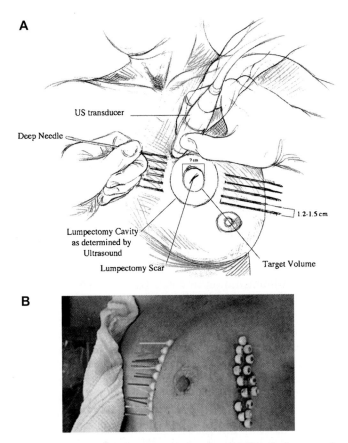

Fig. 1. Interstitial catheter-based brachytherapy. (*A*) Interstitial brachytherapy catheters placed in the tumor bed by the radiation oncologist for planned treatment (*From* Kuske RR. Brachytherapy techniques: the University of Wisconsin/Arizona approach. In: Wazer DE, Vicini FA, editors. Accelerated partial breast irradiation. Berlin: Springer-Verlag; 2006. p. 114.) (*B*) Interstitial brachytherapy catheters in place in the breast. (*From* Cuttino LW, Arthur DW. The Virginia Commonwealth University (VCU) Technique of Interstitial Brachytherapy. In: Wazer DE, Vicini FA, editors. Accelerated partial breast irradiation. Berlin: Springer-Verlag; 2006. p. 84.)

while rarer, have included symptomatic fat necrosis necessitating surgical debridement [21].

The Radiation Therapy Oncology Group (RTOG) 95-17 phase I/II trial is evaluating interstitial catheter-based brachytherapy alone after segmental mastectomy for invasive nonlobular stage I or II breast cancer [22]. Results of a toxicity analysis for low-dose-rate and high-dose-rate APBI have demonstrated acceptable acute and late adverse effects, similar to those after WBI [23]. A phase III multicenter trial designed by the Breast Cancer Working Group of the European Society for Therapeutic Radiology and

Oncology is accruing patients and may provide insight into WBI versus interstitial APBI and local recurrence rates [24].

Advantages of interstitial catheter-based brachytherapy include the short treatment sessions, each lasting as little as 10 minutes, and the overall shorter treatment course. A patient's entire treatment can be completed over 5 days, rather than the 5 to 7 weeks required for WBI. The catheters usually can be removed after 1 week with minimal scarring. This shortened treatment course allows brachytherapy to be completed before chemotherapy (if required) is started, which may have a therapeutic benefit, as delay in initiation of radiotherapy has been observed to result in a higher local recurrence rate [25,26].

Balloon-based intracavitary brachytherapy

Balloon-based intracavitary brachytherapy is the term given to brachytherapy delivered using the MammoSite® Radiation Therapy System (Cytyc Corporation, Palo Alto, California), which was approved by the Food and Drug Administration in 2002. Balloon-based intracavitary brachytherapy has advantages similar to those of interstitial catheter-based brachytherapy. Potential candidates for balloon-based intracavitary brachytherapy include patients aged 50 years or older with a diagnosis of DCIS or invasive ductal carcinoma, tumor diameter no more than 2 cm, negative surgical margins, and negative axillary lymph nodes [27].

The MammoSite® device is essentially a dual-lumen, closed-ended catheter with an inflatable balloon and a port for connecting a remote afterloader to the central lumen for radiotherapy administration (Fig. 2). The MammoSite® device is available in two sizes defined in terms of maximal balloon inflation volume: 70 cm^3 and 125 cm^3. The balloon is placed in the wound cavity at the time of segmental mastectomy or during a separate operative procedure, and the catheter protrudes from the breast through the

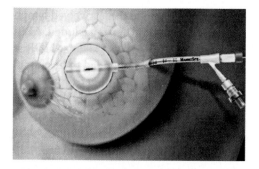

Fig. 2. Balloon-based intracavitary brachytherapy with the MammoSite® system (Proxima Therapeutics, Incorporated.). The MammoSite® device is placed in the wound cavity immediately following segmental mastectomy or during a second procedure. (Courtesy of Cytyc Co. and affiliates, Marlborough, MA; with permission).

incision. The balloon must be placed at least 7 mm from the skin edge. Comparisons of the effects of different device-to-skin distances have shown an increase in the incidence of radiation dermatitis with distances less than 7 mm [28]. Kuerer [29] noted that this spacing is difficult to achieve in many cases, often requiring extensive undermining of the subcutaneous tissue, which may lead to less-than-favorable cosmetic results.

After MammoSite® placement, the balloon at the end of the catheter is filled with saline and expanded to fill the cavity. The balloon may also be filled with a contrast agent to facilitate radiographic visualization to ensure proper device positioning. A radioactive pellet is then inserted through the catheter into the middle of the balloon, and the device is connected to a computer for delivery of the high-dose-rate radiation source. Radiotherapy is delivered twice a day for a total period of 4 to 5 days. Upon completion of the last treatment, the balloon is deflated, and the device is removed.

Postlumpectomy MammoSite® insertion requires a second operative procedure approximately 6 weeks after segmental mastectomy. A postoperative seroma must be identified under US guidance to define the cavity that the balloon will occupy. To ensure optimal skin spacing, the seroma cannot be located directly under the skin. Alternatively, Stolier and colleagues [30] have described the scar-entry technique of MammoSite® insertion, which involves identifying the location and dimensions of the seroma cavity under US guidance 1 week after segmental mastectomy. This technique involves inserting the device through the narrowest portion of the scar under local anesthesia, simultaneously evacuating the seroma as the device is inserted to occupy its cavity.

Balloon-based intracavitary brachytherapy offers many of the same advantages as interstitial catheter-based brachytherapy. In addition, a distinct advantage of the MammoSite® device over traditional indwelling catheters is that the flexible balloon and catheter can be concealed by a bra, potentially leading to greater patient comfort. Balloon-based intracavitary brachytherapy, however, is also associated with distinct concerns and potential complications. Questions regarding cosmesis and final wound appearance arise when patients need to return to the operating room for a second procedure to revise the wound and reposition the device to ensure adequate skin spacing. Persistent seromas after intraoperative placement of the MammoSite® device have also been documented and have required drainage or complete cavity excision, both of which have been linked to an increased rate of postoperative infections [31].

Concern has also been raised that surgeons may remove larger amounts of breast tissue at the time of segmental mastectomy for patients enrolled in the MammoSite® trial to accommodate the balloon. Questions have been posed concerning the compatibility of the MammoSite® device with the use of intracavitary clips to mark the segmental mastectomy cavity. Some institutions have abandoned using these clips altogether, as there have been reports of them causing balloon rupture [32]. Other centers have devised methods to place the clips further into the cavity wall, at least 2 cm away from the balloon [29]. The overall effect of such practices on trial results and final cosmesis remains to be determined.

The fact that MammoSite® applicators are available in only two sizes may exclude many patients from this treatment technique. In a multicenter prospective trial evaluating initial clinical experiences with the Mammo-Site® device in women who had invasive breast cancer and tumors no more than 2 cm in diameter, 23% of the patients initially enrolled in the study were excluded on the basis of cavity nonconformance and inability to achieve adequate skin spacing [18]. As the study progressed, additional patients were excluded on the basis of these same variables, such that only 61% of patients enrolled actually completed their brachytherapy treatment.

A prospective, multicenter phase II trial evaluating clinical experience with the MammoSite® device in 32 patients over a 2-year period [33] found patient tolerance of the device to be quite good and found that placement of the MammoSite® device was easier than placement of interstitial catheter-based implants. The study, however, also documented possible radiation overdoses to the skin; there was a high incidence of late skin damage after just 20 months of follow-up. The authors concluded that the MammoSite® device was best suited for deep-lying tumors in larger breasts. The Mammo-Site® Patient Registry Study, a prospective, nonrandomized phase V trial, is evaluating the efficacy and safety of the device and may help to answer many of these remaining questions.

Three-dimensional conformal radiation therapy

The technique of 3D-CRT uses computer technology to generate a three-dimensional picture of the tumor bed and shape multiple radiation beams to its contour, allowing the administration of the highest possible dose of radiation to this hot spot while sparing the normal surrounding tissue. Intracavitary clips are placed at the time of operation to define the target area. CT or MRI is then used to locate the tumor bed in relation to surrounding vital structures, allowing the prescribed dose of radiation to be delivered from three dimensions to the tumor bed (Fig. 3).

Patients are positioned prone to allow displacement of the breast from the chest wall and reduce motion artifact, thus limiting exposure to intrathoracic structures [34]. One of several fractionation schemes is then implemented, ranging from 30 Gy in five fractions over 10 days to 50 Gy in 25 fractions over 5 weeks, all of which have been found to be biologically equivalent [35].

Whether a patient is a candidate for 3D-CRT depends on breast volume, cavity volume, planning target volume, and clinical target volume, with the ratio of planning target volume to breast volume having the highest correlation with the ability to meet dose–volume constraints [36]. Patients deemed unsuitable for interstitial catheter-based brachytherapy and

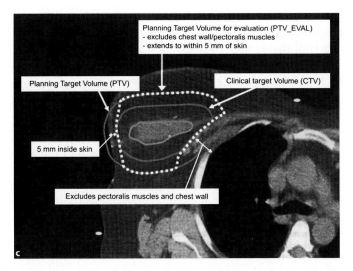

Fig. 3. Three-dimensional conformal radiation therapy. CT image demonstrates the radiation field around the region of the tumor. CTV, clinical target volume; PTV, planning target volume. (*From* Hasan Y, Vicini FA. 3D conformal external beam technique. In: Wazer DE, Vicini FA, editors. Accelerated partial breast irradiation. Berlin: Springer-Verlag; 2006. p. 159.)

balloon-based intracavitary brachytherapy may be eligible for 3D-CRT, allowing them to experience the benefits of APBI.

Advantages of 3D-CRT include dose homogeneity, less fat necrosis, and ultimately, better cosmesis. In addition, no special accommodations need to be made at the time of segmental mastectomy except for clip placement, and hence no special training is required by the surgeon. In addition, the devices needed to deliver 3D-CRT are already in place at multiple radiation centers.

A potential disadvantage of 3D-CRT is that it may require a larger target volume to overcome movement with respiration, other patient movement, and ensure inclusion of the target. Baglan and colleagues [37] found that adding a 5 mm margin to the clinical target volume to create the planning target volume accounted for normal respiratory excursion and that increasing the margin to 10 mm could accommodate for random system error.

The results of RTOG study 0319, published in 2005, demonstrated the technical feasibility and reproducibility across multiple institutions of 3D-CRT as a means of delivering APBI [38]. The study evaluated 42 patients from 17 institutions using strict dosimetric criteria. CT was used to define the clinical and planning target volumes and to image the lumpectomy cavity, which was delineated by surgically placed clips. Optimal conformal plans were devised, and radiation was administered with patients in a supine position 8 weeks after surgery. A total of 38.5 Gy was delivered in 10 fractions over 5 consecutive days. Even with restrictive normal-tissue dose limits, only minimal variations in planning target volumes were observed, suggesting that these results should be reproducible in many other centers.

This phase I/II trial set the groundwork for the inclusion of 3D-CRT as one of the three methods of APBI delivery in a joint NSABP/RTOG phase III multicenter trial that is underway [39].

Single-fraction intraoperative radiation therapy

A potential alternative to interstitial catheter-based and balloon-based intracavitary brachytherapy, single-fraction intraoperative radiation therapy (IORT) entails delivering the entire radiation dose in a single fraction while the patient is in the operating room. Single-fraction IORT is delivered by means of a mobile linear accelerator, several types of which are being tested, or the Intrabeam Photon Radiosurgery System (PRS) (Carl Zeiss Surgical, Oberkochen, Germany), either of which can be transported into the operating room [40]. The mobile linear accelerator can be covered with one of several different applicators ranging in size from 4 to 10 cm, selected to fit the lumpectomy cavity [41]. Likewise, the Intrabeam PRS emits radiation by means of a 3.2 mm diameter probe that can be covered with one of several different applicators ranging in diameter from 2.5 to 5 cm, selected to fit the lumpectomy cavity (Fig. 4A) [42]. With the Intrabeam PRS, radiation doses of 20 Gy at 0.2 cm and 5 Gy at 1 cm are delivered to the breast tissue immediately surrounding the wound cavity [29]. The entire treatment lasts approximately 30 to 35 minutes, with the only required standard procedural deviations being dissection of the breast tissue off the pectoralis fascia to accommodate placement of a lead shield and possibly added time to the procedure to allow for positioning of radiation shields around the operating room before dose administration (Fig. 4B) [29].

A randomized clinical trial that is evaluating the efficacy of IORT as the sole mode of radiation therapy for patients treated with BCT is underway. Designed to compare single-day targeted IORT with conventional

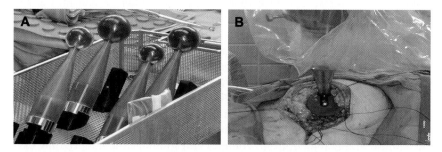

Fig. 4. Single-dose intraoperative radiation therapy. (*A*) Intraoperative radiation therapy applicators for use with the photon radiosurgery system, with diameters ranging from 2.5 to 5.0 cm, are inserted into the lumpectomy cavity. (*B*) The applicator is inserted into the lumpectomy cavity after breast tissue is dissected from the overlying subcutaneous tissue and underlying pectoralis fascia. (*From* Kuerer HM. Surgical considerations for accelerated partial breast irradiation. In: Wazer DE, Vicini FA, editors. Accelerated partial breast irradiation. Berlin: Springer-Verlag; 2006. p. 75.)

postoperative WBI, the TARGIT (TARGeted Intraoperative radiotherapy Trial) aims to determine if the two treatments are equal in terms of local recurrence, disease-free and overall survival, cosmetic outcome, and patient satisfaction. The trial uses the Intrabeam PRS and is being conducted under the guidance of breast surgeons and radiation oncologists. Patients are randomized to receive radiation therapy either as a single complete intraoperative dose or as an intraoperative boost to the wound cavity followed by a complete 7-week postoperative course of conventional WBI [42]. Patient selection criteria include female sex, age of at least 40 years, invasive breast cancer, tumor diameter no more than 3 cm, and eligibility for and desire to undergo BCT. Preliminary results are not yet available.

One advantage of IORT is the potential to complete all components of BCT during a single operative session. This allows for chemotherapy, if indicated, to be commenced sooner, which may confer an oncologic advantage. Likewise, IORT avoids the so-called geographical miss, ensuring that radiation is delivered to the breast tissue immediately surrounding the tumor bed, the most likely site for local recurrence [43].

Disadvantages of IORT include lack of knowledge of the final margin status at the time of radiation administration. IORT also requires unique safety measures during radiation delivery to shield, not only the patient, but the anesthesiologist and other members of the operative crew.

The efficacy of IORT is still under investigation. Questions remain as to the adequacy of a single dose of radiation and the exact dose required.

Ongoing phase III trials of whole-breast irradiation versus accelerated partial breast irradiation and future directions

Early results from published series from several centers evaluating APBI are encouraging, yet follow-up has been modest. Studies have been limited to patients with early-stage disease, wide negative margins, and limited associated intraductal components. Longer-term follow up and consistent results from larger randomized trials will be essential before APBI can be considered an acceptable substitute for WBI.

The NSABP and the RTOG are accruing patients through the National Cancer Institute for a joint study (NSABP-B-39/RTOG-0413) designed to compare WBI versus APBI (Fig. 5) [44]. This phase III randomized, multicenter study is comparing local tumor control (measured in terms of overall survival, recurrence-free survival, and distant disease-free survival), cosmetic outcome, treatment-related side effects, perceived patient convenience, and toxic effects of WBI versus APBI in women who have DCIS or stage I or II breast cancer. The patients in the APBI arm will be assigned randomly after segmental mastectomy to one of three APBI techniques: catheter-based interstitial brachytherapy, balloon-based intracavitary brachytherapy using the MammoSite® device, or 3D-CRT. Because studies from the Joint Center for Radiation Therapy and other institutions suggest that patients with

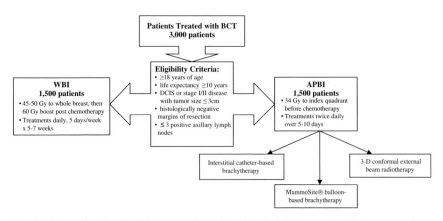

Fig. 5. Scheme for the NSABP-B-39/RTOG-0413 trial of whole-breast irradiation versus three different forms of accelerated partial breast irradiation.

an extensive intraductal component may be at increased risk for locoregional recurrence after BCT [39,45], patients with an extensive intraductal component will be excluded. Eligibility criteria include age 18 years or older, DCIS or stage I or II invasive breast cancer, tumor diameter ≤ 3 cm, histologically negative resection margins, and no more than 3 positive axillary lymph nodes.

The trial has been open since March 21, 2005, and the investigators expect to accrue 1500 patients per treatment arm (3000 total) over 29 months. Preliminary results are not yet available. Data from this trial are needed to establish whether APBI is equivalent to WBI. Results from this trial will not only determine whether APBI is effective as a component of BCT, but also will reveal which of the three techniques of APBI is most effective (see Table 1).

APBI promises shorter treatment duration than WBI and greater patient convenience, and it may be more cost-effective, making BCT a more enticing option for patients who cannot comply with conventional external-beam WBI schedules. It remains to be seen whether APBI will result in lower rates of locoregional recurrence or confer oncologic benefits similar to WBI.

References

[1] Frazier RC, Kestin LL, Kini V, et al. Impact of boost technique on outcome in early stage breast cancer patients treated with breast-conserving therapy. Am J Clin Oncol 2001;24:26–32.

[2] Veronesi U, Salvadori B, Luini A, et al. Breast conservation is a safe method in patients with small cancer of the breast. Long-term results of three randomized trials on 1,973 patients. Eur J Cancer 1995;31:1574–9.

[3] Harris JR, Lippman ME, Veronesi U, et al. Breast cancer. N Engl J Med 1992;327(5):319–28.

[4] Fisher B, Anderson S, Redmond CK, et al. Reanalysis and results after 12 years of follow-up in a randomized clinical trial comparing total mastectomy with lumpectomy with or without irradiation in the treatment of breast cancer. N Engl J Med 1995;333:1456.

[5] Fisher B, Bauer M, Margolese R, et al. Five-year results of a randomized clinical trial comparing total mastectomy and segmental mastectomy with or without radiation in the treatment of breast cancer. N Engl J Med 1985;312:665–73.

[6] Fisher B, Anderson S, Bryant J, et al. Twenty-year follow-up of a randomized trial comparing total mastectomy, lumpectomy, and lumpectomy plus irradiation for the treatment of invasive breast cancer. N Engl J Med 2002;347:1233–41.

[7] Fortin A, Larochelle M, Laverdiere J, et al. Local failure is responsible for the decrease in survival for patients with breast cancer treated with conservative surgery and postoperative radiotherapy. J Clin Oncol 1999;17:101–9.

[8] Veronesi U, Marubini E, Miliani A, et al. Breast-conserving surgery with or without postoperative radiotherapy. Long-term results of a randomized trial. Ann Oncol 2001;12: 997–1003.

[9] Huang E, Buchholz T, Meric F, et al. Classifying local disease recurrences after breast conservation therapy based on location and histology. Cancer 2002;95:2059–67.

[10] Priestman TJ, Bullimore JA, Godden TP, et al. The Royal College of Radiologists' Fractionation Survey. Clin Oncol 1989;1:39–46.

[11] Whelan TJ, Marcellus DC, Clark RM, et al. Adjuvant radiotherapy for early breast cancer. Patterns of practice in Ontario. CMAJ 1993;149:1273–7.

[12] Solin LJ, Fowble BL, Martz KL, et al. Results of the 1983 patterns of care process survey for definitive breast irradiation. Int J Radiat Oncol Biol Phys 1991;20:105–11.

[13] Whelan T, Mackenzie R, Julian J, et al. Randomized trial of breast irradiation schedules after lumpectomy for women with lymph node-negative breast cancer. J Natl Cancer Inst 2002;94:1143–50.

[14] Nattinger AB, Gottlieb MS, Veum J, et al. Geographic variation in the use of breast-conserving treatment for breast cancer. N Engl J Med 1992;326(17):1102–7.

[15] Legorreta AP, Liu X, Parker RG. Examining the use of breast-conserving treatment for women with breast cancer in a managed care environment. Am J Clin Oncol 2000;23(5): 438–41.

[16] Hiotis K, Ye W, Sposto R, et al. Predictors of breast-conservation therapy: size is not all that matters. Cancer 2005;103(5):892–9.

[17] Morrow M, Bucci C, Rademaker A. Medical contraindications are not a major factor in the underutilization of breast-conserving therapy. J Am Coll Surg 1998;186(3): 269–74.

[18] Keisch M, Vicini F, Kuske RR, et al. Initial clinical experience with the MammoSite breast brachytherapy applicator in women with early-stage breast cancer treated with breast-conserving therapy. Int J Radiat Oncol Biol Phys 2003;55:289–93.

[19] Pawlik TM, Bucholz TA, Kuerer HM. The biologic rationale for and emerging role of accelerated partial breast irradiation for breast cancer. J Am Coll Surg 2004;199:479–92.

[20] Vicini FA, Baglan KL, Kestin LL, et al. Accelerated treatment of breast cancer. J Clin Oncol 2001;19:1993–2001.

[21] King TA, Bolton JS, Kuske RR, et al. Long-term results of wide-field brachytherapy as the sole method of radiation therapy after segmental mastectomy for T (is,1,2) breast cancer. Am J Surg 2000;180:299–304.

[22] Trial details. Available at: www.rtog.org. Accessed August 14, 2006.

[23] Kuske RP, Winter K, Arthur DW, et al. Phase II trial of brachytherapy alone after lumpectomy for select breast cancer: toxicity analysis of RTOG 95-17. Int J Radiat Oncol Biol Phys 2006;65:45–51.

[24] Perera F, Yu E, Engel J, et al. Patterns of breast recurrence in a pilot study of brachytherapy confined to the lumpectomy site for early breast cancer with six years' minimum follow-up. Int J Radiat Oncol Biol Phys 2003;57:1239–46.

[25] Buchholz TA, Austin-Seymour MM, Moe RE, et al. Effect of delay in radiation in the combined modality treatment of breast cancer. Int J Radiat Oncol Biol Phys 1993;26(1): 23–35.

[26] Ruo Redda MG, Verna R, Guarneri A, et al. Timing of radiotherapy in breast cancer conserving treatment. Cancer Treat Rev 2002;28:5–10.

[27] Pawlik TM, Perry A, Strom EA, et al. Potential applicability of balloon catheter-based accelerated partial breast irradiation after conservative surgery for breast carcinoma. Cancer 2004;100:490–8.

[28] Jeruss JS, Vicini FA, Beitsch PD, et al. Initial outcomes for patients treated on the American Society of Breast Surgeons MammoSite clinical trial for ductal carcinoma in situ of the breast. Ann Surg Oncol 2006;13:967–76.

[29] Kuerer HM. Surgical considerations for accelerated partial breast irradiation in accelerated partial breast irradiation. Berlin: Springer-Verlag; 2006.

[30] Stolier AJ, Furhman GM, Scroggins TG, et al. Postlumpectomy insertion of the MammoSite brachytherapy device using the scar entry technique: initial experience and technical considerations. Breast J 2005;3:199–203.

[31] Evans SB, Kaufman SA, Price LL, et al. Persistent seroma after intraoperative placement of MammoSite for accelerated partial breast irradiation: incidence, pathologic anatomy, and contributing factors. Int J Radiat Oncol Biol Phys 2006;65:333–9.

[32] Harper JL, Jenrette JM, Vanek KN, et al. Acute complications of MammoSite brachytherapy: a single institution's initial clinical experience. Int J Radiat Oncol Biol Phys 2005;61:169–74.

[33] Niehoff P, Polgar C, Ostertag, et al. Clinical experience with the MammoSite radiation therapy system for brachytherapy for breast cancer: results from an international phase II trial. Radiat Oncol 2006;3:316–20.

[34] Hasan Y, Vicini F. 3D conformal external beam technique in accelerated partial breast irradiation. Berlin: Springer-Verlag; 2006.

[35] Formenti SC. External-beam partial-breast irradiation. Semin Radiat Oncol 2005;15:92–9.

[36] Vicini FA, Remouchamps V, Wallace M, et al. Ongoing clinical experience utilizing 3D conformal external beam radiotherapy to deliver partial-breast irradiation in patients with early-stage breast cancer treated with breast-conserving therapy. Int J Radiat Oncol Biol Phys 2003;57:1247–53.

[37] Baglan KL, Sharpe MB, Jaffray D, et al. Accelerated partial breast irradiation using 3D conformal radiation therapy (3D-CRT). Int J Radiat Oncol Biol Phys 2003;55:302–11.

[38] Vicini F, Winter K, Straube W, et al. A phase I/II trial to evaluate three-dimensional conformal radiation therapy confined to the region of the lumpectomy cavity for stage I/II breast carcinoma: initial report of feasibility and reproducibility of Radiation Therapy Oncology Group (RTOG) Study 0319. Intl J Radiol Oncol Biol Phys 2005;63:1531–7.

[39] Boyages J, Recht A, Connolly JL, et al. Early breast cancer: predictors of breast recurrence for patients treated with conservative surgery and radiation therapy. Radiother Oncol 1990;19:29–41.

[40] Vaidya JS, Tobias JS, Baum M, et al. TARGeted intraoperative radiotherapy (TARGIT): an innovative approach to partial-breast irradiation. Semin Radiat Oncol 2005;2:84–91.

[41] Kuerer HM, Chung M, Giovanna G, et al. The case for accelerated partial-breast irradiation for breast cancer. Contemp Surg 2003;59:508–16.

[42] Trial details. Available at: www.targittrial.com. Accessed August 5, 2006.

[43] Vaidya JS, Tobias J, Baum M, et al. Intraoperative radiotherapy: the debate continues. Lancet Oncol 2004;5(6):339–40.

[44] Trial details. Available at: www.cancer.gov/search/viewclinicaltrials. Accessed August 1, 2006.

[45] Holland R, Connolly JL, Gelman R, et al. The presence of an extensive intraductal component following a limited excision correlates with prominent residual disease in the remainder of the breast. J Clin Oncol 1990;8:113–8.

ELSEVIER
SAUNDERS

SURGICAL
CLINICS OF
NORTH AMERICA

Surg Clin N Am 87 (2007) 499–509

Overview of Adjuvant Systemic Therapy in Early Stage Breast Cancer

Lisa A. Newman, MD, MPH, FACS[a],*,
S. Eva Singletary, MD[b]

[a]Breast Care Center, 1500 East Medical Center Drive, 3308 CGC,
University of Michigan, Ann Arbor, MI 48109, USA
[b]Department of Surgical Oncology, The University of Texas M.D. Anderson Cancer
Center, 1515 Holcombe Boulevard, Box 444, Houston, TX 77030-4095, USA

The benefits of adjuvant systemic therapy in reducing risk of distant relapse from breast cancer have been recognized for several decades. Early detection of breast cancer is essential for improving survival, yet 15% to 20% of patients who have Stage I disease will ultimately experience treatment failure, despite having been diagnosed with small, node-negative lesions. The intent of adjuvant therapy is to eliminate the occult micrometastatic breast cancer burden before it progresses into clinically apparent disease. Successful delivery of effective adjuvant systemic therapy as a complement to surgical management of breast cancer has contributed to the steady declines in breast cancer mortality observed internationally over the past two decades [1]. The National Surgical Adjuvant Breast Project (NSABP) protocols B-13 and B-14 respectively documented the survival advantages associated with adjuvant chemotherapy and endocrine therapy for patients who have node-negative disease, endocrine-resistant disease, or endocrine-sensitive disease [2–5]. Multimodality treatment of invasive breast cancer is therefore essential in optimizing outcomes. Ongoing clinical and translational research in breast cancer seeks to improve the efficacy of systemic agents for use in the conventional postoperative (adjuvant) setting.

The Early Breast Cancer Trialists Collaborative Group (EBCTCG) has published several pooled analyses of the worldwide experience with adjuvant systemic therapy [6–9], and their documentation of an associated 30% to 50% reduction in odds of relapse has provided the foundation for consensus statements regarding selection of cases in which adjuvant therapy is likely to

* Corresponding author.
E-mail address: lanewman@umich.edu (L.A. Newman).

be beneficial. Table 1 [10–12] summarizes the results from these overview analyses of adjuvant systemic chemotherapy as well as endocrine therapy, including ovarian ablation. The ovarian ablation trials have been more common in Europe than in the United States.

Algorithms for adjuvant systemic therapy decisions

As additional prospective clinical trials mature, and as the armamentarium of therapies as well as predictive and prognostic features expands, the algorithms for adjuvant therapy decisions evolve accordingly. Hence, in the 1980s it was commonplace to reserve any systemic therapy for patients who were node-positive, but by the following decade the National Cancer Institute recommended consideration of adjuvant systemic therapy for any woman whose invasive cancer is at least 1 cm in size. Indications for adjuvant therapy have broadened even further as a consequence of studies documenting the persistent risk of distant failure, even in the selected population of T1b/node-negative cancer. The National Surgical Adjuvant Breast Trialists (NSABP) pooled analysis [13] of more than 1250 cases of node-negative cancers up to 1 cm in size (approximately 20% estrogen receptor (ER)-negative) revealed improved survival for cases treated with adjuvant tamoxifen or chemotherapy. The most recent overview analysis [9] documented improved outcomes at 15 years for breast cancer patients receiving polychemotherapy at all ages and regardless of ER status. The majority of invasive breast cancers therefore appear to harbor some risk of distant failure that can be modified by systemic therapy, but the absolute benefit will be a function of the patient's risk of relapse at the time of diagnosis (generally assessed by tumor size and nodal status). The toxicity of adjuvant therapy must be carefully balanced against this relapse risk. For example, adjuvant therapy that provides a 50% odds reduction in recurrence will provide an absolute benefit of 15% to a Stage IIB breast cancer patient who has a 30% relapse risk; in contrast, the absolute benefit will be only 2.5% for patient diagnosed with a 0.5 cm node-negative, ER-positive breast cancer, whose baseline relapse risk is only 5%.

Adjuvant! Online (available at www.adjuvantonline.com) is a Web-based program that provides clinicians a detailed report of outcome risks with versus without systemic therapy, based upon the clinicopathologic profile of the individual patient [14,15]. This program's accuracy has been validated in external datasets [16]. The computer-generated profile presents information on the absolute as well as relative risk benefits of adjuvant therapy. These calculated risks are then shown in pictorial figures that enhance clarity for patients as well as physicians.

The St. Gallen International Consensus Conference [17] defined the primary cancer features that are necessary to assess adjuvant systemic therapy needs as: size of primary tumor invasive component, nodal status, ER expression, progesterone receptor expression, and human epidermal growth

Table 1
Summary of worldwide overview analyses

Treatment analyzed	No. trials analyzed	No. women analyzed	Proportional reduction		Contralateral breast cancer	Comments
			Relapse	Mortality		
Tamoxifen for early-stage breast cancer [8,20]	55	37,000	1 yr: 21% 2 yrs: 29% 5 yrs: 47%	1 yr: 12% 2 yrs: 17% 5 yrs: 26%	1 yr: 13% 2 yrs: 26% 5 yrs: 47%	• Risk of endometrial cancer doubled in trials of 1 or 2 yrs and quadrupled in trials of 5 yrs • Approximately 8000 women had tumors with low/zero ER content; these pts had negligible benefit from tamoxifen for relapse and mortality. They are excluded from relapse and mortality data, but are included in contralateral risk data.
Multi-agent CTX for early breast cancer [7,10]	47	18,000[a]	<50 yo: 35% 50–69 yo: 20%	<50 yo: 27% 50–69 yo: 11%	NR NR	• No significant survival advantage for more than approximately 3 months of polychemotherapy • Anthracycline-containing regimens better than CMF alone
Ovarian ablation for early breast cancer [11,12]	12	2102	18.5%	6.3%	NS	• Benefit of ovarian ablation strongest in women not receiving CTX • Menopausal status not consistently defined in all studies; most limited to women younger than 50 years.

Abbreviations: CMF, cyclophosphamide/methotrexate/fluorouracil; CTX, chemotherapy; ER, estrogen receptor; No, number; NR, not reported; NS, not significantly different; pts, patients; yo, years old; yr, year.

[a] Including 6000 women in 11 trials of longer versus shorter CTX, and 6000 women in 11 trials of doxorubicin-containing CTX versus CMF.

factor receptor-2 (HER-2/neu) expression. Additional characteristics that may influence systemic therapy decisions in borderline cases include histologic grade, presence versus absence of lymphovascular invasion, and primary histology (with metaplastic changes conferring an adverse risk). The data regarding isolated tumor cells in axillary lymph nodes (defined as metastatic foci no larger than 0.2 mm in diameter as per the American Joint Committee on Cancer [AJCC] Sixth Edition Staging System [18], and staged as node-negative) and the presence of circulating tumor cells in peripheral blood or bone marrow were not deemed to be mature enough to warrant taking these features into consideration for selection of adjuvant therapy. The St. Gallen worldwide experts convene on a regular basis and provide updates on adjuvant therapy recommendations for breast cancer patients who have low-; intermediate-; and high-risk disease. The most recent St. Gallen consensus conference recommendations are summarized in Table 1, with modifications that account for additional information related to genetic profiling and HER2/neu status.

The NSABP developed a reverse transcriptase polymerase chain reaction (RT-PCR)-based genetic profile that calculates a recurrence score for ER-positive, node-negative disease, based upon a prospectively-developed, 21-gene assay. This assay (Oncotype DX, Genomic Health, Redwood City, California) is commercially-available for application to paraffin-embedded tumor specimens; it has been shown to be prognostic for risk of relapse and predictive of benefit from chemotherapy in addition to endocrine therapy, independent of primary tumor size and patient age [19]. Preliminary studies reveal that ER-positive, node-negative breast cancer patients who have a low recurrence score can be safely treated with endocrine therapy alone, even if they have a large primary tumor. In contrast, chemotherapy (in addition to endocrine therapy) should be considered for patients who have T1a, node-negative disease if they have a high recurrence score. A prospective randomized clinical trial to evaluate management of patients who have intermediate scores is currently underway. The St. Gallen experts acknowledge the potential value of this genetic profiling, but the test is costly, and it was therefore not included as a routine component of their systemic therapy decision-tree. Table 2 summarizes an algorithm that combines a modified version of the risk stratification scheme of the St. Gallen experts with the associated options for adjuvant systemic therapy.

Selection of patients who can avoid systemic therapy completely

In selected cases, patients who have breast cancer have a sufficiently low risk for distant failure that local treatment alone will be adequate. Optimal characteristics of these low-risk cases include ER/progesterone receptor (PR)-positivity, node-negativity, primary invasive tumor size no larger than 1 cm, and low-grade, with neither lymphovascular invasion nor HER2/neu overexpression. Tubular histology and older age are other favorable feature

Table 2
Systemic adjuvant therapy options for breast cancer patients stratified by risk of relapse

Risk category and associated features		Adjuvant therapy options
Low-risk	Node-negative; AND ER or PR positive; AND T ≤1 cm; AND Grade I; AND no LVI/PVI; AND HER2/neu negative; AND age ≥35 years	• None • Endocrine therapy only • Consider Oncotype Dx to confirm risk assessment via recurrence score
Intermediate risk	Node-negative AND at least one of the following: • T >2 cm; OR • Grade II/III; OR • LVI/PVI present; OR • Age <35 years; OR • HER2/neu positive or amplified	Endocrine-responsive[a,b] • Endocrine therapy alone • CTX followed by ET • Consider Oncotype Dx to evaluate risk via recurrence score (Oncotype Dx appropriate for node-negative cases only)
	Node-positive (1–3 nodes); AND HER2/neu-negative	Not endocrine-responsive[a,b] • CTX
High-risk	Node-positive (1–3 nodes); AND HER2/neu positive	Endocrine-responsive[a,b] • CTX followed by endocrine therapy
	Node-positive (≥4 nodes)	Not endocrine-responsive[a,b] • CTX

This table and the risk categories have been adapted and modified from the risk categories described by Goldhirsch et al [17]; treatment options have been adjusted to reflect data regarding the Oncotype DX genetic profiles, and data regarding adjuvant trastuzamab therapy for HER2/neu overexpressing/amplified tumors. Note that these recommendations acknowledge the existence of varying degrees of risk within both endocrine-sensitive and endocrine-resistant breast cancer subtypes. Application of the algorithm suggested by this table therefore requires that the patient's disease is first assessed by nodal status, and then by primary clinicopathologic features (age, histopathologic descriptors, molecular markers, and so forth).

Abbreviations: CTX, chemotherapy; ER, estrogen receptor; LVI, lymphovascular invasion; PR, progesterone receptor; PVI, perivascular invasion.

[a] Include trastuzamab therapy if HER2/neu-positive or amplified (however, note that trastuzamab is generally only offered to patients deemed to be at high enough risk that CTX is indicated).

[b] Consider postmastectomy irradiation or extended-field-regional field irradiation if primary tumor larger than 5 cm or if 1–3 nodes are positive for metastatic disease.

that justify a modified approach to systemic adjuvant therapy recommendations. Hormone receptor-negative disease usually does not fall into this category unless it is associated with only a microinvasive, node-negative lesion.

Systemic therapy for endocrine-responsive breast cancer

Breast cancer is expected to be sensitive to endocrine therapy if immunohistochemistry staining reveals at least 10% staining for the estrogen receptor within the invasive component. ER-negative tumors are also considered endocrine-responsive if they stain positive for the progesterone receptor, because expression of the PR marker is dependent upon the presence of intact ER machinery.

Endocrine therapy for postmenopausal cases

Tamoxifen has been the mainstay of endocrine therapy for hormone receptor-positive breast cancer over the past 30 years. Tamoxifen was originally developed as an antifertility medication, and alternative uses in the oncology field were sought as a result of its dismal failure in this area because of tamoxifen's ovulatory effects. As a very effective antagonist of estrogen receptors on mammary tissue, however, it has remained extremely powerful as first-line adjuvant systemic therapy in breast cancer management. Tamoxifen's selective estrogen receptor activity also yields estrogen agonist activity on the uterus, cardiovascular, cerebrovascular, and osseous tissues; this results in the mixed benefits and risks of uterine cancer, lowered cholesterol levels, vasomotor symptoms, and protection against osteoporosis. Tamoxifen will decrease the odds of relapse in endocrine-responsive breast cancer by 3% to 50% [8,9,20]. Tamoxifen also decreases the incidence of contralateral new primary tumors, and this benefit has resulted in its applications for chemoprevention in high-risk women [21,22]. The NSABP B-14 trial [23] randomized early-stage breast cancer patients to receive 5 versus 10 years of tamoxifen postoperatively, and found that extended therapy resulted in higher rates of adverse events that were not outweighed by added protection.

Recent advances in the development of aromatase inhibitors (AIs) have expanded the options for postmenopausal women who have endocrine-responsive disease. AIs result in near-complete shutdown of estrogen production by blocking peripheral conversion of adrenal gland-derived estrogen precursors by the enzyme aromatase. Following natural or induced menopause with loss of ovarian estrogen production, the majority of circulating estrogen is produced by adipocytes in body fat stores, because this is the primary source of aromatase. The Arimidex and Tamoxifen: Alone or in Combination (ATAC) trial was one of the first prospective randomized clinical trials to study an AI as adjuvant therapy for early-stage breast cancer. The ATAC trial randomized 9366 postmenopausal women to receive anastrazole versus tamoxifen versus the combination of anastrazole and tamoxifen. With a median follow-up of 3 years, anastrozole proved to be superior to both tamoxifen and the combination arm of the study [24].

Other large prospective randomized clinical trials have evaluated alternative AIs such as letrozole and exemestane, and have studied sequential therapy, with the AI given after 2 to 5 years of adjuvant tamoxifen therapy [25–27]. These trials have consistently demonstrated added value for use of an AI in postmenopausal, ER-positive breast cancer; however, there is no consensus regarding which AI is superior, what the optimal sequence should be for tamoxifen and AI therapy, or whether an AI should completely replace tamoxifen.

The growing experience with AI therapy has been very promising for improved outcomes in endocrine-responsive breast cancer, but the toxicity profile of AIs must still be considered. Unlike tamoxifen, AI therapy will not affect the uterus, but vasomotor symptoms will occur in approximately

40% of cases; the most concerning risk associated with AI therapy is the potential for osteoporosis. Nonetheless, the American Society of Clinical Oncology has recommended inclusion of AI therapy as a component of managing postmenopausal endocrine-responsive breast cancer, either alone or in addition to tamoxifen [28].

Endocrine therapy for premenopausal cases

Tamoxifen is the standard of care in managing endocrine-responsive breast cancer among women who have functioning ovaries. Ongoing multi-center clinical trials are studying the potential benefits of ovarian suppression in combination with aromatase inhibition in premenopausal women; the optimal duration and long-term effects of ovarian suppression are presently undefined. Oophorectomy has been advocated as well, but concerns regarding the cardiovascular and osteoporotic risks of premature, permanent menopause have limited its popularity.

Adjuvant chemotherapy in addition to endocrine therapy
for endocrine-sensitive breast cancer

Patients who have node-positive breast cancer face a substantial increase in risk for disease relapse, and these women are therefore recommended to receive chemotherapy in addition to their endocrine treatment. Tamoxifen is known to be cytostatic (as opposed to cytotoxic), which potentially can interfere with chemotherapy effect on rapidly proliferating cancer cells. Tamoxifen therapy is therefore usually sequenced to follow chemotherapy, and concurrent treatment is discouraged. AI therapy is generally recommended to follow chemotherapy as well. As noted previously, use of the Oncotype DX recurrence score may also facilitate decision-making regarding need for chemotherapy in endocrine-sensitive, node-negative breast cancer.

Systemic therapy for endocrine-resistant breast cancer

Fewer options exist for this category of disease. Invasive breast cancers that are negative for both ER and PR can only be offered chemotherapy as adjuvant therapy, and trastuzumab (discussed below) should be considered for those cases that overexpress HER2/neu. All node-positive cases are considered candidates for adjuvant chemotherapy and many node-negative cases (unless the disease is microinvasive). Tumors that overexpress the HER2/neu marker and that have been deemed appropriate candidates for chemotherapy will be referred for trastuzamab therapy as well.

Selection and dosing of chemotherapy regimen

Several different chemotherapy regimens are accepted as being comparable for management of breast cancer. The earliest studies of chemotherapy for breast cancer involved perioperative administration of medications that are considered inferior to the effective agents currently available, and the goal of these early investigations was to eliminate dissemination of cancer cells that might have occurred in conjunction with surgical manipulation of tumors. The NSABP B-01 [29] trial (conducted nearly 40 years ago) therefore involved intravenous thiotepa versus placebo administered at the time of radical mastectomy and over the first couple of days postoperatively. Not surprisingly, this regimen failed to produce any improvements in outcome for the entire group of treated patients, but the subset of highest-risk women (those who have four or more metastatic nodes) did experience some overall survival advantages. Subsequent trials conducted during the 1970s and 1980s revealed the power of cyclophosphamide and combination cyclophosphamide (CTX) regimens in reducing breast cancer relapse rates as well as mortality risks.

Until recently, the two regimens of cyclophosphamide/methotrexate/fluorouracil (CMF), and cyclophosphamide/doxorubicin/fluorouracil (CAF), delivered in every 3-week cycles, were the most commonly-employed regimens for adjuvant therapy of breast cancer. During the late 1990s the taxanes emerged as an alternative and highly effective agent against breast cancer. Furthermore, the development of active and tolerable bone marrow-supportive therapy in the form of granulocyte colony-stimulating factors has opened the door to dose-dense regimens allowing safe delivery of higher cumulative CTX doses within shorter time frames. Collectively, the randomized controlled trial data show that adjuvant CTX regimens that include a taxane as well as doxorubicin are most reasonable for node-positive breast cancer patients. This conclusion is supported by findings from the Cancer and Leukemia Group B (CALGB) 9344 trial [30], NSABP B-28 trial [31], and Breast Cancer International Research Group (BCIRG) 001 trial [32] Phase III studies. These three trials all randomized node-positive patients to receive doxorubicin-based combinations versus doxorubicin CTX plus a taxane, and all three demonstrated an outcome advantage for the taxane arms. The CALGB 9741 [33,34] and 9344 [30] trials also revealed superiority of dose-dense therapy (9741), but no outcome advantage for increased doses of doxorubicin (9344). Questions regarding superiority of one taxane versus the other (paclitaxel versus docetaxol) remain unanswered.

Targeted therapy for breast cancer with trastuzamab (herceptin)

Overexpression of the HER2/neu molecular marker is a well-recognized adverse primary tumor prognostic factor in breast cancer. The development of a trastuzamab, a monoclonal antibody that is administered intravenously and targets the HER2/neu marker, has proven to be effective in the management of metastatic breast cancer, and recently-reported prospective randomized clinical trials have demonstrated its value as adjuvant therapy for early-stage disease as well [35,36]. These trials have revealed 30% to 50% reductions in odds of recurrence for these high-risk cancers. Breast cancer patients whose disease warrants chemotherapy will usually be offered 1 year of trastuzamab if the cancer overexpresses HER 2/neu. A Phase III clinical trial comparing 1 versus 2 years of adjuvant trastuzamab is ongoing [35].

Adjuvant systemic therapy for breast cancer: summary and practical considerations

Any invasive breast cancer is associated with some risk of distant organ micrometastatic disease, and the risk of breast cancer mortality is reduced by delivery of systemic therapy as adjuvant treatment after primary surgery. The absolute benefit from adjuvant therapy will depend on the patient's underlying risk of relapse. Patients who have node-positive breast cancer therefore have the largest-magnitude benefit from adjuvant therapy. Conversely, patients who have small, node-negative cancers must balance the toxicity of systemic therapy against the estimated risk of metastatic disease, because some of these patients will have an excellent outcome with primary surgery alone. Web-based computerized programs such as Adjuvant! Online provide patients and clinicians with a summary of calculated risks versus benefits from systemic therapy based upon primary clinicopathologic features. Genetic profiling and assignment of a recurrence score via the Oncotype DX test can be helpful in determining benefit from adjuvant chemotherapy in addition to endocrine therapy for ER-positive, node-negative cases.

ER-responsive breast cancer (ER- or PR-positive disease) will usually require tamoxifen or an aromatase inhibitor if the patient is postmenopausal. Chemotherapy is recommended for high-risk endocrine-responsive disease (eg, node-positive breast cancer), and for any endocrine-resistant breast cancer that is deemed appropriate for systemic treatment. Trastuzamab is indicated as targeted therapy to follow chemotherapy for HER-2/neu-overexpressing cancers.

References

[1] Peto R, Boreham J, Clark M, et al. UK and USA breast cancer deaths down 25% in year 2000 at ages 20–69 years. Lancet 2000;355(9217):1822.

[2] Fisher B. Highlights from recent National Surgical Adjuvant Breast and Bowel Project studies in the treatment and prevention of breast cancer. CA Cancer J Clin 1999;49(3):159–77.

[3] Fisher B, Costantino J, Redmond C , et al. A randomized clinical trial evaluating tamoxifen in the treatment of patients with node-negative breast cancer who have estrogen-receptor-positive tumors. N Engl J Med 1989;320(8):479–84.

[4] Fisher B, Dignam J, Bryant J, et al. Five versus more than five years of tamoxifen therapy for breast cancer patients with negative lymph nodes and estrogen receptor-positive tumors. J Natl Cancer Inst 1996;88(21):1529–42.

[5] Fisher B, Dignam J, Mamounas EP, et al. Sequential methotrexate and fluorouracil for the treatment of node-negative breast cancer patients with estrogen receptor-negative tumors: eight-year results from National Surgical Adjuvant Breast and Bowel Project (NSABP) B-13 and first report of findings from NSABP B-19 comparing methotrexate and fluorouracil with conventional cyclophosphamide, methotrexate, and fluorouracil. J Clin Oncol 1996; 14(7):1982–92.

[6] Effects of adjuvant tamoxifen and of cytotoxic therapy on mortality in early breast cancer. An overview of 61 randomized trials among 28,896 women. Early Breast Cancer Trialists' Collaborative Group. N Engl J Med 1988;319(26):1681–92.

[7] Polychemotherapy for early breast cancer: an overview of the randomised trials. Early Breast Cancer Trialists' Collaborative Group. Lancet 1998;352(9132):930–42.

[8] Tamoxifen for early breast cancer: an overview of the randomised trials. Early Breast Cancer Trialists' Collaborative Group. Lancet 1998;351(9114):1451–67.

[9] Effects of chemotherapy and hormonal therapy for early breast cancer on recurrence and 15-year survival: an overview of the randomised trials. Lancet 2005;365(9472):1687–717.

[10] Multi-agent chemotherapy for early breast cancer. Cochrane Database Syst Rev 2002;1: CD000487.

[11] Ovarian ablation in early breast cancer: overview of the randomised trials. Early Breast Cancer Trialists' Collaborative Group. Lancet 1996;348(9036):1189–96.

[12] Ovarian ablation for early breast cancer. Cochrane Database Syst Rev 2000;3:CD000485.

[13] Fisher B, Dignam J, Tan-Chiu E, et al. Prognosis and treatment of patients with breast tumors of one centimeter or less and negative axillary lymph nodes. J Natl Cancer Inst 2001; 93(2):112–20.

[14] Ravdin PM, Siminoff LA, Davis GJ, et al. Computer program to assist in making decisions about adjuvant therapy for women with early breast cancer. J Clin Oncol 2001;19(4):980–91.

[15] Adjuvant! On line: Available at: www.adjuvantonline.com. Accessed June 15, 2006.

[16] Olivotto IA, Bajdik CD, Ravdin PM, et al. Population-based validation of the prognostic model ADJUVANT! for early breast cancer. J Clin Oncol 2005;23(12):2716–25.

[17] Goldhirsch A, Glick JH, Gelber RD, et al. Meeting highlights: international expert consensus on the primary therapy of early breast cancer 2005. Ann Oncol 2005;16(10):1569–83.

[18] Singletary SE, Allred C, Ashley P, et al. Revision of the American Joint Committee on Cancer staging system for breast cancer. J Clin Oncol 2002;20(17):3628–36.

[19] Paik S, Shak S, Tang G, et al. A multigene assay to predict recurrence of tamoxifen-treated, node-negative breast cancer. N Engl J Med 2004;351(27):2817–26.

[20] Tamoxifen for early breast cancer. Cochrane Database Syst Rev 2001;(1):CD000486.

[21] Fisher B, Powles TJ, Pritchard KJ. Tamoxifen for the prevention of breast cancer. Eur J Cancer 2000;36(2):142–50.

[22] Fisher B, Costantino JP, Wickerham DL, et al. Tamoxifen for prevention of breast cancer: report of the National Surgical Adjuvant Breast and Bowel Project P-1 Study. J Natl Cancer Inst 1998;90(18):1371–88.

[23] Fisher B, Dignam J, Bryant J, et al. Five versus more than five years of tamoxifen for lymph node-negative breast cancer: updated findings from the National Surgical Adjuvant Breast and Bowel Project B-14 randomized trial. J Natl Cancer Inst 2001;93(9):684–90.

[24] Baum M, Budzar AU, Cuzik J, et al. Anastrozole alone or in combination with tamoxifen versus tamoxifen alone for adjuvant treatment of postmenopausal women with early breast cancer: first results of the ATAC randomised trial. Lancet 2002;359(9324):2131–9.

[25] Goss P, Ingle J, Martino S, et al. Updated analysis of the NCIC CTG MA.17 randomized placebo-controlled trial of letrozole after five years of tamoxifen in postmenopausal women with early stage breast cancer. Presented at the American Society of Clinical Oncology 2004 Annual Meeting. New Orleans (LA), (Post-Meeting Edition). Vol 22, No 14S (July 15 Supplement), 2004:847.

[26] Goss PE, Ingle JN, Martino S, et al. A randomized trial of letrozole in postmenopausal women after five years of tamoxifen therapy for early-stage breast cancer. N Engl J Med 2003;349(19):1793–802.

[27] Coombes RC, Hall E, Gibson LJ, et al. A randomized trial of exemestane after two to three years of tamoxifen therapy in postmenopausal women with primary breast cancer. N Engl J Med 2004;350(11):1081–92.

[28] Winer EP, Hudis C, Burstein HJ, et al. American Society of Clinical Oncology technology assessment working group update: use of aromatase inhibitors in the adjuvant setting. J Clin Oncol 2003;21(13):2597–9.

[29] Fisher B, et al. Surgical adjuvant chemotherapy in cancer of the breast: results of a decade of cooperative investigation. Ann Surg 1968;168(3):337–56.

[30] Henderson IC, Berry DA, Demetri GD, et al. Improved outcomes from adding sequential paclitaxel but not from escalating doxorubicin dose in an adjuvant chemotherapy regimen for patients with node-positive primary breast cancer. J Clin Oncol 2003;21(6):976–83.

[31] Mamounas EP, et al. Paclitaxel after doxorubicin plus cyclophosphamide as adjuvant chemotherapy for node-positive breast cancer: results from NSABP B-28. J Clin Oncol 2005; 23(16):3686–96.

[32] Martin M, Pienkowski T, Mackey J, et al. Adjuvant docetaxel for node-positive breast cancer. N Engl J Med 2005;352(22):2302–13.

[33] Citron ML. Dose density in adjuvant chemotherapy for breast cancer. Cancer Invest 2004; 22(4):555–68.

[34] Citron ML, Berry DA, Cirrincione C, et al. Randomized trial of dose-dense versus conventionally scheduled and sequential versus concurrent combination chemotherapy as postoperative adjuvant treatment of node-positive primary breast cancer: first report of Intergroup Trial C9741/Cancer and Leukemia Group B Trial 9741. J Clin Oncol 2003;21(8):1431–9.

[35] Piccart-Gebhart MJ, Proctor M, Leyland-Jones B, et al. Trastuzumab after adjuvant chemotherapy in HER2-positive breast cancer. N Engl J Med 2005;353(16):1659–72.

[36] Romond EH, Perez EA, Bryant J, et al. Trastuzumab plus adjuvant chemotherapy for operable HER2-positive breast cancer. N Engl J Med 2005;353(16):1673–84.

ELSEVIER
SAUNDERS

SURGICAL
CLINICS OF
NORTH AMERICA

Surg Clin N Am 87 (2007) 511–526

Postmastectomy Radiation Therapy: Indications and Controversies

Marie Catherine Lee, MD[a],*,
Reshma Jagsi, MD, DPhil[b]

[a]Department of Surgery, University of Michigan Hospitals, 1500 East Medical Center Drive,
3216A Cancer Center/Box 0932, Ann Arbor, MI 48109, USA
[b]Department of Radiation Oncology, University of Michigan Hospitals, 1500 East Medical
Center Drive, Room B2C490, Ann Arbor, MI 48109, USA

Surgery and radiation share the common goals of addressing and controlling the locoregional manifestations of breast cancer. The most recent update of the comprehensive meta-analysis conducted by the Oxford Early Breast Cancer Trialists Collaborative Group (EBCTCG) has now definitively established the critical impact of locoregional control upon the ultimate survival of patients with breast cancer [1]. Therefore, while the prevailing paradigm of breast cancer progression in recent years has presumed that systemic therapy to control distant organ disease is the dominant determinant of outcome, the importance of controlling primary disease cannot be disputed.

For some early-stage breast cancer patients, local therapy in the form of mastectomy alone or lumpectomy coupled with radiation therapy to the breast will be "curative." In contrast, selected cases of breast cancer are associated with a sufficiently high risk of failure that more aggressive therapy is warranted. Indeed, in some patients who undergo mastectomy, occult, microscopic disease may remain beyond the boundaries of the surgical field and may not be adequately controlled by adjuvant systemic therapy, potentially leading to morbid locoregional recurrences and providing a reservoir to seed (or re-seed) distant sites. Radiation therapy, therefore, plays an important role in the locoregional management of some patients treated with mastectomy.

The issue of postmastectomy radiation therapy (PMRT) has generated extensive controversy during the past few decades. Although there is substantial evidence, as shown in Table 1 [1–3], to suggest that radiation

* Corresponding author.
E-mail address: mariecat@med.umich.edu (M.C. Lee).

Table 1
Randomized trials of postmastectomy irradiation in patients treated with axillary lymph node dissection and adjuvant systemic therapy for which subset analyses based on extent of nodal metastases were available

Study		Year	Number of patients	Median follow-up (months)	Locoregional failure (%)[c]		Overall survival (%)[d]	
					No PMRT	PMRT	No PMRT	PMRT
DBCG 82b [18]	All	1997	1708	114	32	9	45	54
	1–3 positive nodes		1061	114	30	7[a]	54	62
	≥4 positive nodes		510	114	42	14	20	32
DBCG 82c [19]	All	1999	1375	123	35	8	36	45
	1–3 positive nodes		794	123	31	6	44	55
	≥4 positive nodes		448	123	46	11	17	24
Glasgow [1]	All	1986	219	63	25	11	57	61
	1–3 positive nodes		141	63	NR	NR	68	76
	≥4 positive nodes		72	63	NR	NR	46	54
BC [20]	All	1997	318	150	33	13	46	54
	1–3 positive nodes		183	150	33	13	NR	NR
	≥positive nodes		112	150	46	21	NR	NR
DFCI [2][a]	1–3 positive nodes	1987	83	53	5	2	85	77
	≥4 positive nodes		123	45	20	6	63	59
SECSG [3][b]	≥4 positive nodes	1992	295	120	23	13	44	55

Abbreviations: BC, British Columbia; dBCG, Danish Breast Cancer Group; DFCI, Dana Farber Cancer Institute; eCOG, eastern Cooperative Oncology Group; German BCG, German Breast Cancer Group; NR, not reported; PMRT, postmastectomy radiation therapy; SECSG, Southeast Cancer Study Group.

[a] DFCI trial patients who had one to three positive nodes received cyclophosphamide, methotrexate, fluorouracil adjuvant chemotherapy: patients who had four or more positive nodes received doxorubicin cyclophosphamide adjuvant chemotherapy.

[b] All SECSG trial patients had at least four positive nodes.

[c] Differences in locoregional failure between No PMRT and PMRT arms were statistically significant (*P* < .05) in the DBCG 82b, DBCG 82c, Glasgow, BC, and DFCI trials.

[d] Differences in overall survival were significant in the DBCG 82b and DBCG 82c trials.

therapy can reduce the risk of locoregional failure after mastectomy (by approximately two thirds), debate remains regarding the specific subgroups who have sufficient risks of residual microscopic locoregional disease after mastectomy with or without systemic therapy to warrant further locoregional therapy with radiation. In theory, the improvements in local control clearly afforded by PMRT should translate into improved breast cancer-specific survival for all patients receiving this treatment. Nevertheless, when the baseline risk of recurrence is low, the magnitude of any cause-specific survival advantage may be relatively small and may be offset by potential treatment-related mortality. Therefore, a number of studies have sought to define more clearly the impact of PMRT on overall survival.

Several meta-analyses have attempted to determine the effects of PMRT on survival. The EBCTCG publishes periodic updates of a systematic meta-analysis of individual patient data from randomized trials [1–3]. Earlier reports of the EBCTCG have revealed a reduction in breast cancer mortality associated with adjuvant radiation therapy that was offset by increases in non-breast cancer-related mortality. Of note, higher radiation doses were delivered to the heart and lungs in the older studies included in the meta-analysis than are delivered with modern techniques, probably resulting in greater toxicity to these critical structures and accounting for at least some of the non–breast cancer mortality offsetting the benefits of radiation therapy. The meta-analyses of Cuzick and colleagues [4,5] demonstrate this issue well. Their initial 1987 report revealed an overall survival disadvantage for patients receiving PMRT [4]; a follow-up study reported in 1994, however, confirmed that PMRT was indeed associated with improved breast cancer cause-specific survival, but this benefit was offset by non–breast cancer events [5].

Another meta-analysis conducted by Whelan and colleagues [6] pooled the results from 18 trials reported between 1967 and 1999. Collectively, these studies involved 6367 patients who had breast cancer (most node positive), all of whom were treated by mastectomy, axillary dissection, and systemic therapy and assigned randomly to PMRT or no PMRT. Radiation was shown to reduce the risk of local recurrence (odds ratio, 0.25; 95% confidence interval, 0.19–0.34) as well as overall mortality (odds ratio, 0.83; 95% confidence interval, 0.74–0.94). Similarly, a meta-analysis by Van de Steene and colleagues [7] revealed an approximately 20% reduction in mortality odds in favor of adjuvant radiation, provided that contemporary fractionation techniques were used to minimize cardiovascular toxicity.

Finally, most recently, in its landmark 2005 publication, which includes greater follow-up of patients from earlier trials as well as analysis of data from patients enrolled on trials initiated through 1995, the EBCTCG has now documented a clear overall survival advantage due to the use of PMRT in node-positive patients. Among 8340 women treated with mastectomy and axillary clearance for node-positive disease and enrolled in trials of PMRT (generally to the chest wall and regional lymph nodes), the five-year local recurrence risk was reduced from 22.8% to 5.8%, with 15-year breast cancer mortality risks of 54.7% vs 60.1% (reduction 5.4%, $2p = 0.0002$) and overall mortality reduction of 4.4% (64.2% vs 59.8%, $2p = 0.0009$).

These studies together provide compelling evidence in support of PMRT. Questions remain, however, regarding appropriate patient selection for PMRT, particularly because contemporary systemic therapy is improved compared to the regimens utilized in some of the older studies included in the meta-analysis and because the results were not analyzed by subsets defined by extent of nodal metastases.

Current practice: the 2001 American Society of Clinical Oncology guidelines

The conflicting data described above motivated several professional societies to develop practice guidelines regarding the use of PMRT. The American Society of Clinical Oncology (ASCO) Health Services Research Committee commissioned a multidisciplinary panel of breast cancer experts for an in-depth review of worldwide data on locoregional failure from breast cancer and the ability of PMRT to reduce risk of locoregional as well as distant relapse [8,9]. When evidence-based data were inadequate, the expert panel was charged with using their expert opinion to assess the utility of PMRT. The panel's systematic, graded review of all published evidence regarding PMRT was assembled into a clinical practice guideline as summarized in Table 2 [8].

The language used in the guideline has very specific implications. "Recommendations" are based on level I or level II data. Level I data are derived from meta-analyses of multiple well-designed, controlled studies or from highly powered, randomized trials. Level II data are based on at least one well-designed experimental trial and low-powered randomized trials. "Suggestions" are based on data from levels III, IV, or V. Data in these levels are weaker, so these guidelines are based in some part on consensus from the ASCO panel. "Insufficient evidence" denotes a lack of either evidence or panel consensus regarding the population in question.

The ASCO PMRT practice guideline includes recommendations for the routine use of PMRT in cases of highest-risk breast cancer, defined as disease with at least four metastatic lymph nodes. PMRT was suggested for cases of T3 and operable stage 3 disease. The panel concluded that data regarding net benefits of PMRT in cases of T1/T2 tumors and one to three metastatic nodes were insufficient to warrant its routine use. Similarly, the panel assessed the available evidence on using patient factors (such as age or menopausal status) and primary tumor features (such as lymphovascular invasion) as being insufficient criteria for using PMRT. The majority of the panel favored routine use of PMRT in breast cancer cases receiving neoadjuvant chemotherapy because patients who have relatively more advanced clinical stages of disease comprise the population most likely to be referred for this treatment sequence. The panel acknowledged the paucity of clinical trial data to address this issue, however, and concluded that no definitive recommendation could be offered for this patient population. Furthermore, neoadjuvant chemotherapy is used increasingly for patients who have T2 tumors as a strategy for improving lumpectomy eligibility, and this treatment sequence is no longer restricted to cases of locally advanced disease.

Similar guidelines were developed by the American Society for Therapeutic Radiology and Oncology [10], the American College of Radiology [11], and the Canadian Committee on Clinical Practice Guidelines for the Care and Treatment of Breast Cancer [12]. Of note, all expert panels recommended the use of PMRT in patients with 4 or more positive axillary nodes. They also all acknowledged the lesser clarity surrounding patients with 1-3 positive axillary nodes. Of note, the ASTRO experts stated, "The data regarding patient selection for survival advantage are less clear, but the most recent evidence suggests that the greatest survival benefit is seen in node-positive patients with low tumor burdens (ie, fewer positive nodes or smaller tumors). Radiation therapy in these patients for survival benefit is worthy of consideration, pending more definitive data.... Consultation with a radiation oncologist should occur in node-positive patients treated with mastectomy to help patients assess the risks and benefits of PMRT." The ACR recommendations echo this statement.

As clinical studies continue to mature, the oncology community continues to debate the potential value of PMRT for categories of intermediate-risk breast cancer, in which data were insufficient to warrant definitive recommendations by the ASCO panel. Indeed, a survey of radiation oncologists found that although the vast majority (>98%) reported that they would offer radiation at least to the chest wall in patients who had four or more involved lymph nodes, there was less consensus in the cases of T3N0 disease (in which 88.3% would offer PMRT to the chest wall), and even less so for cases in which one to three lymph nodes were involved (85.2% would offer PMRT to the chest wall if extracapsular extension was noted, and 61.7% would offer PMRT if extracapsular extension were absent) [13]. The issues fueling these debates are summarized in the following sections.

Current practice: controversy regarding postmastectomy radiation therapy for patients who have one to three metastatic axillary nodes

The question of whether to irradiate women who have T1-T2 lesions and one to three positive axillary nodes remains unanswered 5 years after the ASCO panel publication and the decision about whether to pursue PMRT in this group requires detailed discussion between the oncologist and patient regarding the expected risk of locoregional recurrence in the

Table 2
2001 American Society of Clinical Oncology practice guidelines for the use of postmastectomy radiation therapy

Patient characteristics	Guideline recommendation or suggestion
Patients who have four or more positive axillary nodes	PMRT is recommended for patients who have four or more positive axillary lymph nodes.
Patients who have one to three positive axillary nodes	There is insufficient evidence to make recommendations regarding patients who have T1/T2 tumors and one to three positive axillary nodes.
Patients who have T3 or stage 3 tumors	PMRT is suggested for patients who have T3 tumors with positive axillary nodes and patients who have operable stage 3 tumors.
Patients undergoing preoperative systemic therapy	There is insufficient evidence to make recommendations whether patients initially treated with preoperative systemic therapy should be given PMRT after surgery.
Modification of these guidelines for special patient subgroups	There is insufficient evidence for modifying these guidelines based on other tumor-related, patient-related, or treatment-related factors.
Chest wall irradiation	In patients given PMRT, the panel suggests that adequately treating the chest wall is mandatory.
Details of chest wall irradiation	There is insufficient evidence for the panel to recommend aspects of chest wall irradiation such as total dose, fraction size, bolus use, and scar boosts.
Axillary nodal irradiation	The panel suggests that full axillary radiotherapy not be given routinely to patients undergoing complete or level I/level II axillary dissection. There is insufficient evidence to suggest whether some patient subgroups may benefit from axillary irradiation.
Supraclavicular nodal irradiation for patients who have four or more positive axillary nodes	The incidence of clinical supraclavicular failure is sufficiently great in patients who have four or more positive axillary nodes that the panel suggests supraclavicular field radiation in all such patients.
Supraclavicular irradiation for patients who have one to three positive axillary nodes	There is insufficient evidence to state whether supraclavicular radiation should or should not be used in patients who have one to three positive axillary nodes.

Internal mammary nodal irradiation	There is insufficient evidence to make recommendations oas to whether deliberate internal mammary nodal irradiation should or should not be used in any patient subgroup.
Sequencing of PMRT and systemic therapy	There is insufficient evidence to recommend the optimal sequencing of chemotherapy, tamoxifen, and PMRT. The panel does suggest, given the available evidence regarding toxicities, that doxorubicin not be administered concurrently with PMRT.
Integration of PMRT and reconstructive surgery	There is insufficient evidence to make recommendations with regard to the integration of PMRT and reconstructive surgery.
Long-term toxicities	The potential long-term risks of PMRT include lymphedema, brachial plexopathy, radiation pneumonitis, rib fractures, cardiac toxicity, and radiation-induced second neoplasms. There is sufficient evidence for the panel to suggest that, in general, the risk of serious toxicity of PMRT (when performed using modern techniques) is low enough that such considerations should not limit its use when otherwise indicated. However, follow-up in patients treated with current radiotherapy techniques is insufficient to rule out the possibility of very late cardiac toxicity.
Toxicity consideration for special patient subgroups	There is insufficient evidence to make recommendations that PMRT should not be used for some subgroups of patients because of increased rates of toxicity (such as radiation carcinogenesis) compared with the rest of the population.

Abbreviation: PMRT, postmastectomy radiation therapy.

From Recht A, Edge SB, Solin LJ, et al. Postmastectomy radiotherapy: Guidelines of the American Society of Clinical Oncology. J Clin Oncol 2001;19(5):1542; with permission from the American Society of Clinics Oncology.

absence of radiation therapy, the proportionate and absolute risk reductions afforded by PMRT, and the expected impact upon mortality from breast cancer and overall survival. A number of studies have quantified the risk of locoregional recurrence in the absence of PMRT in patients with 1-3 positive nodes.

A large retrospective study by the British Columbia Cancer Agency reviewed the long-term outcomes (mean follow-up, 7.7 years) of 847 mastectomy patients who had T1-T2 lesions and one to three positive axillary nodes [14]. None of these patients received PMRT; the goal of the study was to identify characteristics associated with an increased risk of LRR. In this population, the overall baseline risk of developing LRR was 13% to 16% at 10 years. Age less than 45 years, the presence of more than 25% positive nodes, medial tumor location, and estrogen receptor (ER)-negative tumor status were all independently significant factors for LRR and increased the risk from the baseline; the authors suggest that women who have any individual or a combination of these attributes be considered for PMRT, but the risk–benefit ratio for patients who do not have any positive risk factors is low.

Ten-year risk of locoregional failure related to extent of nodal positivity after mastectomy and chemotherapy (without radiation) also has been reported in retrospective analyses of clinical trials conducted by the Eastern Cooperative Oncology Group (ECOG) [15], the National Surgical Adjuvant Breast and Bowel Project (NSABP) [16], and the MD Anderson Cancer Center [17]. Recht and colleagues reported locoregional failure rates as a function of clinicopathologic features in more than 2000 patients who had breast cancer treated by mastectomy and chemotherapy in four ECOG trials. Locoregional failure occurred in 13% of patients who had one to three metastatic nodes, compared with 29% of patients who had at least four metastatic nodes. Taghian and colleagues [16] reported locoregional failures among more than 5000 patients treated on NSABP trials of mastectomy followed by chemotherapy, with rates of 13%, 24%, and 32% for patients who had one to three, four to nine, and 10 or more metastatic nodes, respectively. Katz and colleagues [17] observed locoregional failures rates of 4%, 10%, 21%, and 22% among more than 1000 patients treated in five MD Anderson Cancer Center trials in whom axillary dissection revealed zero, one to three, four to nine, and 10 or more metastatic nodes, respectively.

The Danish Breast Cancer Group conducted two large, prospective clinical trials involving 1708 premenopausal [18] and 1375 postmenopausal [19] patients who had breast cancer treated by mastectomy and systemic therapy (tamoxifen for the postmenopausal patients and chemotherapy for the premenopausal patients) and who were assigned randomly to receive PMRT or no PMRT. As shown in Table 1, this study reported improved overall survival as well as locoregional control for patients randomly assigned to receive PMRT. Of note, these benefits were seen for patients who had one to three metastatic nodes and also for patients who had four or more metastatic nodes. This trial, however, has been criticized for a number of reasons, including the surgical treatment rendered. The average number of nodes retrieved from the axillary lymph node dissection specimens (seven) was somewhat lower than would be expected in a standard level I and II dissection, prompting concern that inadequate regional surgery may have contributed to an increased incidence of locoregional failures or led to the underestimation of the true extent of axillary disease in these patients.

The British Columbia group randomly assigned 318 patients who had node-positive breast cancer to PMRT or no PMRT in addition to mastectomy and chemotherapy [20,21]. This trial resulted in findings similar to those of the Danish studies. In both the Danish and British Columbia studies, the LRR rates in the control arms (no PMRT) for patients who had one to three metastatic nodes were substantially higher (30%–33%) than the locoregional failure rates that have been observed historically for these patients when treated by surgery and mastectomy alone. As noted earlier, the MD Anderson Cancer Center, ECOG, the NSABP, and the British Columbia Cancer Agency reported locoregional failure rates of 10% to 16% in patients who had one to three metastatic nodes. The US Intergroup Trial S9927 [22] was designed specifically to address the question of PMRT in mastectomy patients who have one to three metastatic axillary nodes by randomly assigning patients to PMRT or to observation (in addition to systemic therapy as indicated), but the ASCO guidelines in 2001 cite studies indicating that locoregional recurrence rates are high in patients with T3 disease, even when node-negative [23,24]. Since then, additional studies have been reported regarding the need for PMRT in patients with node-negative breast cancer, suggesting that rates of locoregional recurrence may be lower than expected, at least among patients with T3N0 disease that does not reach extremely large size. A unfortunately this phase III trial was terminated early because of poor accrual. This important therapeutic question therefore remains unanswered. Nevertheless, given the findings of the meta-analyses and the two most recent large trials of PMRT, all patients with node-positive disease warrant referral for consultation with a radiation oncologist to discuss in detail whether they wish to pursue PMRT based upon the current evidence regarding their risks and the risk reduction afforded by PMRT.

Current practice: controversy regarding postmastectomy radiation therapy for patients who have T3, node-negative breast cancer

Recent retrospective study [23] of 70 patients treated at three institutions by mastectomy and systemic therapy (but not PMRT) for T3N0 disease with mean tumor size of 6 cm revealed a 5-year LRR rate of only 7.6% [24]. Another recent study [25] examined the long-term outcomes of 313 node-negative patients who had tumors larger than 5 cm who underwent mastectomy but not PMRT in five NSABP trials. The investigators found that the overall 10-year cumulative incidence of isolated locoregional failure was 7.1%, and the incidence of locoregional failure with or without distant failure in this population was 10.0%. They were unable to identify any statistically significant prognostic factors for locoregional failure. With such low incidences of locoregional failure over an extended follow-up period, the authors strongly recommended that patients who have negative axillae not undergo PMRT, in spite of the size of the initial tumor [26]. It is important to note, however, that these were small, retrospective series, and the median size of the tumors in these studies was on the smaller end of the spectrum for T3 tumors, so that relatively fewer tumors of extremely large size were included. Patients with T3N0 tumors still warrant consultation with a radiation oncologist, who may discuss these data with the patient as well as the older data suggesting high rates of failure in patients with large tumor size, in order to help guide the patient's decision regarding PMRT.

On the other hand, other studies have identified a number of risk factors for recurrence in broader populations of node-negative patients who had tumors of all sizes and have suggested that patients who have multiple risk factors may be at higher risk for locoregional failure. A retrospective analysis of 1275 node-negative patients treated in the International Breast Cancer Study Group trials suggested that although overall LRR rates were low, certain subgroups who had multiple risk factors, including vascular invasion and tumor size greater than 2 cm in premenopausal patients and vascular invasion in postmenopausal patients, may have higher risk [27]. A retrospective analysis of 877 node-negative postmastectomy patients treated at the Massachusetts General Hospital confirmed a relatively low overall 6.0% cumulative incidence of LRR at 10 years [28]. It also identified a number of risk factors for locoregional failure, including (1) tumor size greater than 2 cm, (2) premenopausal status, (3) margins less than 2 mm, and (4) evidence of lymphovascular invasion. Similarly, a series of 1505 women who had T1-2N0 breast cancer treated with mastectomy alone in British Columbia [29] found a 10-year LRR rate of 7.8% overall but higher rates in subgroups who had multiple risk factors, including grade, lymphovascular invasion, tumor stage, and absence of systemic therapy. Thus, it seems appropriate at least to consider PMRT in some node-negative patients, even with lesions that may not exceed 5 cm in size, but with multiple other adverse features, as well as in patients with tumors that are extremely large in size.

Current practice: controversy regarding postmastectomy radiation therapy for patients treated with neoadjuvant chemotherapy

The number of patients who have advanced disease being treated with preoperative systemic chemotherapy is growing, because this strategy is used increasingly for relatively early-stage breast cancer as a means of improving lumpectomy eligibility. Since 2001, two retrospective studies from the MD Anderson Cancer Center have addressed the use of PMRT in patients treated with neoadjuvant chemotherapy. As retrospective studies, they cannot be categorized as level I or level II evidence, but they do offer some interesting information that may prove useful in the treatment of this expanding population.

The first study, published in 2004, examined the outcomes of 542 patients treated with neoadjuvant chemotherapy, mastectomy, and PMRT. A 10-year retrospective review compared these patients with a control group of 134 patients not treated with PMRT. At 10 years, local-regional recurrence rates were significantly lower for irradiated patients (11% versus 22%). Patients who presented with clinical stage 3 disease and who subsequently achieved a complete pathologic response to systemic therapy also had a significantly lower LRR rate than patients not treated with PMRT. At 10 years, these patients had a 3% LRR rate, versus 33% in nonirradiated patients. Postmastectomy radiation also improved cause-specific survival in patients who had stage 3b disease, clinical T4 tumors, and more than four positive lymph nodes [30]. The authors suggested that PMRT should be considered for patients in all of these subsets, regardless of their response to preoperative systemic chemotherapy.

A follow-up retrospective review of the same series of 542 patients was published in 2005 examining the risk factors associated with LRR. The authors remarked on the importance of disease staging both before and after neoadjuvant chemotherapy, because several risk factors were associated with either the pretreatment or posttreatment extent of disease. Supraclavicular nodal involvement on presentation was associated with a higher risk of LRR after treatment. On postneoadjuvant chemotherapy assessment, evidence of skin or nipple involvement and extracapsular invasion also were correlated strongly with LRR. Lack of tamoxifen use postoperatively also was associated with increased LRR, but, because of the preponderance of ER-negative patients who had increased LRR, this finding was considered to be of little clinical significance. Of note, ER receptor–negative disease was the strongest predictor of LRR in this group. Patients who had one or none of these factors had a 4% 10-year LRR rate, but this rate jumped to 28% with the presence of three or more risk factors [31].

The NSABP B-18 trial offered a powerful opportunity to study patterns of locoregional failure in patients receiving neoadjuvant chemotherapy. This protocol randomly assigned women who had stage 1–3 breast cancer to receive four cycles of doxorubicin and Cytoxan chemotherapy in the preoperative or postoperative sequence. Use of PMRT was specifically excluded. Among patients undergoing mastectomy, risk factors for LRR were the same in both the pre- and postoperative chemotherapy arms: age less than 50 years, four or more metastatic nodes, and increasing primary tumor size. A critical component of these findings was that locoregional failure rates were similar in the pre- and postoperative chemotherapy patient subsets as stratified by these various categories of disease stage, indicating that downstaging by neoadjuvant therapy did not compromise locoregional control. In any case, given the complexities of assessing risks based on prechemotherapy clinical data and postchemotherapy pathology in patients treated with neoadjuvant chemotherapy, treatment in a multidisciplinary context with radiation oncology consultation before any treatment commences would be especially prudent in these cases.

Current practice: controversy regarding postmastectomy radiation therapy for margin control

The use of radiation therapy for mastectomy patients who have microscopically positive or close margins is another area of concern, and in these patients PMRT may offer some benefit. A small retrospective study at Fox Chase Cancer Center examined the outcomes of women with stage 1-2 breast cancer treated with mastectomy whose tumors were less than 5 cm in size, involved zero to three positive lymph nodes, and who had close (less than 1 cm from the margin of resection) or positive margins postoperatively. They found that the likelihood of having a positive or close margin after mastectomy was low but was more common in younger patients. Furthermore, patients aged 50 years or younger who had T1 or T2 lesions and close or positive postoperative margins had an 8-year cumulative incidence of chest wall recurrence of 28% despite the use of adjuvant systemic therapy in the majority; therefore, younger women in this select population should be strongly considered for PMRT [32].

A second, slightly larger series investigating the use of PMRT in patients who have positive postmastectomy margins was published in 2003 [33]. Similar to the Fox Chase study of patients who had close or positive margins and the studies of node-negative patients discussed earlier, the rates of LRR in the overall population of node-negative patients who had positive margins were low both with and without PMRT. Patients in this study treated with mastectomy but not with PMRT had a local relapse rate of 9.4% and a regional relapse rate of 5.7%. Patients treated with PMRT had a LRR rate of 2.4%. Although the power of the study was limited by the sample size, the authors also noted several trends associated with increased LRR, including age under 50 years, T2 tumor size, grade 3 histology, and evidence of lymphovascular invasion; patients with these risk factors had a LRR rate approaching 20%. Again, this study suggested that having close or positive margins alone is not a strong indication for PMRT; however, younger patients and patients who have larger tumors or more aggressive tumor histology may benefit from PMRT. Unfortunately, the small number of patients involved in these studies indicates the need for further investigation in this population. Most radiation oncologists continue to consider positive margins to be a standard general indication for radiotherapy, and patients with close or positive margins merit referral for radiation oncology consultation and further discussion.

Complications and adverse effects of postmastectomy radiation therapy

The benefits of any therapeutic strategy must be weighed against the risk for toxicity, and the adverse effects of PMRT therefore must be balanced against the potential for improved outcomes. The risk of lymphedema in patients treated with PMRT is variable but is greater than in patients treated with axillary dissection alone [9,34–36]. A retrospective review performed at Roswell Park investigated the incidence of lymphedema in patients treated with PMRT. This study cited a 27% incidence of lymphedema in 105 patients treated with PMRT. Total dose and posterior axillary boost doses also were significantly associated with the development of lymphedema [34]. Other studies have suggested that the risk of lymphedema increases with the extent of surgical dissection [37].

Cardiac toxicity is also a consideration [38–41], especially in older patients and in light of the growing use of cardiotoxic systemic agents such as anthracyclines and trastuzumab in patients who have breast cancer. With advances in the administration of radiation therapy, the risks of radiation pneumonitis, brachial plexopathy, and rib fractures is reduced but is not eliminated [9]. One small series of patients undergoing PMRT at the University of Louisville noted one patient who developed radiation pneumonitis among 273 treated with PMRT [42]. Also, the rare complication of secondary cancers developing in the irradiated field is a risk that should be discussed with all patients [43–45].

Summary

The indications for and benefits of PMRT continue to evolve. Advances in systemic adjuvant therapy and targeted therapy for breast cancer are likely to play an increasingly important role in control of locoregional as well as distant disease, and patterns of chest wall failure will require ongoing scrutiny to define the net benefit derived from PMRT. There are clear indications for the use of PMRT, based on multiple randomized clinical trials and meta-analyses, in patients who have four or more positive axillary lymph nodes. Delivery of PMRT in these patients results in decreased LRR rates and improved overall survival. Subsets of patients who have breast cancer for whom the benefits of PMRT are less well defined include patients who have T1/T2 primary tumors and one to three metastatic nodes; patients who have node-negative breast cancer but multiple other adverse prognostic features, and patients whose cancers have been substantially downstaged by neoadjuvant chemotherapy. Ultimately, some of these ambiguities may be clarified by the results of the ongoing British SUPREMO randomized trial of chest wall radiation in patients who have T1-2N1 or high-risk T2N0 disease. In the meantime, for these intermediate indications of PMRT, other clinicopathologic features, such as age less than 50 years, ER-negative tumor status, and lymphovascular invasion, may be useful in the final decision-making process. If participation in a randomized trial is not available for patients in these ambiguous groups, patients should be carefully informed of their estimated risk of recurrence in the absence of PMRT and the proportional and absolute reductions in risk of recurrence and improvements in survival—if any—that can be expected from the use of PMRT based on that level of risk, Such discussions are optimally held in a multidisciplinary setting in which surgeons, radiation oncologists, and medical oncologists can collaborate in guiding the patient through the complicated issues discussed here.

References

[1] Early Breast Cancer Trialists' Collaborative Group. Effects of radiotherapy and of differences in the extent of surgery for early breast cancer on local recurrence and 15-year survival: an overview of the randomised trials. Lancet 2005;366(9503):2087–106.

[2] Early Breast Cancer Trialists' Collaborative Group. Effects of radiotherapy and surgery in early breast cancer: an overview of the randomised trials. N Engl J Med 1995;333:1444–55.

[3] Early Breast Cancer Trialists' Collaborative Group. Favourable and unfavourable effects on long-term survival of radiotherapy for early breast cancer: an overview of the randomised trials. Lancet 2000;355(9217):1757–70.

[4] Cuzick J, et al. Overview of randomized trials of postoperative adjuvant radiotherapy in breast cancer. Cancer Treat Rep 1987;71(1):15–29.

[5] Cuzick J, et al. Cause-specific mortality in long-term survivors of breast cancer who participated in trials of radiotherapy. J Clin Oncol 1994;12(3):447–53.

[6] Whelan TJ, et al. Does locoregional radiation therapy improve survival in breast cancer? A meta-analysis. J Clin Oncol 2000;18(6):1220–9.

[7] Van de Steene J, Soete G, Storme G. Adjuvant radiotherapy for breast cancer significantly improves overall survival: the missing link. Radiother Oncol 2000;55(3):263–72.

[8] Recht A, Edge SB. Evidence-based indications for postmastectomy irradiation. Surg Clin North Am 2003;83(4):995–1013.

[9] Recht A, et al. Postmastectomy radiotherapy: clinical practice guidelines of the American Society of Clinical Oncology. J Clin Oncol 2001;19(5):1539–69.

[10] Harris JR, et al. Consensus statement on postmastectomy radiation therapy. Int J Radiat Oncol Biol Phys 1999;1999(44):5.

[11] Taylor ME, et al. Postmastectomy radiotherapy. American College of Radiology. ACR Appropriateness Criteria. Radiology 2000; (215 Suppl): p. 1153–70.

[12] Truong PT, et al. Clinical practice guidelines for the care and treatment of breast cancer: 16. Locoregional post-mastectomy radiotherapy. CMAJ 2004;170(8):1263–73.

[13] Ceilley E, et al. Radiotherapy for invasive breast cancer in North America and Europe: results of a survey. Int J Radiat Oncol Biol Phys 2005;61(2):365–73.

[14] Truong PT, et al. Selecting breast cancer patients with T1-T2 tumors and one to three positive axillary nodes at high postmastectomy locoregional recurrence risk for adjuvant radiotherapy. Int J Radiat Oncol Biol Phys 2005;61(5):1337–47.

[15] Recht A, et al. Locoregional failure 10 years after mastectomy and adjuvant chemotherapy with or without tamoxifen without irradiation: experience of the Eastern Cooperative Oncology Group. J Clin Oncol 1999;17(6):1689–700.

[16] Taghian A, et al. Patterns of locoregional failure in patients with operable breast cancer treated by mastectomy and adjuvant chemotherapy with or without tamoxifen and without radiotherapy: results from five National Surgical Adjuvant Breast and Bowel Project randomized clinical trials. J Clin Oncol 2004;22(21):4247–54.

[17] Katz A, et al. Locoregional recurrence patterns after mastectomy and doxorubicin-based chemotherapy: implications for postoperative irradiation. J Clin Oncol 2000;18(15):2817–27.

[18] Overgaard M, et al. Postoperative radiotherapy in high-risk premenopausal women with breast cancer who receive adjuvant chemotherapy. Danish Breast Cancer Cooperative Group 82b Trial. N Engl J Med 1997;337(14):949–55.

[19] Overgaard M, et al. Postoperative radiotherapy in high-risk postmenopausal breast-cancer patients given adjuvant tamoxifen: Danish Breast Cancer Cooperative Group DBCG 82c randomised trial. Lancet 1999;353(9165):1641–8.

[20] Ragaz J, et al. Adjuvant radiotherapy and chemotherapy in node-positive premenopausal women with breast cancer. N Engl J Med 1997;337(14):956–62.

[21] Ragaz J, et al. Locoregional radiation therapy in patients with high-risk breast cancer receiving adjuvant chemotherapy: 20-year results of the British Columbia randomized trial. J Nat Cancer Inst 2005;97(2):116–26.

[22] Pierce LJ. Treatment guidelines and techniques in delivery of postmastectomy radiotherapy in management of operable breast cancer. J Natl Cancer Inst Monogr 2001;(30): 117–24.

[23] Mignano JE, et al. Local recurrence after mastectomy in patient with T3N0 breast carcinoma treated without postoperative irradiation. Breast Cancer Res Treat 1996;41:255 (abstract).

[24] Helinto M, et al. Post-mastectomy radiotherapy in pT3N0M breast cancer: is it needed? Radiother Oncol 1999;52:213–7.

[25] Floyd SR, et al. Low local recurrence rate without postmastectomy radiation in node-negative breast cancer patients with tumors 5 cm and larger. Int J Radiat Oncol Biol Phys 2006; 66(2):358–64.

[26] Taghian AG, et al. Low locoregional recurrence rate among node-negative breast cancer patients with tumors 5 cm.

[27] Wallgren A, et al. Risk factors for locoregional recurrence among breast cancer patients: results from International Breast Cancer Study Group Trials I through VII. J Clin Oncol 2003;21(7):1205–13.

[28] Jagsi R, et al. Locoregional recurrence rates and prognostic factors for failure in node-negative patients treated with mastectomy: implications for postmastectomy radiation. Int J Radiat Oncol Biol Phys 2005;62(4):1035–9.

[29] Truong PT, et al. Patient subsets with T1-T2, node-negative breast cancer at high locoregional recurrence risk after mastectomy. Int J Radiat Oncol Biol Phys 2005;62(1):175–82.

[30] Huang EH, et al. Postmastectomy radiation improves local-regional control and survival for selected patients with locally advanced breast cancer treated with neoadjuvant chemotherapy and mastectomy. J Clin Oncol 2004;22(23):4691–9.

[31] Huang EH, et al. Predictors of locoregional recurrence in patients with locally advanced breast cancer treated with neoadjuvant chemotherapy, mastectomy, and radiotherapy. Int J Radiat Oncol Biol Phys 2005;62(2):351–7.

[32] Freedman GM, et al. A close or positive margin after mastectomy is not an indication for chest wall irradiation except in women aged fifty or younger. Int J Radiat Oncol Biol Phys 1998;41(3):599–605.

[33] Truong PT, et al. A positive margin is not always an indication for radiotherapy after mastectomy in early breast cancer. Int J Radiat Oncol Biol Phys 2004;58(3):797–804.

[34] Hinrichs CS, et al. Lymphedema secondary to postmastectomy radiation: incidence and risk factors. Ann Surg Oncol 2004;11(6):573–80.

[35] Pierce LJ. The use of radiotherapy after mastectomy: a review of the literature. J Clin Oncol 2005;23(8):1706–17.

[36] Coen JJ, et al. Risk of lymphedema after regional nodal irradiation with breast conservation therapy. Int J Radiat Oncol Biol Phys 2003;55(5):1209–15.

[37] Larson D, et al. Edema of the arm as a function of the extent of axillary surgery in patients with Stage I–II carcinoma of the breast treated with primary radiotherapy. Int J Radiat Oncol Biol Phys 1986;12:1575–82.

[38] Paszat LF, et al. Mortality from myocardial infarction after adjuvant radiotherapy for breast cancer in the surveillance, epidemiology, end-results cancer registries. J Clin Oncol 1998;16: 2625–31.

[39] Harris EE, et al. Late cardiac mortality and morbidity in early-stage breast cancer patients after breast-conservation treatment. J Clin Oncol 2006;24(25):4100–6.

[40] Marks LB, et al. The incidence and functional consequences of RT-associated cardiac perfusion defects. Int J Radiat Oncol Biol Phys 2005.

[41] Amin-Zimmerman F, et al. Postmastectomy chest wall radiation with electron-beam therapy: outcomes and complications at the University of Louisville. Cancer J 2005;11(3):204–8.

[42] Taghian A, et al. Long-term risk of sarcoma following radiation treatment for breast cancer. Int J Radiat Oncol Biol Phys 1991;21(2):361–7.

[43] McArdle CS, et al. Adjuvant radiotherapy and chemotherapy in breast cancer. Br J Surg 1986;73(4):264–6.

[44] Griem KL, et al. The 5-year results of a randomized trial of adjuvant radiation therapy after chemotherapy in breast cancer patients treated with mastectomy. J Clin Oncol 1987;5(10): 1546–55.

[45] Velez-Garcia E, et al. Postsurgical adjuvant chemotherapy with or without radiotherapy in women with breast cancer and positive axillary nodes: a South-Eastern Cancer Study Group (SEG) Trial. Eur J Cancer 1992;28A(11):1833–7.

ELSEVIER
SAUNDERS

Surg Clin N Am 87 (2007) 527–538

SURGICAL
CLINICS OF
NORTH AMERICA

Locoregional Resection in Stage IV Breast Cancer: Tumor Biology, Molecular and Clinical Perspectives

Julie E. Lang, MD, Gildy V. Babiera, MD*

Department of Surgical Oncology, The University of Texas M. D. Anderson Cancer Center, P.O. Box 301402, Houston, TX 77230-1402, USA

Surgical treatment of the intact primary in patients diagnosed with Stage IV breast cancer is generally reserved for palliative indications—bleeding, tumor ulceration, infection and hygienic considerations. In 1943, Haagensen and Stout [1] published their criteria of inoperability for carcinoma of the breast, which hold true today when considering a resection for curative intent. These criteria include tumor fixation to the chest wall, ulceration and peau d'orange, features considered to be grave prognostic signs. Surgical treatment alone is unlikely to prolong life in patients who possess these grave signs. Because of improvements in breast cancer screening and awareness, fewer patients present with inoperable breast cancer. In modern breast cancer treatment, we are faced with a different dilemma, because some patients are found on imaging studies to have oligometastatic or stable metastatic disease with an intact operable primary. This article considers the role of surgical treatment of the intact primary as part of multimodal treatment for Stage IV breast cancer patients because several recent challenges have arisen to previous dogma to never operate on Stage IV breast cancer patients except with palliative intent.

Background

Three dominant theories of breast cancer tumor progression have evolved: (1) the Halsted paradigm, (2) the Fisher paradigm, and (3) the

---

* Corresponding author. Department of Surgical Oncology, The University of Texas M. D. Anderson Cancer Center, P.O. Box 301402, 1515 Holcombe Blvd., Unit 444, Houston, TX 77230-1402.

E-mail address: gvbabiera@mdanderson.org (G.V. Babiera).

0039-6109/07/$ - see front matter © 2007 Elsevier Inc. All rights reserved.
doi:10.1016/j.suc.2007.01.001
surgical.theclinics.com

Spectrum paradigm. The first, the Halsted paradigm, states that breast cancer follows an orderly progression, from primary tumor to axillary lymph nodes, and then finally on to metastatic sites. Intuitively, therefore, aggressive locoregional resection of tumor and regional metastases would be paramount to achieving superior survival benefits over less minimal surgery. However, the National Surgical Adjuvant Breast and Bowel Project breast carcinoma B-04 study (NSABP-B-04) proved that no benefit exists for radical mastectomy over less radical surgical treatments [2], dispelling the notion that more radical surgery could prove to be a more efficacious cure. Furthermore, the impact of axillary nodal dissection on patients' overall survival is controversial; the NSABP-B-04 study found that axillary nodal dissection provided a 4% improvement in survival rate versus no dissection, but the study was underpowered to detect a statistically significant difference in survival [2]. Gervasoni and colleagues [3] reviewed the literature on axillary dissection and concluded that it does not impact overall survival, although nodal status is an essential staging element and prognostic marker. In a conflicting report, Krag and Single [4] analyzed the Surveillance, Epidemiology, and End Results (SEER) data (72,102 patients) and found that the removal of axillary lymph nodes, even when such nodes are pathologically negative, significantly improves patient survival. They found a hazard ratio of death of approximately 8% to 9% less for each additional five nodes removed for the node-positive group; for the node-negative group they found a hazard ratio of death of approximately 5% less for each five nodes removed, a benefit on par with that of systemic chemotherapy. No randomized controlled trials comparing overall survival for patients who underwent sentinel lymph node dissection versus those who underwent axillary nodal dissection are currently available. Currently, axillary lymph node dissections are the standard of care for patients who have positive nodal disease; however, if the therapeutic role of axillary dissection for local control is controversial, it is not surprising that the role of resection of the intact primary in Stage IV breast cancer is that much more controversial.

Clinicians have recognized that even Stage I breast cancer patients over long-term follow-up (20 years) carry a 20% risk of metastatic disease. Clearly, in many cases locoregional control of breast cancer is necessary but not sufficient to achieve cure. The second theory, the Fisher paradigm, contends that breast cancer is a systemic disease at its inception and the only hope for definitive cure is by addressing the micrometastatic burden of occult cancer. The third and a more moderate, generally accepted viewpoint, however, is the Spectrum paradigm, which is essentially a compromise between the Halsted and Fisher paradigms: breast cancer may be but is not universally systemic at its inception. Locoregional treatments are important because often a primary tumor or nodal deposits occur before dissemination of metastases. Clearly, the best chance for cure is achieved via locoregional and systemic treatment through a multimodal approach for breast cancer patients of all stages.

Rationale for resection of the intact primary tumor

The precise effect of locoregional resection of the intact primary tumor in the metastatic setting is unknown. Theoretical advantages to removal of the intact primary tumor in Stage IV breast cancer include cessation of further seeding of the blood with the micrometastatic population of cells shed by the primary lesion. Additionally, surgical intervention may permit decreasing the overall tumor burden, with potential for prolongation of metastatic progression-free survival. The role of metastatectomy for distant metastases of breast cancer is evolving, but clearly some Stage IV patients do benefit from surgical control of distant metastatic sites [5]. This same approach could be applied to Stage IV breast cancer patients who have an intact primary tumor in a properly designed randomized controlled trial to study this issue. Resection of primary tumor and metastases also would supply cancer researchers with much needed tissue for their tumor banks—enabling the advancement of our understanding of the molecular derangements associated with metastatic potential.

Metastatic progression at the cellular and molecular level

Understanding of the biology of metastasis is crucial when considering whether surgical intervention is appropriate treatment for these patients. Important advances in molecular profiling of metastases, tumor immunology and tumor growth kinetics are reviewed below. These areas of research inform new hypotheses on mechanisms of metastasis in breast cancer, which are listed here:

- Possible mechanisms of metastasis—newer theories
  Parallel evolution/circulating tumor cells
  Gene expression of the primary tumor predicts metastasis
  Breast cancer stem cell
- Metastasis and host interactions: feedback regulatory mechanisms
  Primary tumor and immunologic effects
  Tumor dormancy theory

A critical appraisal of the relevant basic science and clinical evidence is presented to provide insight into the controversy of surgical resection of the intact primary for Stage IV patients.

New molecular-based hypotheses of metastasis in breast cancer

The principle that metastasis is a late event in tumorigenesis has been challenged by recent molecular evidence, which has resulted in three new models of metastasis in breast cancer: (1) the parallel evolution (or circulating tumor cell) model, (2) the gene expression of the primary tumor predicts metastasis model, and (3) the breast cancer stem cell model [6].

The parallel evolution hypothesis suggests that circulating tumor cells (found in blood) or disseminated tumor cells (found in bone marrow and secondary organs such as liver, bone, or lung) are found early in tumorigenesis, and are independent of the primary tumor characteristics [7]. In a pooled analysis of nine studies including 4703 breast cancer patients who had Stage I through III disease, Braun and colleagues [8] found bone marrow micrometastases in 30.6% of breast cancer patients. The presence of micrometastasis in the bone marrow at the time of diagnosis was associated with poor overall survival and breast cancer disease free survival; however, limitations of this study included differing assays used for assessment of micrometastases and meta-analysis study design. Conceptually, patients viewed as early stage by conventional staging who are found to harbor micrometastatic disease are not very different from Stage IV breast cancer patients with minimal metastatic burden or Stage IV, no evidence of disease (NED) breast cancer patients. If surgical treatment is the standard of care for these early-stage breast cancer patients who have micrometastatic disease, then it may seem reasonable to perform surgical intervention for the Stage IV patients who have an intact primary.

A second new hypothesis of metastatic progression proposes that intrinsic molecular characteristics of the primary tumor predict risk of subsequent metastasis. Data derived from gene expression microarrays and comparative genomic hybridization provide important information on the molecular progression from primary tumor to metastasis. Studies of single-cell comparative genomic hybridization of disseminated tumor cells derived from bone marrow show that, surprisingly, these cells have significantly fewer chromosomal anomalies compared with either primary tumors or distant visceral metastases [7]. This suggests that systemic progression of circulating tumor cells may be a relatively early event in breast cancer. Several gene expression signatures of primary tumors have been reported to be associated with increased risk of metastasis, suggesting that the capacity to metastasize might be an early step in oncogenesis [9,10]. This again underscores the premise that breast cancer is both a local and systemic disease that requires multimodal therapies inclusive of effective local control. According to this model, resection of the primary tumor with modern, individualized chemotherapy regimens to target the circulating tumor cell burden should be the suggested treatment goal for these patients.

The third new hypothesis is the breast cancer stem cell theory, a relatively new area of breast cancer research that has recently received growing interest. This theory contends that specialized tumor-initiating cancer cells have the exclusive potential to proliferate and form new sites of tumor metastasis [11]. In murine studies, as few as 100 breast cancer stem cells implanted into the mammary fat pad were able to form tumors, whereas thousands of cancer cells lacking this stem cell phenotype were unable to produce tumor growth [12]. Proponents of this theory contend that targeted therapies directed at the stem cell population are requisite to achieve effective cures for breast cancer. Similar to the parallel evolution model, extirpation of the primary tumor followed by effective targeted chemotherapy to wipe out the stem cell population would be the goal in this model.

Metastasis and host interactions: feedback regulatory mechanisms

Metastasis and immunologic effects

Metastatic cancer cells have numerous effects on the immune system. They elaborate multiple neoantigens that act as proinflammatory signals that activate both the innate and adaptive immunity pathways [13]. Additionally, established malignancies use induction of immune tolerance to avoid immune surveillance. A recent study used a mouse model to show that surgical removal of the primary tumor in mice who have metastatic breast cancer reverses tumor-induced immunosuppression, restoring both B and T cell-mediated immune function, even when disseminated metastatic disease was present [14]. Another recent study showed that breast cancer patients' T lymphocytes produce lower amounts of cytokines (interleukin [IL]-2, interferon [IFN]-gamma, tumor necrosis factor [TNF]-alpha and IL-4) compared with healthy controls [15]. Interestingly, dysregulation of T-cell response correlated with the number of micrometastases present in the bone marrow.

Tumor dormancy theory

The tumor dormancy theory, based on retrospective series [16], proposes that at the time of primary breast cancer resection the occult micrometastatic burden may rest dormant for up to 20 to 30 years. This theory is based on Gompertzian growth kinetics—exponential growth when small numbers of cancer cells are present, with slower growth when larger numbers of cancer cells are present. Studies using animal models have demonstrated that removal of the primary tumor resulted in proliferation of macrometastases by increasing angiogenesis and reduction of apoptosis [17]. Some proponents of this theory parallel this finding to the Lewis lung model, in which removal of the primary tumor stimulates profound angiogenesis and proliferation [18]. This theory is a potential argument against resection of the intact primary in Stage IV breast cancer patients, although only anecdotal data exist to substantiate that surgery hastens metastatic progression in these patients. This has only rarely been observed in clinical practice, with only level 4 evidence to support this theory. Certainly our patients deserve better scientific evidence to guide clinical judgment on this question than what exists at the present time.

Stage IV presentations and breast cancer survival

In general, metastatic breast cancer is an incurable disease with a median prognosis of 18 to 24 months [19]; however, location of disease recurrence correlates with differing 5-year survival rates: soft tissue, 41%; bone, 23%; and visceral metastases, 13% [20]. Furthermore, several studies have noted variations in survival depending on the time period of treatment, with improved survival over time. In a multivariate analysis of 834 women who developed recurrent breast cancer from 1974 to 2000, Giordano and colleagues [20] demonstrated that year of recurrence was associated with a trend toward improved survival. Andre and colleagues [19] confirmed this finding in a study of 724 breast cancer patients who had newly diagnosed metastatic disease; overall 3-year survival for patients treated from 1987 to 1993 was 27%, whereas for patients treated from 1994 to 2000 was 44%. The findings from these two studies suggest that improvement in adjuvant therapy is resulting in demonstrable improvements in survival for patients who have Stage IV breast cancer.

Rarely (1%–3%), Stage IV breast cancer patients can achieve a complete remission, with survival sometimes beyond 20 years after chemotherapy [21,22]. These unusual long-term survivors who have Stage IV disease are typically young, have oligometastatic disease and excellent performance status; therefore this subgroup challenges the notion that Stage IV breast cancer is universally fatal and supports the possibility of inducing a prolonged remission [21].

Another subgroup deserving special consideration is breast cancer patients who develop an isolated distant recurrence that may be treated by either curative surgical resection, radiation, or both, and are rendered Stage IV-NED. Fewer than 10% of metastatic breast cancer patients fall into the category of Stage IV-NED. Rivera and colleagues [23] compared three different adjuvant treatment regimens to locoregional therapy alone for Stage IV-NED breast cancer. They found a benefit in 3-year overall survival (84% versus 55%) and disease-free survival (66% versus 11%) for patients who received doxorubicin-based adjuvant chemotherapy compared with those who received locoregional therapy alone. These excellent results demonstrate the combined effect of multimodal therapy. The sites of recurrence included soft tissue (91%), bone (2%), visceral (5%), and brain (2%) [23]. The treatment arm that yielded the most beneficial overall results for Stage IV-NED breast cancer patients included chemotherapy plus 80% of the patients treated with surgical treatment of recurrences, 2% radiation therapy alone, and 18% both surgical and radiation therapy [23]. Clearly, these improved results for Stage IV-NED patients are predicated on adequate surgical resection for locoregional control. Given the improved efficacy of modern chemotherapy and the benefits gained from locoregional treatment with surgery, it only seems logical to re-evaluate the role of surgical excision of the intact primary in Stage IV patients who have minimal metastatic burden because these patients may in a similar fashion be converted to Stage IV-NED patients.

Resection of the intact primary in Stage IV breast cancer

Very limited data exist to guide surgeons on locoregional treatment of the intact primary tumor in Stage IV breast cancer. In fact, only four retrospective studies are available in the literature to address this issue (Table 1). These four studies are summarized below. The studies include level 3 and level 4 study designs (retrospective cohorts evaluated with or without control groups).

The first study to question the role of aggressive surgical extirpation of the intact primary in Stage IV breast cancer is by Khan and colleagues [24]. This study retrospectively analyzed data from the National Cancer database of the American College of Surgeons collected between the years 1990 and 1993 for women presenting with Stage IV disease. This database accumulates information from cancer registries across the county—as a result, although treatment rendered may differ dramatically between centers, the database reflects a cross-section of cancer treatment around the country. A total of 16,023 patients who had Stage IV disease were identified in this database during the study period; most had either T1 or T2 disease. Of these, 9162 (57.2%) underwent either partial (3513) or total mastectomy (5649). Patients who had only a single metastatic focus were more likely to receive local treatment than those who had more than one site of metastatic disease ($P < .0001$). A multivariate analysis was performed to examine the impact of surgery on the primary endpoint of time to death. The multivariate proportional hazards model factored in number of metastatic sites, type of metastatic burden (visceral, soft tissue, or bone) and the extent of resection of the primary tumor as significant independent variables. Women treated surgically with clear margins had a superior prognosis than women not treated surgically, as reflected by a hazard ratio of 0.61. Independent of margin status, partial mastectomy conferred a hazard ratio of 0.88. whereas total mastectomy conferred a hazard ratio of 0.74 compared with no surgical excision. An advantage of this study is the large number of patients examined. One obvious limitation is that there is no molecular subclassification of cancers in this study (for example, estrogen receptor, progesterone receptor, human epidermal growth factor receptor 2 [HER2/neu] status), nor is there information on timing of surgery or tumor grade, and the distribution of more indolent and more aggressive tumors within this series is unknown. Also, the clinical biases that resulted in some patients having surgical excision while others received no surgical treatment cannot be controlled for in a large multi-institutional retrospective database study such as this. No information is available regarding other treatment regimens in terms of chemotherapy or endocrine therapy for the study patients.

Table 1
Studies on resection of the intact primary tumor in metastatic breast cancer

Author	Year	Number treated operatively	Number treated non-operatively	Follow-up duration	Primary endpoint	Statistical analysis
Khan et al [24]	2002	9162	6861	NA	Time to death	HR = 0.61 for resection (95% CI = 0.58–0.65), P value not reported[a]
Carmichael et al [25]	2002	20	0	23 months	Local control	None—case series only
Rapiti et al [26]	2006	127	173	NA	Risk of mortality	HR = 0.6 for resection (95% CI = 0.4–1.0, P = .49)[a]
Babiera et al [27]	2006	82	142	32.1 months	1) Overall survival 2) Metastatic progression-free survival	1) RR = 0.5 (95% CI = 0.21–1.19, P = .12)[a] 2) RR = 0.54 (95% CI = 0.38–0.77, P = .0007)[a]

Abbreviations: HR, hazard ratio; RR, relative risk.
[a] Cox model

Additionally, this study is subject to all of the limitations of retrospective, population-based studies, particularly in the sense of analyzing data collected by numerous different individuals from different centers with differing treatment practices. That being said, this study did find a survival advantage for patients treated with resection of the intact primary, and appropriately stated the conclusion that resection of the intact primary in Stage IV breast cancer merits consideration with a prospective, randomized controlled study.

Carmichael and colleagues [25] reported a retrospective, small, single institution case series of 20 Stage IV breast cancer patients who underwent local surgery. They reported a median survival after breast surgery of 23 months. Ten of the patients (50%) were alive with no evidence of local disease at 20 months median follow-up. The study authors concluded that surgical resection does have a role in the management of limited Stage IV breast cancer with an intact primary tumor. This study has some limitations, especially given that no control group was implemented in the study design, questioning the significance of these findings. No receptor status of tumors, grade, or rationale for surgical treatment was provided. No details of the specific multimodal treatment regimen were provided. Single-center institutional reports are important when attempting to prove that any treatment may yield improved results at independent centers; this report, however, simply demonstrates proof of principle that further study is necessary to address this question.

Rapiti and colleagues [26] reported a retrospective study of 300 metastatic breast cancer patients recorded in the Geneva Cancer Registry from 1977 to 1996. This included multiple institutions, both public university hospitals and private clinics. Overall, 173 patients (58%) received no surgical treatment, whereas 127 (42%) underwent surgery for the intact primary. Complete excision with clear margins imparted a 40% reduced risk of death on multivariate analysis compared with no surgical treatment ($P = .49$). Patients who had surgical excision with clear margins had 5-year disease-free survival of 27%, compared with 16% for patients who had surgical excision with positive margins, and 12% for patients who did not have surgery. This effect was particularly evident in patients who had bone metastasis only ($P = .001$). Unsurprisingly, tumor characteristics were better delineated for patients who underwent surgical excision. This study attempted to rule out potential selection biases associated with the surgical excision group by performing additional subset analyses (excluding certain populations, stratifying for effect of axillary dissection, and stratifying for effect of large tumors or nodal disease), which again demonstrated that surgery remained strongly associated with survival. Criticisms of this retrospective population-based study are identical to those described above for Khan and colleagues. Limited information on receptor status of tumors and grade is provided in this study, but is absent for the majority of study patients. Limited information on adjuvant chemotherapy and radiation therapy is provided. Although subset analysis of patterns of metastasis and stage was performed, there is no analysis by either performance status or comorbidities. This study is similar in design to that of Khan and colleagues, but is significantly smaller in study population. In contrast to Khan and colleagues, more patients who had T3 and T4 tumors were included in this study population; unfortunately, there are as yet no data available to guide clinical judgment on whether resection of the intact primary is any more beneficial for larger or smaller primary tumors in the setting of metastatic disease and the effect on progression of metastasis. Similar to Khan and colleagues, this study concludes that a prospective, randomized controlled trial will be necessary to truly prove the benefit for surgery of the primary tumor in metastatic breast cancer; however, evidence provided by the study does suggest that surgical extirpation of the intact primary is beneficial to survival.

Babiera and colleagues [27] reported a retrospective single institution cohort of 224 patients who had Stage IV breast cancer and an intact primary tumor. Eighty-two went on to have surgical resection of their primary tumor. Of these, 11 patients underwent additional resection of metastatic foci with intention to cure. Significant differences were noted between the surgical and nonsurgical patients; the patients treated by resection of the intact primary were younger, had less nodal disease, had fewer sites of metastasis, were more likely to have HER2/neu gene amplification, and more likely to have received chemotherapy as first-line treatment. On multivariate analysis, surgical treatment was associated with a trend toward improvement in overall survival ($P = .12$) and a significant improvement in metastatic progression-free survival ($P = .0007$). The advantages of this study are that the study population is well-characterized (for example, type of surgery, receptor status, and HER2/neu status are known) and comprises a group of patients treated by physicians with a uniform practice philosophy. Limitations of the study include short duration of follow-up (less than 3 years) and the conclusion of only a trend toward a survival advantage. It is concerning that only a trend toward a survival advantage was demonstrated, despite clear clinical selection bias favoring patients who had less advanced metastasis receiving surgical intervention; however, this result could certainly be different with a larger study population with longer-term follow-up.

Summary

The four existing clinical studies examining the effect of resection of the primary tumor in Stage IV breast cancer conclude that local therapy for these patients may translate into a measurable survival advantage in favor of surgery for the intact primary. The dogma to never operate in the setting of metastatic disease certainly has been dispelled in favor of critical evaluation of whether surgically achieved local control can lead to improved survival as part of multimodality treatment. The message is clear that this is a question worthy of a prospective, randomized controlled trial. Surgical intervention for these patients should be viewed as more than just for palliative indications—surgery may well benefit some of these patients to the same extent as systemic chemotherapy, and this deserves to be carefully studied in well-designed clinical trials. These trials will also enable the advancement of our knowledge of the tumor biology of metastasis, and will directly determine whether the tumor dormancy theory is valid. By challenging the current paradigm of nonoperative treatment for these patients, we may discover that surgery is an important tool that offers hope for prolonged survival for these Stage IV patients in the setting of comprehensive multidisciplinary breast cancer treatment.

References

[1] Haagensen C, Stout A. Carcinoma of the breast: criteria of inoperability. Am Surg 1943;118: 859.

[2] Fisher B, Wolmark N, Redmond C, et al. Findings from NSABP protocol No. B-04: comparison of radical mastectomy with alternative treatments. II. The clinical and biologic significance of medial-central breast cancers. Cancer 1981;48(8):1863–72.

[3] Gervasoni JE Jr, Taneja C, Chung MA, et al. Axillary dissection in the context of the biology of lymph node metastases. Am J Surg 2000;180(4):278–83.

[4] Krag DN, Single RM. Breast cancer survival according to number of nodes removed. Ann Surg Oncol 2003;10(10):1152–9.

[5] Singletary SE, Walsh G, Vauthey JN, et al. A role for curative surgery in the treatment of selected patients with metastatic breast cancer. Oncologist 2003;8(3):241–51.

[6] Weigelt B, Peterse JL, van 't Veer LJ. Breast cancer metastasis: markers and models. Nat Rev Cancer 2005;5(8):591–602.

[7] Schmidt-Kittler O, Ragg T, Daskalakis A, et al. From latent disseminated cells to overt metastasis: genetic analysis of systemic breast cancer progression. Proc Natl Acad Sci U S A 2003;100(13):7737–42.

[8] Braun S, Vogl FD, Naume B, et al. A pooled analysis of bone marrow micrometastasis in breast cancer. N Engl J Med 2005;353(8):793–802.

[9] Sorlie T, Perou CM, Tibshirani R, et al. Gene expression patterns of breast carcinomas distinguish tumor subclasses with clinical implications. Proc Natl Acad Sci U S A 2001;98(19): 10869–74.

[10] van de Vijver MJ, He YD, van't Veer LJ, et al. A gene-expression signature as a predictor of survival in breast cancer. N Engl J Med 2002;347(25):1999–2009.

[11] Al-Hajj M, Clarke MF. Self-renewal and solid tumor stem cells. Oncogene 2004;23(43): 7274–82.

[12] Al-Hajj M, Wicha MS, Benito-Hernandez A, et al. Prospective identification of tumorigenic breast cancer cells. Proc Natl Acad Sci U S A 2003;100(7):3983–8.

[13] Pardoll D. Does the immune system see tumors as foreign or self? Annu Rev Immunol 2003; 21:807–39.

[14] Danna EA, Sinha P, Gilbert M, et al. Surgical removal of primary tumor reverses tumor-induced immunosuppression despite the presence of metastatic disease. Cancer Res 2004;64(6): 2205–11.

[15] Campbell MJ, Scott J, Maecker HT, et al. Immune dysfunction and micrometastases in women with breast cancer. Breast Cancer Res Treat 2005;91(2):163–71.

[16] Karrison TG, Ferguson DJ, Meier P. Dormancy of mammary carcinoma after mastectomy. J Natl Cancer Inst 1999;91(1):80–5.

[17] Demicheli R, Retsky MW, Swartzendruber DE, et al. Proposal for a new model of breast cancer metastatic development. Ann Oncol 1997;8(11):1075–80.

[18] Baum M, Demicheli R, Hrushesky W, et al. Does surgery unfavourably perturb the "natural history" of early breast cancer by accelerating the appearance of distant metastases? Eur J Cancer 2005;41(4):508–15.

[19] Andre F, Slimane K, Bachelot T, et al. Breast cancer with synchronous metastases: trends in survival during a 14-year period. J Clin Oncol 2004;22(16):3302–8.

[20] Giordano SH, Buzdar AU, Smith TL, et al. Is breast cancer survival improving? Cancer 2004;100(1):44–52.

[21] Hortobagyi GN. Can we cure limited metastatic breast cancer? [comment]. J Clin Oncol 2002;20(3):620–3.

[22] Greenberg PA, Hortobagyi GN, Smith TL, et al. Long-term follow-up of patients with complete remission following combination chemotherapy for metastatic breast cancer. J Clin Oncol 1996;14(8):2197–205.

[23] Rivera E, Holmes FA, Buzdar AU, et al. Fluorouracil, doxorubicin, and cyclophosphamide followed by tamoxifen as adjuvant treatment for patients with Stage IV breast cancer with no evidence of disease. Breast J 2002;8(1):2–9.

[24] Khan SA, Stewart AK, Morrow M. Does aggressive local therapy improve survival in metastatic breast cancer? Surgery 2002;132(4):620–6 [discussion: 6–7].

[25] Carmichael AR, Anderson ED, Chetty U, et al. Does local surgery have a role in the management of Stage IV breast cancer? Eur J Surg Oncol 2003;29(1):17–9.

[26] Rapiti E, Verkooijen HM, Vlastos G, et al. Complete excision of primary breast tumor improves survival of patients with metastatic breast cancer at diagnosis. J Clin Oncol 2006;24(18):2743–9.

[27] Babiera GV, Rao R, Feng L, et al. Effect of primary tumor extirpation in breast cancer patients who present with Stage IV disease and an intact primary tumor. Ann Surg Oncol 2006;13(6):776–82.

SURGICAL
CLINICS OF
NORTH AMERICA

Surg Clin N Am 87 (2007) 539–550

Radiofrequency, Cryoablation, and Other Modalities for Breast Cancer Ablation

Keiva L. Bland, MD[a], Jennifer Gass, MD[b],
V. Suzanne Klimberg, MD[a,c,*]

[a]Division of Breast Surgical Oncology, Department of Surgery, University of Arkansas
for Medical Sciences, 4301 West Markham, Slot 725, Little Rock, AR 72205-7199, USA
[b]Departments of Surgery and Oncology, Women & Infant's Breast Health Center,
101 Dudley Street, Providence, RI 02905, USA
[c]Department of Pathology, University of Arkansas for Medical Sciences,
4301 West Markham, Slot 725, Little Rock, AR 72205-7199, USA

Radiofrequency ablation (RFA) is accomplished by heat generated from high-frequency alternating currents distributed by means of a single prong or an array of prongs deployed from a probe (Fig. 1). The friction-generated heat from ion movement in the tissues causes increasing levels of cell damage with the rise in temperature. The tissues are heated by gradually increasing the frequency until the desired temperature is reached or resistance or impedance is met [1]. Cell injury begins at 42°, and by 60°, cell death occurs. The histological result is protein denaturation and coagulation leading to necrosis [2].

The medical literature contains a comprehensive collection of articles indicating the routine use and ongoing investigation of RFA for managing solid tumors. The use of RFA for managing breast cancers is a relatively novel technique. Its first use in human breast tissue was reported in 1999, and its effectiveness is being investigated [3].

Percutaneous ablation

The studies of percutaneous ablation of breast cancer with RFA are small, and results have been less than 100% successful (Table 1). The series

Supported by the Susan G. Komen Breast Cancer Clinical Fellowship and the Arkansas Breast Cancer Act.

* Corresponding author. Division of Breast Surgical Oncology, Department of Surgery, University of Arkansas for Medical Sciences, 4301 West Markham, Slot 725, Little Rock, AR 72205-7199.

E-mail address: klimbergsuzanne@uams.edu (V.S. Klimberg).

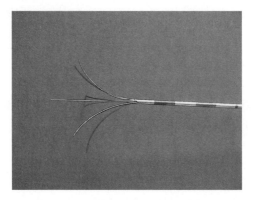

Fig. 1. Radiofrequency ablation probe.

to attempt complete ablation are divided between immediate and delayed resection. They almost uniformly use ultrasound (US) for localization and
have focused primarily on T1 disease. Immediate resection can underesti-
mate assessment of cell death.

Jeffrey and colleagues [3] reported on the first series of patients having RFA
in the breast, and they demonstrated that RFA could be used effectively and

Table 1
Trials of percutaneous radiofrequency ablation

Author	N	Mean tumor size (range)	Percent complete ablation (by viability stain)	Postablation treatment	Complications
Jeffery et al 1999 [3]	5	4–7 cm	80% (4/5)	Immediate resection	No complications
Izzo et al 2001 [2]	26	1.8 cm (0.7–3 cm)	94% (25/26)	Immediate resection	Full-thickness burn (4%)
Elliott et al 2002 [9]	1	1.6 cm	100% (1/1)	1 month delayed resection	Stereotactic placement
Hayashi et al 2003 [8]	22	0.9 cm (0.5–2.6 cm)	86% (19/22)	1–2 week delayed resection	Five patients had disease distant to ablation zone
Burak et al [7] 2003	10	1.2 cm (0.8–1.6 cm)	90% (9/10)[b]	1–3 week delayed resection	Pre- and post-radiofrequency ablation MRI
Fornage et al 2004 [5]	21[a]	≤2 cm	100%	Immediate resection	One patient had disease distant to ablation zone
Noguchi et al 2006 [4]	10	1.1 cm (0.5–2 cm)	100%	Immediate resection	No complications

[a] 20 patients, 21 tumors.
[b] CK 8/18 used for staining.

safely. Ablation zones of 0.8 to 1.8 cm were achieved and confirmed by immediate excision and pathologic analysis using nicotinamide adenine dinucleotide–diaphorase (NADH-diaphorase) staining. All but one of the ablated portions of the tumors demonstrated complete destruction.

Izzo and colleagues [2] reported a series of 26 percutaneous ablations on patients who had T1 and T2 tumors ranging from 0.7 to 3 cm (mean 1.8 cm) followed by immediate resection. Twenty-five of the 26 tumors (96%) were ablated completely. In one case a single microscopic focus of blue staining on NADH-diaphorase evaluation was identified near the probe track. The authors discounted its validity based on negative repeat NADH staining and improbability of cell survival at the needle track where temperatures surpass 100°.

In a 10-patient series reported by Noguchi and colleagues [4] of invasive ductal carcinomas ranging 0.5 to 2 cm, patients underwent percutaneous RFA immediately followed by wide excision or mastectomy. The cells in the ablated tissue demonstrated a range of histological responses from marked necrosis to near normalcy when examined by hematoxylin and eosin (H&E) staining. No viable cells were identified by NADH-diaphorase stain, however, indicating complete ablation. In this series, stereotaxis was used for radiofrequency (RF) probe placement in one case, as the lesion was ultrasonographically occult.

Fornage and colleagues [5] reported on 21 tumors less than 2 cm that underwent US-guided RFA in the operating room before immediate resection. All tumors demonstrated no cell viability in the zone of ablation by NADH-diaphorase staining. In one case, however, there was extensive US and mammographically occult invasive tumor beyond the ablation zone. It was thought that in this single patient, neoadjuvant chemotherapy had reduced the initial mass, with pathology demonstrating viable tumor within a 4 cm area around the 1 cm target lesion. This report was part of a larger multicenter trial with participation from the John Wayne Cancer Center and the New York Weill Cornell Medical Center [6]. Summary of the preliminary data reported complete ablation in 25 of 29 (86.2%) tumors treated [6].

In subsequent series reported here, excision was delayed for varying amounts of time after RFA. Burak and colleagues [7] reported on 10 patients who had a mean tumor size of 1.2 cm (0.8 to 1.8 cm) undergoing percutaneous RFA paired with delayed excision using lumpectomy or mastectomy 1 to 3 weeks later. Cytokeratin 8/18 (CK 8/18) staining revealed 9 of 10 tumors were successfully ablated. Unique to this study was the use of MRI to evaluate the lesions before and after ablation. Postablation MRI correctly predicted that eight of nine patients had no residual disease. The one lesion with postablation MRI enhancement was found to have a small focus of residual cancer attributed to poor probe placement [7].

Hayashi and colleagues [8] series reported on a group of 22 patients who underwent percutaneous RFA ablation followed by delayed surgical excision at 1 to 2 weeks. Patients had tumors with a mean size of 0.9 cm (0.5 to 2.6 cm). Nineteen of the 22 patients (86%) had successful ablation. Of the three incomplete ablations, two had microscopic foci at the margins, and one had 50% ablation of the tumor. In this latter patient, the RFA probe did not deploy fully; this was attributed to increased breast density. In addition, five specimens contained viable tumor distant to the target lesion that was not identified on preoperative imaging.

Problems and limitations

Insufficient ablation in most studies

Only one series, Noguchi, demonstrated 100% ablation of 10 breast tumors. Incomplete ablations have been attributed to technical difficulties such as improper placement of the probe, equipment malfunction, or underestimation of tumor size by imaging [7,8]. The increased use of MRI in preoperative assessment of breast cancer likely will diminish this pitfall.

Lack of real-time imaging

One of the unresolved issues of RFA use in breast cancer treatment is real-time visual monitoring of the tumor for evidence of ablation. With US monitoring of ablation, a very hyperechoic image develops, with significant shadowing that obscures visualization of the entire tumor [2,7,8]. In a case report, Fornage and colleagues reported on two tumors that showed a decrease in pre- versus postablation peripheral vascularity. Preliminary work at University of Arkansas has demonstrated that by using Doppler US, the ablation zone can be monitored during RFA ablation (Fig. 2).

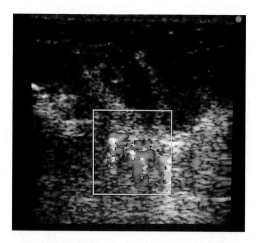

Fig. 2. Doppler image during radiofrequency ablation of breast lesion demonstrating the effective ablation zone at the site of a tumor.

Small subgroup of patients

Because RFA is suited best for localized, discretely visualized disease, patients who have an extensive intraductal component or invasive lobular carcinoma are not ideal candidates for this procedure. Although ablation zones have been reported as large as 4.5 cm, it appears that patients having large tumors are not suitable for this procedure [7]. In the reported studies, tumors selected were 3 cm or less [1,2,6–8]. The tumor size was limited to ablate the tumor and an additional 0.5 to 1 cm margin of surrounding normal tissue [2]. Patients having undergone neoadjuvant chemotherapy (NACT) are also not ideal candidates for this procedure. Neoadjuvant chemotherapy resulting in tumor reduction can result in imaging occult tumor. Fornage and colleagues reported that in one case, although the target lesion was ablated successfully, there was a 4 cm diameter area of mammogram and US occult invasive tumor surrounding the target lesion. This patient had undergone neoadjuvant chemotherapy. As a result, the authors' institution has excluded patients having completed NACT from RFA protocols that use US guidance.

Complications

Few complications are reported in any of the studies. Minor burn and minimal bruising encompass the spectrum of complications outside of failure of complete ablation. RFA seems to be tolerated well by patients. In the study evaluating pain medication use, only three (13.6%) patients took pain medication (up to two acetaminophen with codeine tablets) in the week following ablation, and 95% of the participants indicated that they would be willing to undergo RFA again [8]. Only one study reported a patient with mild swelling at 1 week follow-up after RFA and some tenderness and induration at 2 weeks [9]. No infections or hematomas were reported in any of the studies.

Inadequate ablation or complications were reported in studies in which the tumor was too close to the skin or chest wall. Izzo and colleagues [2] reported the first complication with RFA in a patient who had a 2.5 cm full thickness burn where the tumor was "immediately beneath the skin." Hayashi and colleagues [8] had insufficient ablation in a patient who had a tumor located very near the chest wall. The ablation had to be interrupted because of patient discomfort. Subsequent studies established exclusion criteria for tumors that were less than 1 cm from the skin or chest wall [6].

Imaging expertise required

The studies to date predominantly have been performed under US guidance. Therefore, proficiency with US and US-guided procedures has been very important to the success of this therapy. There have been two instances reported in the literature, however, on stereotaxis for RFA probe placement. The case reported by Elliott and colleagues [9] used stereotactic placement of the RFA probe, and the procedure was performed on the stereotactic table. The procedure, performed under local anesthetic with sedation, was tolerated well by the patient, with no discomfort being reported. Noguchi used stereotactic guidance for placement of the probe for a mass that was not visible by US. In this instance, however, the ablation was performed in the operating room. No technical difficulties were reported with the ablations as a result of this maneuver, and there were no viable tumors identified in the specimens.

Burak and colleagues [7] performed postablation MRIs to determine extent of ablation. To date, no instance of breast RFA under MRI guidance has been reported as MRI-compatible probes only recently have been made commercially available. There have been reports, however, of solid tumor ablation using MRI guidance and/or monitoring from as early as 1998 [10–15].

Pathological assessment of ablation zone

One of the major disadvantages to percutaneous radiofrequency ablation without resection is that the extent and completeness of ablation cannot be evaluated fully in situ. This contributes to the hesitation to leave ablated tissue in place and follow with biopsies and radiologic studies.

On gross pathology, the resulting lesion typically consists of a whitish, central area (where the probe was located) surrounded by yellowish coagulated tissue, further surrounded by a hyperemic ring of tissue [16].

On histology, H&E staining demonstrates a wide range of cellular changes in the zone of ablation, from normal-appearing cells to severely damaged-appearing cells with cytoskeleton destruction and nuclear changes. In addition to evaluating structural changes in cells following RFA, cell viability also can be assessed. In most studies reported, such as those by Jeffrey, Izzo, and Fornage, NADH-diaphorase was used to evaluate for cell viability. Triphenyl tetrazolium chloride (TTC), an enzyme viability dye sometimes referred to as NADH, can be used also to identify the boundary between viable and nonviable tissue following ablation macroscopically. It stains viable tissue red-orange, and dead tissue in the ablated area does not stain [17]. Burak and colleagues [7] used CK8/18 to assess viability, as it was suggested in earlier studies that it is degraded earlier during apoptosis, and therefore nonviable tissues would not stain [18]. Proliferating cell nuclear antigen (PCNA) staining is also an option for ascertaining cell death. It determines the presence of actively dividing DNA [19,20].

Although RFA shows significant promise as an effective means of tumor destruction, there have been no data demonstrating long-term effects of ablation without subsequent excision. Trials are planned for RFA followed by biopsy and/or imaging surveillance [6,7].

Excision followed by radiofrequency ablation or open ablation

Lumpectomy with radiation is used widely as a form of breast cancer management. At least 75% of recurrences occur at the previous lumpectomy site, and positive margins are found in 20% to 55% of lumpectomy specimens [21]. Excision followed by RFA (eRFA) uses the effectiveness of lumpectomy combined with RFA of the margins to ablate residual disease [19]. This procedure is designed to increase the margin in primary lumpectomy cavities without further excision, thereby avoiding additional tissue resection and maintaining optimum cosmesis in breast-conserving surgery (Fig. 3).

In a pilot trial to evaluate eRFA, 41 patients underwent lumpectomy followed by intraoperative RFA. Eleven of 41 patients had inadequate margins; however, only one required re-excision for a grossly positive margin. Seventeen of the 41 patients had postoperative radiation therapy. During the median follow-up of 24 months, there were no local recurrences. Two of the patients have had recurrence distant to the operative site [19]. Ongoing trials in Europe and a multi-institutional trial in the United States will evaluate this procedure further.

Cryoablation

Fibroadenomas

Cryoablation creates an elliptical ice ball as argon gas flows through the needle percutaneously placed into the lesion of interest (Fig. 4A). The duration of freezing depends on the size of the lesion and local factors such as vascularity. The freezing process along with proximity to the skin and

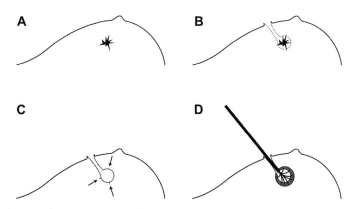

Fig. 3. Illustration of excision followed by radiofrequency ablation (RFA). The tumor is depicted in (A) with the resection of the tumor by means of lumpectomy depicted in (B) and (C). (D) depicts possible remaining tumor following standard resection. With the application of RFA following excision, the remaining missed tumor is ablated.

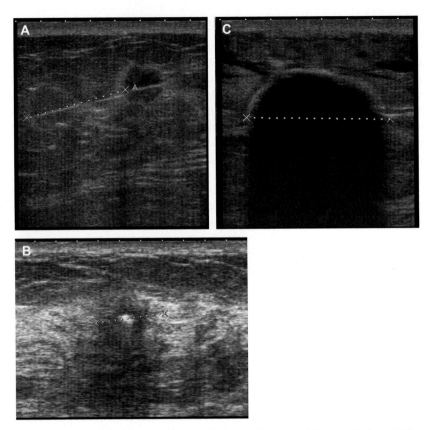

Fig. 4. (*A*) Ultrasound of tumor with cryoablation needle centered in tumor before ablation. (*B*) Ultrasound of tumor demonstrating needle centered in lesion. (*C*) Ultrasound of tumor with fully developed ice ball of cryoablation.

muscle are easily visualized with real-time US (Fig. 4B, C). The only Food and Drug Administration (FDA)-approved use of cryoablation is the treatment of core biopsy-proven fibroadenomas. Cryoablation effectively and safely treats fibroadenoma in an office setting with local anesthesia. Kaufman and colleagues [22] reported on 37 treated fibroadenomas (84% palpable) with a mean diameter of 2.1 cm (0.8 to 4.2 cm) with a median volume reduction of 99% observed by US. Sixteen percent of all the treated masses remained palpable during the average follow-up of 2.6 years. Of the fibroadenomas measuring less than 2 cm before treatment, 6% remained palpable during the average follow-up period. The largest series consisting of 444 patients from FibroAdenoma Cryoablation Treatment (FACT) registry reported by Nurko and colleagues [23] with a mean tumor size of 1.8 cm demonstrated reduced palpability at 6 and 12 months follow-up. On initial evaluation, 75% of the fibroadenomas were palpable. The degree of palpability was decreased to 46% at months and 35% at 12 months. Following treatment, lesions get smaller over time and may take at least 12 months to completely resolve. Patient satisfaction with the procedure was rated 88% to 97% [23].

Breast cancer

Trials of cryoablation in small invasive breast cancers have yielded varying results. In a feasibility trial conducted by Pfleiderer and colleagues [24], all invasive cancers no more than 16 mm in diameter were ablated completely, while no tumors at least 23 mm in diameter sustained complete destruction. There were no complications reported. Sabel and colleagues [25] reported on cryoablation of 27 breast cancers with a mean size of 1.2 cm (0.6 to 2 cm). Twenty-three of the tumors were ablated completely on microscopic evaluation. Complete ablation was achieved in all tumors under 1.0 cm and also in tumors between 1.0 and 1.5 cm provided there was nonlobular histology and lack of extensive intraductal component The presence of ductal carcinoma in situ limits the success of US-guided cryoablation in treating breast cancer. At present, the maximum iceball achievable is 4.0, limiting therapy to small cancers. There were no complications reported in this study.

Tafra and colleagues [26] first reported the use of cryosurgery to improve accuracy and decrease positive margins in breast cancer cases. Cryoprobe-assisted lumpectomy (CAL) was performed on 24 patients in a feasibility study. This procedure entailed inserting a cryoprobe under US guidance in into the center of the desired lesion and creating an iceball with a desired margin of at least 5 mm around the tumor. Four of the 24 (16.7%) patients underwent re-excision of the margins. The group concluded that CAL provided a superior alternative to needle wire localization (NWL). This led to the prospective multicenter CAL trial [26]. In this study, 17 sites participated enrolling 310 patients in a 2:1 randomization between CAL and NWL. The study was limited to invasive ductal carcinomas under 1.7 cm. The primary endpoint, overall negative margin status, was not significantly different for the two arms of the study; 28% CAL and 31% NWL. When the margin for invasive cancer was distinguished, however, the results were significant, showing 11% for CAL and 20% for NWL. Secondary endpoints such as volume of resected tissue, breast cosmesis and procedure time were significantly lower when cryoassistance was used. Therefore, the FDA has approved use of the cryoprobe for localization of tumors. Nonetheless, DCIS remains the Achilles heel of US-guided cryoablation, even in this series limited to small nonlobular cancers.

American College of Surgeon's Oncology Group has explored a prospective trial incorporating magnetic resonance breast imaging of small ductal carcinomas before subsequent planned cryoablation with then 2 to 4 week delayed reimaging and resection. This trial would expand on the Sabel trial looking at the effectiveness of cryotechnology for definitive ablation.

Imaging expertise required

As with RFA, US guidance is currently the most widely used method for placement of the cryoprobe. The formation and extent of the iceball is visualized clearly real-time with US, as the treatment zone is anechoic. Skin injury can result during iceball formation if it is not monitored closely. This can be prevented by dripping saline on the skin, injecting saline under the skin, or placing warm gauze pads on the skin during the procedure [25]. None of the patients in the multicenter trial sustained skin injury. In distinction to RFA or other heat-generating modalities of tissue destruction, cryoablation is anesthetic and therefore able to be moved to the office setting.

Focused ultrasound

Focused US (FUS) is a noninvasive thermal ablation technique that uses focused US beams to penetrate through soft tissues to targeted lesions, resulting in destruction of the lesion while sparing surrounding tissues. Using this technique with magnetic resonance guidance (MRgFUS) allows for imaging and tissue temperature monitoring during the ablation, as well as controlling the direction of the FUS beam. The magnetic resonance apparatus is set up so that the patient is in a prone position with the breast supported by a plastic-enclosed water bath that is set upon the US transducer [27].

Fibroadenomas

Hynynen and colleagues [28] reported on 11 fibroadenomas treated with MRgFUS. The mean volume of tumors of 1.9 cm^3 was decreased to 1.1 cm^3 ($P = .01$), and 73% of tumors were "partially or nearly totally successfully treated." Overall, there was minimal discomfort, and one patient had edema of the ipsilateral pectoralis muscle.

Breast cancer

Furusawa and colleagues [29] reported on the use of MRgFUS to ablate breast cancers Twenty-eight patients with invasive cancers less than 3.5 cm, had tumors ablated with a mean necrosis of 96.9% (78% to 100%) of the tumor volume. Of the tumors ablated, only three had necrosis less than 95%. The authors reported one full-thickness skin burn and one allergic reaction but otherwise minimal complaints of pain.

Wu and colleagues [30] reported the successful ablation of 23 breast cancers ranging in size from 2 to 4.7 cm. They focused on the histopathologic evaluation of FUS-ablated tumors. The ablated tumors were grayish in color with a red hemorrhagic ring at the periphery on gross inspection. On microscopic evaluation, the normal cellular architecture was maintained on H&E staining. On NADH-diaphorase staining, however, there was no evidence of cellular viability.

Summary

The ablative techniques reported demonstrate promise as less invasive treatments for breast cancer. None is 100% effective, however, and more investigation is needed before these techniques can be used alone as treatment for cancers. Specifically, a superior template of the extent of the disease will be needed to deliver the ideal percutaneous ablative technique to the target area. At present, the leading technologies, RFA and cryo-technology, seem more ideally suited to small ($\leq$) nonlobular carcinomas without extensive intraductal component. eRFA is an emerging ablative technique with excellent initial results whether RFA is delivered after percutaneous excision or open biopsy. The results of ongoing trials will establish efficacy and specific uses of the various technologies.

References

[1] Mirza AN, Fornage BD, Sneige N, et al. Radiofrequency ablation of solid tumors. Cancer J 2001;7(2):95–102.

[2] Izzo F, Thomas R, Delrio P, et al. Radiofrequency ablation in patients with primary breast carcinoma: a pilot study in 26 patients. Cancer 2001;92(8):2036–44.

[3] Jeffrey SS, Birdwell RL, Ikeda DM, et al. Radiofrequency ablation of breast cancer: first report of an emerging technology. Arch Surg 1999;134(10):1064–8.

[4] Noguchi M, Earashi M, Fujii H, et al. Radiofrequency ablation of small breast cancer followed by surgical resection. J Surg Oncol 2006;93(2):120–8.

[5] Fornage BD, Sneige N, Ross MI, et al. Small (< or = 2 cm) breast cancer treated with US-guided radiofrequency ablation: feasibility study. Radiology 2004;231(1):215–24.

[6] Singletary SE. Radiofrequency ablation of breast cancer. Am Surg 2003;69(1):37–40.

[7] Burak WE Jr, Agnese DM, Povoski SP, et al. Radiofrequency ablation of invasive breast carcinoma followed by delayed surgical excision. Cancer 2003;98(7):1369–76.

[8] Hayashi AH, Silver SF, van der Weshuizen NG, et al. Treatment of invasive breast carcinoma with ultrasound-guided radiofrequency ablation. Am J Surg 2003;185(5):429–35.

[9] Elliott RL, Rice PB, Suits JA, et al. Radiofrequency ablation of a stereotactically localized nonpalpable breast carcinoma. Am Surg 2002;68(1):1–5.

[10] Boss A, Clasen S, Kuczyk M, et al. Magnetic resonance-guided percutaneous radiofrequency ablation of renal cell carcinomas: a pilot clinical study. Invest Radiol 2005;40(9): 583–90.

[11] Clasen S, Boss A, Schmidt D, et al. Magnetic resonance imaging for hepatic radiofrequency ablation. Eur J Radiol 2006;59(2):140–8.

[12] Teichgraber V, Aube C, Schmidt D, et al. Percutaneous MR-guided radiofrequency ablation of recurrent sacrococcygeal chordomas. AJR Am J Roentgenol 2006;187(2):571–4.

[13] Nour SG. MRI-guided and monitored radiofrequency tumor ablation. Acad Radiol 2005; 12(9):1110–20.

[14] Lewin JS, Connell CF, Duerk JL, et al. Interactive MRI-guided radiofrequency interstitial thermal ablation of abdominal tumors: clinical trial for evaluation of safety and feasibility. J Magn Reson Imaging 1998;8(1):40–7.

[15] Lewin JS, Nor SG, Connell CF. Phase II clinical trial of interactive MR imaging-guided interstitial radiofrequency thermal ablation of primary kidney tumors: initial experience. Radiology 2004;232(3):835–45.

[16] Huston TL, Simmons RM. Ablative therapies for the treatment of malignant diseases of the breast. Am J Surg 2005;189(6):694–701.

[17] Fishbein MC, Meerbaum S, Rit J, et al. Early phase acute myocardial infarct size quantifi-cation: validation of the triphenyl tetrazolium chloride tissue enzyme staining technique. Am Heart J 1981;101:593–600.

[18] Bloom KJ, Dowlat K, Assad L. Pathologic changes after interstitial laser therapy of infiltrat-ing breast carcinoma. Am J Surg 2001;182:384–8.

[19] Klimberg VS, Kepple J, Shafirstein G, et al. eRFA: excision followed by RFA—a new tech-nique to improve local control in breast cancer. Ann Surg Oncol 2006;13(1):1422–33.

[20] Korourian S, Klimberg S, Henry-Tillman R, et al. Assessment of proliferating cell nuclear antigen activity using digital image analysis in breast carcinoma following magnetic resonance-guided interstitial laser photocoagulation. Breast J 2003;9(5):409–13.

[21] Fisher ER, Anderson S, Tan-Chiu E. Fifteen-year prognostic discriminants for invasive breast carcinoma: National Surgical Adjuvant Breast and Bowel Project Protocol-06. Can-cer 2001;91(8 Suppl):1679–87.

[22] Kaufman CS, Littrup PJ, Freeman-Gibb LA, et al. Office-based cryoablation of breast fibroadenomas with long-term follow-up. Breast J 2005;11(5):344–50.

[23] Nurko J, Mabry CD, Whitworth P, et al. Interim results from the FibroAdenoma Cryoabla-tion Treatment Registry. Am J Surg 2005;190(4):647–51.

[24] Pfleiderer SO, Freesmeyer MG, Marx C, et al. Cryotherapy of breast cancer under ultrasound guidance: initial results and limitations. Eur Radiol 2002;12(12):3009–14.

[25] Sabel MS, Kaufman CS, Whitworth P, et al. Cryoablation of early-stage breast cancer: work-in-progress report of a multi-institutional trial. Ann Surg Oncol 2004;11(5):542–9.

[26] Tafra L, Fine R, Whitworth P, et al. Prospective randomized study comparing cryo-assisted and needle-wire localization of ultrasound visible breast tumors. Am J Surg 2006;192: 462–70.

[27] Huber PE, Jenne JW, Rastert R, et al. A new noninvasive approach in breast cancer therapy using magnetic resonance imaging-guided focused ultrasound surgery. Cancer Res 2001; 61(23):8441–7.

[28] Hynynen K, Pomeroy O, Smith DN, et al. MR imaging-guided focused ultrasound surgery of fibroadenomas in the breast: a feasibility study. Radiology 2001;219(1):176–85.

[29] Furusawa H, Namba K, Thomsen S, et al. Magnetic resonance-guided focused ultrasound surgery of breast cancer: reliability and effectiveness. J Am Coll Surg 2006;203(1):54–63.

[30] Wu F, Wang ZB, Cao YD, et al. Heat fixation of cancer cells ablated with high-intensity focused ultrasound in patients with breast cancer. Am J Surg 2006;192(2):179–84.

SURGICAL
CLINICS OF
NORTH AMERICA

Surg Clin N Am 87 (2007) 551–568

Investigating the Phenotypes and Genotypes of Breast Cancer in Women with African Ancestry: The Need for More Genetic Epidemiology

Awori J. Hayanga, MD[a],
Lisa A. Newman, MD, MPH, FACS[b],*

[a]Department of Surgery, University of Michigan, 1500 East Medical Center Drive,
Ann Arbor, MI 48109, USA
[b]Breast Center, University of Michigan Comprehensive Cancer Center,
1500 East Medical Center Drive, Ann Arbor, MI 48109, USA

Breast cancer in African American women

The breast cancer burden of African American women is characterized by several poorly understood features when compared with breast cancer in white American women:

1. Lower lifetime incidence
2. Higher mortality
3. Younger age distribution
4. More advanced stage distribution
5. Increased frequency of endocrine-resistant, high-grade tumors.

The population-based Surveillance, Epidemiology and End Results (SEER) program documents an age-adjusted breast cancer incidence of 119 per 100,000 African American women and 141 per 100,000 white American women. In contrast, mortality rates for breast cancer patients are reported at 35 per 100,000 African American women and 26 per 100,000 white American women [1]. The median age at diagnosis of breast cancer is 62 years for white American women and is only 57 years for African American women; for women younger than age 45 years, the incidence of breast cancer is

* Corresponding author.
  E-mail address: lanewman@umich.edu (L.A. Newman).

0039-6109/07/$ - see front matter © 2007 Published by Elsevier Inc.
doi:10.1016/j.suc.2007.01.003

higher for African American than for white American women [1]. The increased frequency of poorly differentiated, estrogen- and progesterone receptor-negative tumors has been documented by several single-institution studies as well by the SEER program [1–4].

The prevalence of socioeconomic disadvantages that impede access to health care, such as poverty and lack of insurance, is approximately twofold higher for African Americans than for white Americans, and these features certainly contribute to disparities in breast cancer survival [5,6]. Available studies that have accounted for socioeconomic status and comorbidities among breast cancer patients have failed to demonstrate that these issues completely explain the observed outcome differences, however [7–9]. Newman and colleagues [7] conducted a meta-analysis of survival in more than 13,000 African American and more than 70,000 white American patients who had breast cancer based on data from studies published between 1980 and 2005. The pooled analysis revealed that after adjusting for socioeconomic status, African American ethnicity was associated with a statistically significant 28% increase in mortality risk. Tammemagi and colleagues [8] found that comorbidities accounted substantially for the overall survival differences in African American and white American patients who had breast cancer, but African American ethnicity continued to affect survival adversely even after controlling for comorbidity in the breast cancer–specific survival analyses. Furthermore, although socioeconomic resources and comorbidities might influence the stage at which a breast cancer is diagnosed and the likelihood of completing successful treatment, it is not at all clear that these disadvantages account for the endocrine responsiveness or the age distribution of breast cancer in African American women.

Other paradoxical associations are observed in relation to ethnic/racial variations in breast cancer burden. As noted previously, African American women have a lower lifetime incidence of breast cancer than white American women; as Anderson and colleagues [10] have shown, this difference is largely a consequence of their reduced incidence rates of estrogen receptor–positive breast cancer. In contrast, incidence rates for estrogen receptor–negative breast cancer in African American women are similar to or higher than those in white American women at all deciles of age [10]. Several investigators have correlated circulating endogenous estrogen/hormone levels and risk of breast cancer [11], and this association seems to be strongest for predicting risk of estrogen receptor–positive breast cancer [12,13]. Data on measured sex hormone levels in African American women are scarce, but surrogate markers such as bone mineral density and obesity rates suggest that endogenous estrogen levels would be elevated for this population subset, because African American have lower rates of osteoporosis [14–16] and higher rates of obesity [5,17–19] than white American women. A single study focusing on circulating hormones in premenopausal women reported increased levels in African Americans [20], but data on postmenopausal African American women are largely inferential and are based on surrogate parameters. The collective information is provocative, nonetheless: the evidence of elevated estrogen exposure would be expected to result in an increased risk of estrogen receptor–positive breast cancer, but African American women have diminished incidence rates of endocrine-sensitive disease.

Women carrying a mutation in the *BRCA1* breast cancer susceptibility gene are more likely to be diagnosed with estrogen receptor–negative, high-grade tumors that are detected at young ages [21–23]. As discussed previously, these features are prominent among African American women who have breast cancer [2], and these parallels motivate questions regarding the extent of hereditary risk in African American women. Studies of hereditary cancer risk among African American women have been limited [24–27], although some *BRCA1* and *BRCA2* founder mutations and other unique (but not necessarily deleterious) genotype patterns have been identified [28–31]. It is unlikely that a single high-penetrance, major breast cancer susceptibility mutation will be identified that explains the breast cancer patterns of African American women, because these types of genetic abnormalities are rare. On the other hand, it is quite plausible that low- and moderate-risk genetic variants exist that collectively contribute to the breast cancer burden of particular populations [32,33].

Reproductive history has been proposed as an explanation for ethnicity-associated variations in age distribution [34]. Multiple pregnancies result in diminished lifetime exposure of the breasts to estrogen, yielding a lower breast cancer incidence in multiparous than in nulliparous women, although the risk of breast cancer is increased briefly in the early postpartum period. Because early childbearing is more common among African American women, it is biologically plausible that a dual effect of parity on breast cancer risk might be observed at a population level, with multiple pregnancies at young ages causing an increased risk of premenopausal disease but a lower lifetime incidence. This theory was supported in an analysis of breast cancer risk among the Black Woman's Health Study [35], a prospective study of self-reported health and lifestyle issues among African American women subscribers to the magazine *Essence*. More than 50,000 women completed a follow-up questionnaire, representing more than 214,000 person-years of follow-up between 1995 and 1999. Evaluation of breast cancer events revealed that multiparity was associated with an increased incidence rate ratio (IRR) among women younger than 45 years (IRR, 2.4; 95% confidence interval [CI], 1.1–5.1) but was protective against breast cancer among women age 45 years and older (IRR, 0.5; 95% CI, 0.3–0.9).

In contrast, investigators from the Women's Contraceptive and Reproductive Experience (CARE) study found no differences in effect of parity on age-related risk of breast cancer [36]. The Women's CARE study was a population-based, multicenter case-controlled study of more than 3000 African American women and nearly 6000 white American women (approximately 50% of both subsets had a history of breast cancer), and this study was designed specifically to analyze the impact of endogenous as well as exogenous hormonal factors on breast cancer risk in a large, biracial/ethnic dataset. Ursin and colleagues [36] reported that parity was associated with similar degrees of reduction of the risk of breast cancer among younger (age 35–49 years) versus older (age 50–64 years) women in both African American and white American subsets. Risk reduction proportions were 13% and 10% for younger and older white Americans, respectively, and were 10% and 6% for younger and older African Americans, respectively.

Advances in medical technology have strengthened the understanding of the genetic aberrations that accumulate with breast tumors, defining the risk for distant organ metastasis and mortality. Gene expression analyses have characterized luminal breast cancer subtypes versus the more virulent basal subtype. The basal breast cancer subtype is characterized by elevations in basement membranous genes (eg, selected cytokeratins), and it has become known commonly as the "triple-negative" subtype because of its negativity for estrogen receptor, progesterone receptor, and *Her2/neu*. Recent studies are revealing provocative ethnicity-associated differences in the frequency of this aggressive breast cancer subtype. Carey and colleagues [37] reported on the frequency of basal breast cancers among the African American and white American participants in the Carolina Breast Cancer Study (CBCS), a population-based dataset of breast cancer cases and controls in North Carolina. They observed a significantly higher prevalence of basal-type tumors among premenopausal African American women than in postmenopausal African American and non–African American women of all ages (39% versus 14% and 16%, respectively; $P < .001$).

Breast cancer in African women

Large-scale, population-based databases that document the cancer burden of Africa are lacking because of limited financial support for the health care and research system. The World Health Organization estimates that the Americas account for 10% of the global burden of disease and have 37% of the world's health workers spending more than 50% of the world's health financing, whereas Africa has 24% of the global disease burden but possesses only 3% of health workers using less than 1% of world health expenditure [38]. These limited resources leave little for investment into cancer and tumor registries in Africa. Available data on the epidemiology of breast cancer in Africa, however, reveal some provocative similarities to breast cancer in African American women, thereby strengthening the case for conducting genetic research investigating cancer susceptibility in women of African ancestry.

Fig. 1 demonstrates breast cancer incidence and mortality data for women in Africa, based on the Globocan program [39]. In general, women of Africa are at low risk of being diagnosed with breast cancer. Although the breast cancer mortality rates are similarly low in comparison with Western nations,

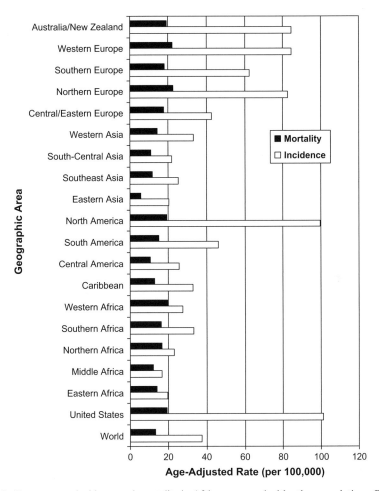

Fig. 1. Breast cancer incidence and mortality in Africa compared with other populations. Rates shown are age adjusted, per 100,000 population.

the ratio of mortality to incidence tends to be higher. The lifestyle and repro-ductive history of African women contributes to an overall protective risk-factor profile. Childbearing is initiated at relatively younger ages; fullterm pregnancies are multiple; postpartum lactation frequently is extended; and menarche may be delayed [40–42]. Diminished access to health care and lack of breast cancer screening programs results in delayed diagnoses, ad-vanced stage disease at diagnosis, and higher mortality rates [42,43]. Studies correlating risk factors with incidence of breast cancer and correlating tumor features with disease outcome, however, have been inconsistent in ruling out the possibility that African women may have some inherent predisposition for developing more biologically aggressive breast tumors [43–51].

As discussed by Fregene and Newman [42], contemporary generations of African American and sub-Saharan African women are likely to have some shared ancestry as a consequence of the colonial-era slave trade posts. These sites were clustered along the southwestern coast of Africa, within present-day Ghana, Nigeria, Senegal, and Gambia. Comparisons of breast cancer in these various populations of women therefore are warranted.

Comparisons of breast cancer in women of African ancestry

Table 1 [52] summarizes patterns of breast cancer incidence and outcome for African American, white American, and native sub-Saharan African women. Indeed, frequencies of larger tumors, high-grade cancer, estrogen receptor–negative cancer, and early-onset disease are highest for African women, intermediate for African American women, and lowest for white American women. Ikpatt and colleagues [49] conducted one particularly impressive clinicopathologic analysis of 148 Nigerian patients who had breast cancer and reported the following features: 67% of cases were premenopausal; mean age was 44 years; mean tumor size was 4.2 cm; 78% of cases were grade 2 or 3; only 23% were estrogen receptor–positive; and *Her2/neu* overexpression was observed in 19%.

It is therefore worthy of speculation that some genotypic variant(s), perhaps related to estrogen metabolism and/or the estrogen receptor pathway and associated with African ancestry, might exert some oncogenic effects on mammary tissue that result in a lower lifetime risk for endocrine-sensitive breast cancer while increasing the risk for endocrine-resistant, early-onset disease. These patterns might be most apparent in native sub-Saharan African populations, but 4 centuries of genetic admixture might result in an intermediate expression of this pattern of disease among African Americans.

Table 1
Summary of breast cancer epidemiology in sub-Saharan African, African American, and white American women

Feature	African	African American	White American
Incidence (per 100,000)	30	119	141
Mortality (per 100,000)	18	35	26
Mortality: incidence ratio	1:2	1:3	1:5
Median age (in years)	45	57	62
Percentage with high-grade tumors	> 50	43	32
Percentage with stage III/IV disease	75	19	11
Percentage with estrogen receptor–negative disease	75	40	22

Data from refs. [39,49,52].

Estrogen receptor, genetic association studies, and breast cancer risk

The complex mechanisms associated with estrogen, the estrogen receptor genes (*ESR1* and *ESR2*), and expression of the estrogen receptor proteins (ERα and ERβ) have been summarized by Hall and colleagues [53], Sand and colleagues [54], and others. The steroid hormone 17β estradiol (E_2) regulates tissue function in several organ systems, including the breast, cardiovascular, reproductive, and skeletal systems. These tissue effects are mediated by the interactions of E_2 with the nuclear receptors ERα and ERβ. Although the understanding of ER signaling remains incomplete, more is known about ERα than ERβ, and it has been postulated that the ratio of these two proteins determines overall estrogenic effects on tissues that express both receptors [55]. In general, however, ER activation and signaling occur through several different pathways: (1) classical ligand-dependent, (2) ligand-independent, (3) DNA binding-independent, and (4) cell-surface (nongenomic) signaling. Studies of variants in the genes that code for ERα and ERβ are motivated by the assumption that these variants can result in alterations of any of these signaling pathways. These altered mechanisms might result in modified risk for breast, cardiovascular, and/or bone disease. These diseases are all notable for the significant differences observed in their impact on African American and white American populations.

Single-nucleotide polymorphisms (SNPs) and haplotypes for these receptors have been associated with the risk of developing and surviving all of these diseases. Furthermore, limited evidence suggests an association between particular haplotypes and specific ethnicity-stratified populations [56]. Variants in *ESR1* that have been studied most extensively include

1. c.454-397 T>C (also known as IVS1-397 T/C; rs2234693; and PvuII restriction site) located on intron 1
2. c.454-351 A>G (also known as IVS1-351 A/G; rs9340799; and XbaI restriction site) located on intron 1
3. c.975 C>G
4. GT repeat polymorphism 2.8 kb 5' to exon 1D
5. c.478 G>T on exon 2
6. c.729 C>T on exon 3
7. c.908 A>G on exon 4
8. c.926 C>T on exon 4
9. c.933 G>A on exon 4

The methodology for statistical evaluation of genotyping studies continues to evolve. Genotyping error can be minimized by performing an initial data check establishing that the frequencies of individual alleles conform to Hardy-Weinberg equilibrium. Statistical analysis is somewhat more straightforward in studies of single SNPs than in studies of multiple-loci variants and haplotypes. Statistical tests are available that provide estimates of linkage disequilibrium between SNPs; if multiple SNPs seem to be closely linked in chromosomal location, then one SNP can be selected for correlation with the disease state. Analyses of the SNPs as homozygous versus heterozygous variants (versus absence of the SNP) can be incorporated into logistic regression analyses that adjust for other risk factors for breast cancer, yielding odds ratios as the measure of association. These analyses frequently are reported as the odds ratio for disease among patients who have 0, 1, or 2 copies of the SNP; alternatively the analysis may show the odds ratio of disease among patients who have no copies of the SNP versus those who have at least one copy.

When multiple loci or haplotypes are studied, additional uncertainty and potential bias is introduced into the point estimation (statistical association) process by cases that are heterozygous at multiple sites. These cases have ambiguous haplotypes (phase), and individual-level haplotypes must be estimated by assignments made on the basis of the most commonly observed patterns in the group. The likelihood of introducing bias with this method is minimized when the alleles within the haplotype are located close together, indicating a lesser risk for recombination between the allelic loci. Tests of linkage disequilibrium can guide this assessment. Sensitivity analyses also can be conducted in which alternative haplotype assignments are made and the odds ratios are computed. One then can see directly how much of difference results from the different haplotype assignments for the ambiguous cases.

A potentially powerful research program would involve comparing genotyping studies in African populations with studies in African American and other populations. The Human Genome Project has ushered in a new era that will permit studies of population stratification in a way that can improve the understanding of cancer risk. Such studies, however, must be performed with appropriate scientific and statistical rigor and with appropriate attention to patient education, culture, and ethics. These principles are emphasized accordingly by the Human Genome Project program on Ethical, Legal and Social issues (ELSI) [57], which represents the world's largest bioethics program. ELSI emphasizes that, because 99.9% of the DNA between any two individuals is identical, genetically distinct "races" cannot be distinguished. The variation that does exist between populations can influence risk from many diseases, however, including diabetes, hypertension, and cancer. Therefore continued research is warranted. Association studies involving the hormone receptors and other proteins involved in their pathways are promising targets as explanations are sought for the unique pattern of disease that is prevalent among patients of African ancestry who have breast cancer.

Genotyping data for the estrogen receptor and other molecules involved in the estrogen receptor pathway are now emerging, and interesting associations with the risk of breast cancer are becoming apparent. As shown in Tables 2 and 3, however, few of the genotyping studies conducted thus far have included significant numbers of women of African ancestry. Some notable exceptions include the CBCS; the Multiethnic Cohort; and the Breast and Prostate Cancer Cohort Consortium (BPC3). These three case-control datasets were established as large programs addressing previously understudied minority ethnicity populations.

The Multiethnic Cohort Study was created in 1993, based in Hawaii and California. A nested breast cancer case-control study was derived from this cohort in 1995 and includes samples of women from five major ethnic/racial groups: white American, African American, Japanese, Latino, and Native Hawaiian [58]. This cohort has been used to evaluate SNPs in several genes involved in the estradiol/estrone pathway. The overall frequencies of these variants differed between ethnic subsets, and the investigators reported an inverse association between *CYP1A2*1F* and risk for hormone receptor–negative breast cancer [58]. The CBCS is a population-based, case-control study of breast cancer conducted in 24 counties of central and eastern North Carolina. This group, in conjunction with investigators at Vanderbilt University, identified a polymorphism in mitochondrial DNA (mtDNA10398A) that was associated with breast cancer risk in African American women [59]. The largest multiethnic breast cancer association study group is the BPC3 [60], which includes case-control participants from the Nurses Health Study, the American Cancer Society Cancer Prevention Study, the European Prospective Investigation into Cancer and Nutrition, and the Multiethnic Cohort. This group studied the *HSD17B1* gene, which encodes 17β-hydroxysteroid dehydrogenase1, the protein that catalyzes the conversion of estrone to the more biologically active hormone estradiol. Again, interethnic variation in frequency of alleles was observed, and a variant of *HSD17B1* was associated with risk of estrogen receptor–negative disease [60]. Gold and colleagues [56] identified haplotypes in *ESR1* and *ESR2* that were associated with risk of breast cancer.

As noted in Tables 2 and 3 [61–82], several ethnicity-related variations in genotype patterns and genotype-associated cancer risk have indeed been identified, confirming the value of continued study. Data on the estrogen receptor genotypes in African Americans are notably lacking. Furthermore, although numerous genotyping association studies have involved international populations, none have included evaluations of the risk of breast cancer in African populations.

Summary

Genetic association studies will become increasingly prominent in the risk assessment of breast cancer. This technology may provide useful clues to explain disparities in breast cancer epidemiology and outcome in women of African versus European ancestry. Creation of datasets that will be informative regarding genotypes and breast tumor phenotypes among African, African American, and white American women therefore is necessary.

Table 2
Selected studies of estrogen receptor genotyping and breast cancer risk

Study	Type	Polymorphism	Study size Overall (Nationality)	African Americans	Findings
Zuppan [61], 1991	Linkage analysis	c.454-351 A>G	11 Families (American)	None	Linkage in one family
Hill [62], 1989	Case control (tumor and normal tissue samples)	c.454-397 C>T	188 Tumors; 53 reference samples	NR	C allele associated with risk of ER-negative disease
Parl [63], 1989	Case only	c.454-397 C>T c.454-351 A>G	59 (American)	3	Younger age for cases with TT genotype
Yaich [64], 1992	Case only	c.454-397 C>T	257 (American)	NR	Younger age for cases with TT genotype
Andersen [65], 1994	Case control	c.454-397 C>T c.454-351 A>G	360/672 (Norwegian)	None	Increased risk associated with c.454-351 A>G G allele
Roodi [66], 1995	Case only	c. 975 C>G c.729 C>T	188 (American)	NR	c. 975 C>G: G associated with family history of breast cancer
Iwase [67], 1996	Case only	c. 975 C>G	57/30 (British)	None	c. 975 C>G: G associated with increased risk of breast cancer
Southey [68,69], 1998	Case control	c. 975 C>G	388/294 (Australian)	None	c. 975 C>G: GG versus CC associated with increased risk of early-onset breast cancer

Study	Design	Polymorphism	Sample (population)		Findings
Schubert [70], 1999	Case control	c. 975 C>G c.729 C>T	105/151 (American)	Yes	c. 975 C>G: no association with familial breast cancer
Curran [71], 2001	Cross-sectional, association	c. 975 C>G	125/125 (Australian)	None	c. 975 C>G: trend for allele C associated with breast cancer risk
Vasconcelos [72], 2002	Case control	c. 975 C>G	70/69 (Portuguese)	None	c. 975 C>G: G or GG associated with increased breast cancer risk
Kang [73], 2002	Case control	c. 975 C>G	110/45 (Korean)	None	c. 975 C>G: trend for G allele associated with ER-positive/PR-positive tumors
Comings [74], 2003	Case control	c.454-351 A>G	67/145 (American)	Yes	No association
Shin [75], 2003	Case control	c.454-397 C>T c.454-351 A>G	205/205 (Korean)	None	c.454-351 A>G: A allele associated with decreased risk of breast cancer
Cai [76], 2003	Case control	c.454-397 C>T c.454-351 A>G	1069/1166 (Shanghai Chinese)	None	c.454-397 C>T: TC and CC genotypes associated with increased risk of breast cancer
Kang [73], 2002	Case control	478 G>T 908 A>G 926 C>T 933 G>A 975 G>C +15 G>A	110/45 (Korean)	None	975 G>C associated with PR/ER expression

(continued on next page)

Table 2 (*continued*)

Study	Type	Polymorphism	Study size Overall (Nationality)	African Americans	Findings
Han [77], 2003	Case control	Whole *ESR1* gene sequencing	100/100 (Korean)	None	975 G>C: GG and 1782 G>A: AA associated with decreased risk of breast cancer
Cai [78], 2003	Case control	GTn (promoter region)	947/993 (Shanghai Chinese)	None	GT17 or GT18 allele carriers had reduced risk of breast cancer than did GT16 homozygotes
Wedren [79], 2004	Case control	Tan (exon 1) c.454-397 C>T c.454-351 A>G c.729 C>T c.975 C>G	Approx 1500/1500 (Swedish)	None	No association with SNPs; haplotype c.454-351 A>G or c.454-397 C>T and c975 C>G associated with increased risk of breast cancer, especially in high women with high body mass indices
Boyapati [80], 2005	Case only	Pvu II Xba I GTn	1069 (Shanghai Chinese)	None	PvuII PP versus pp associated with increased mortality in women who had ER-negative tumors

Gold [56], 2004	Case control	SNPs selected through Celera data-mining and limited resequencing ESR1 ESR2 PGR	1011/615	92/57 AA	Three *ESR1* haplotypes associated with decreased risk of breast cancer. One *ESR1* haplotype associated with increased risk. No associations identified for **PR** variants; some *ESR1* and *ESR2* haplotypes uniquely associated with risk in Ashkenazi women
Yu [81], 2006	Case control	rs2228480	468/470	None	Strongest ER SNP effect in presence of clinical risk factors

Abbreviations: AA, African American; ER, estrogen receptor; NR, not reported; PR, progesterone receptor; SNP, single-nucleotide polymorphism.

Table 3
Selected studies of other genotypes possibly associated with risk of breast cancer

Study	Type	Genes evaluated	Study size Overall (Nationality)	African Americans	Findings
LeMarchand [58], 2005	Case control (multiethnic cohort study)	Genes involved with estrogen metabolism: CYP SULT AHR	1339/1370	259/389	Inverse association between CYP1A2*1F and risk of breast cancer
Yu [81], 2006	Case control	Genes involved with estrogen receptor pathway: MTA3 Snail E-cadherin MTA1	468/470 (Chinese)	None	Strongest genotype SNP effect in presence of clinical risk factors
Millikan [82], 2005	Case control (CBCS)	Genes involved with DNA repair: XRCC3 NBS1 RXCC2 BRCH2	894/788 (American)	Yes (335/332)	Increased risk of breast cancer seen in patients who have multiple variants and history of increased volume ionizing radiation
Feigelson [60], 2006	Case control (BPC3)	Estradiol biosynthesis gene: HSD17B1	5370/7480 (American; European)	Yes (340/435)[a]	HSD17B1 associated with risk of ER-negative breast cancer

Abbreviations: BPC3, Breast and Prostate Cancer Cohort Consortium; CBCS, Carolina Breast Cancer Study; ER, estrogen receptor; SNP, single-nucleotide polymorphism.

[a] Estimate based upon data provided in Feigelson HS, et al. Haplotype analysis of the *HSD17B1* gene and risk of breast cancer: a comprehensive approach to multicenter analyses of prospective cohort studies. Cancer Res 2006;66(4):2468–75.

References

[1] Ries L, Eisner M, Kosary C, et al. SEER cancer statistics review, 1975–2002. Vol 2006: NCI; 2005.

[2] Newman LA. Breast cancer in African–American women. Oncologist 2005;10(1):1–14.

[3] Elledge RM, Clark GM, Chamness GC, et al. Tumor biologic factors and breast cancer prognosis among white, Hispanic, and black women in the United States. J Natl Cancer Inst 1994;86(9):705–12.

[4] Eley JW, Hill HA, Chen VW, et al. Racial differences in survival from breast cancer. Results of the National Cancer Institute Black/White Cancer Survival Study. JAMA 1994;272(12): 947–54.

[5] Ward E, Jemal A, Cokkinides V, et al. Cancer disparities by race/ethnicity and socioeconomic status. CA Cancer J Clin 2004;54(2):78–93.

[6] US Census Bureau. Current population survey, 2002 to 2004. Annual Social and Economic Supplements. 2004.

[7] Newman LA, Griffith KA, Jatoi I, et al. Meta-analysis of survival in African American and white American patients with breast cancer: ethnicity compared with socioeconomic status. J Clin Oncol 2006;24(9):1342–9.

[8] Tammemagi CM, Nerenz D, Neslund-Dudas C, et al. Comorbidity and survival disparities among black and white patients with breast cancer. JAMA 2005;294(14):1765–72.

[9] Field TS, Buist DS, Doubeni C, et al. Disparities and survival among breast cancer patients. J Natl Cancer Inst Monographs 2005;35:88–95.

[10] Anderson WF, Chatterjee N, Ershler WB, et al. Estrogen receptor breast cancer phenotypes in the Surveillance, Epidemiology, and End Results database. Breast Cancer Res Treat 2002; 76(1):27–36.

[11] Key T, Appleby P, Barnes I, et al. Endogenous sex hormones and breast cancer in postmenopausal women: reanalysis of nine prospective studies. J Natl Cancer Inst 2002;94(8): 606–16.

[12] Missmer SA, Eliassen AH, Barbieri RL, et al. Endogenous estrogen, androgen, and progesterone concentrations and breast cancer risk among postmenopausal women. J Natl Cancer Inst 2004;96(24):1856–65.

[13] Cummings SR, Lee JS, Lui LY, et al. Sex hormones, risk factors, and risk of estrogen receptor-positive breast cancer in older women: a long-term prospective study. Cancer Epidemiol Biomarkers Prev 2005;14(5):1047–51.

[14] Nelson DA, Pettifor JM, Barondess DA, et al. Comparison of cross-sectional geometry of the proximal femur in white and black women from Detroit and Johannesburg. J Bone Miner Res 2004;19(4):560–5.

[15] Cauley JA, Lui LY, Ensrud KE, et al. Bone mineral density and the risk of incident nonspinal fractures in black and white women. JAMA 2005;293(17):2102–8.

[16] Kleerekoper M, Nelson DA, Peterson EL, et al. Reference data for bone mass, calciotropic hormones, and biochemical markers of bone remodeling in older (55–75) postmenopausal white and black women. J Bone Miner Res 1994;9(8):1267–76.

[17] Allison DB, Edlen-Nezin L, Clay-Williams G. Obesity among African American women: prevalence, consequences, causes, and developing research. Women Health 1997;3: 243–74.

[18] Moorman PG, Jones BA, Millikan RC, et al. Race, anthropometric factors, and stage at diagnosis of breast cancer. Am J Epidemiol 2001;153(3):284–91.

[19] Masi CM, Olopade OI. Racial and ethnic disparities in breast cancer: a multilevel perspective. Med Clin North Am 2005;89(4):753–70.

[20] Pinheiro SP, Holmes MD, Pollak MN, et al. Racial differences in premenopausal endogenous hormones. Cancer Epidemiol Biomarkers Prev 2005;14(9):2147–53.

[21] Robson ME, Boyd J, Borgen PI, et al. Hereditary breast cancer. Curr Probl Surg 2001;38(6): 387–480.

[22] Newman LA, Kuerer HM, Hunt KK, et al. Educational review: role of the surgeon in hereditary breast cancer. Ann Surg Oncol 2001;8(4):368–78.

[23] Thull DL, Vogel VG. Recognition and management of hereditary breast cancer syndromes. Oncologist 2004;9(1):13–24.

[24] Hall M, Olopade OI. Confronting genetic testing disparities: knowledge is power. JAMA 2005;293(14):1783–5.

[25] Thompson HS, Valdimarsdottir HB, Duteau-Buck C, et al. Psychosocial predictors of BRCA counseling and testing decisions among urban African-American women. Cancer Epidemiol Biomarkers Prev 2002;11(12):1579–85.

[26] Lee R, Beattie M, Crawford B, et al. Recruitment, genetic counseling, and BRCA testing for underserved women at a public hospital. Genet Test 2005;9(4):306–12.

[27] Nanda R, Schumm LP, Cummings S, et al. Genetic testing in an ethnically diverse cohort of high-risk women: a comparative analysis of BRCA1 and BRCA2 mutations in American families of European and African ancestry. JAMA 2005;294(15):1925–33.

[28] Olopade O, Fackenthal J, Dunston G, et al. Breast cancer genetics in African Americans. Cancer 2002;97(1 Suppl):236–45.

[29] Gao Q, Neuhausen S, Cummings S, et al. Recurrent germ-line BRCA1 mutations in extended African American families with early-onset breast cancer. Am J Hum Genet 1997; 60(5):1233–6.

[30] Gao Q, Tomlinson G, Das S, et al. Prevalence of BRCA1 and BRCA2 mutations among clinic-based African American families with breast cancer. Hum Genet 2000;107(2): 186–91.

[31] Matthews A, Cummings S, Thompson S, et al. Genetic testing of African Americans for susceptibility to inherited cancers: Use of focus groups to determine factors contributing to participation. J Psychosoc Oncol 2000;18:1–19.

[32] Antoniou AC, Pharoah PD, McMullan G, et al. Evidence for further breast cancer susceptibility genes in addition to BRCA1 and BRCA2 in a population-based study. Genet Epidemiol 2001;21(1):1–18.

[33] Gilliland FD. Ethnic differences in cancer incidence: a marker for inherited susceptibility? Environ Health Perspect 1997;105(Suppl 4):897–900.

[34] Pathak DR, Osuch JR, He J. Breast carcinoma etiology: current knowledge and new insights into the effects of reproductive and hormonal risk factors in black and white populations. Cancer 2000;88(5 Suppl):1230–8.

[35] Palmer JR, Wise LA, Horton NJ, et al. Dual effect of parity on breast cancer risk in African-American women. J Natl Cancer Inst 2003;95(6):478–83.

[36] Ursin G, Bernstein L, Wang Y, et al. Reproductive factors and risk of breast carcinoma in a study of white and African-American women. Cancer 2004;101(2):353–62.

[37] Carey LA, Perou CM, Livasy CA, et al. Race, breast cancer subtypes, and survival in the Carolina Breast Cancer Study. JAMA 2006;295(21):2492–502.

[38] World Health Organization. The World Health Report 2006—working together for health. Available at: http://www.who.int/whr/2006/en/index.html. Accessed April 11, 2006.

[39] Ferlay J, Bray F, Pisani P, et al. Globocan 2002: cancer incidence, mortality and prevalence worldwide. IARC CancerBase No. 5 version 2.0. Lyon (France): IARC Press; 2004.

[40] Anyanwu SN. Breast cancer in eastern Nigeria: a ten year review. West Afr J Med 2000;19(2): 120–5.

[41] Muguti GI. Experience with breast cancer in Zimbabwe. J R Coll Surg Edinb 1993;38(2): 75–8.

[42] Fregene A, Newman LA. Breast cancer in sub-Saharan Africa: how does it relate to breast cancer in African-American women? Cancer 2005;103(8):1540–50.

[43] Hassan I, Onukak EE, Mabogunje OA. Breast cancer in Zaria, Nigeria. J R Coll Surg Edinb 1992;37(3):159–61.

[44] Adebamowo CA, Adekunle OO. Case-controlled study of the epidemiological risk factors for breast cancer in Nigeria. Br J Surg 1999;86(5):665–8.

[45] Adebamowo CA, Ogundiran TO, Adenipekun AA, et al. Obesity and height in urban Nigerian women with breast cancer. Ann Epidemiol 2003;13(6):455–61.

[46] Ademuyiwa FO, Neuhausen S, Adebamowo CA, et al. Early onset breast cancer in black women of African ancestry: Genetic or environmental influence? [abstract no. 3225]. Presented at the American Association for Cancer Research. Anaheim, CA; May, 2005.

[47] Amir H, Makwaya CK, Aziz MR, et al. Breast cancer and risk factors in an African population: a case referent study. East Afr Med J 1998;75(5):268–70.

[48] Ijuin H, Douchi T, Oki T, et al. The contribution of menopause to changes in body-fat distribution. J Obstet Gynaecol Res 1999;25(5):367–72.

[49] Ikpatt O, Xu J, Kramtsov A, et al. Hormone receptor negative and basal-like subtypes are overrepresented in invasive breast carcinoma from women of African ancestry [abstract no. 2550]. American Association for Cancer Research; May, 2005.

[50] Ikpatt OF, Kuopio T, Collan Y. Proliferation in African breast cancer: biology and prognostication in Nigerian breast cancer material. Mod Pathol 2002;15(8):783–9.

[51] Ikpatt OF, Kuopio T, Ndoma-Egba R, et al. Breast cancer in Nigeria and Finland: epidemiological, clinical and histological comparison. Anticancer Res 2002;22(5):3005–12.

[52] Li CI, Malone KE, Daling JR. Differences in breast cancer stage, treatment, and survival by race and ethnicity. Arch Intern Med 2003;163(1):49–56.

[53] Hall JM, Couse JF, Korach KS. The multifaceted mechanisms of estradiol and estrogen receptor signaling. J Biol Chem 2001;276(40):36869–72.

[54] Sand P, Luckhaus C, Schlurmann K, et al. Untangling the human estrogen receptor gene structure. J Neural Transm 2002;109(5–6):567–83.

[55] Hall JM, McDonnell DP. The estrogen receptor beta-isoform (ERbeta) of the human estrogen receptor modulates ERalpha transcriptional activity and is a key regulator of the cellular response to estrogens and antiestrogens. Endocrinology 1999;140(12):5566–78.

[56] Gold B, Kalush F, Bergeron J, et al. Estrogen receptor genotypes and haplotypes associated with breast cancer risk. Cancer Res 2004;64(24):8891–900.

[57] Hill AD, Mann GB, Borgen PI, et al. Sentinel lymphatic mapping in breast cancer. J Am Coll Surg 1999;188(5):545–9.

[58] Le Marchand L, Donlon T, Kolonel LN, et al. Estrogen metabolism-related genes and breast cancer risk: the multiethnic cohort study. Cancer Epidemiol Biomarkers Prev 2005;14(8): 1998–2003.

[59] Canter JA, Kallianpur AR, Parl FF, et al. Mitochondrial DNA G10398A polymorphism and invasive breast cancer in African-American women. Cancer Res 2005;65(17): 8028–33.

[60] Feigelson HS, Cox DG, Cann HM, et al. Haplotype analysis of the HSD17B1 gene and risk of breast cancer: a comprehensive approach to multicenter analyses of prospective cohort studies. Cancer Res 2006;66(4):2468–75.

[61] Zuppan P, Hall JM, Lee MK, et al. Possible linkage of the estrogen receptor gene to breast cancer in a family with late-onset disease. Am J Hum Genet 1991;48(6):1065–8.

[62] Hill SM, Fuqua SA, Chamness GC, et al. Estrogen receptor expression in human breast cancer associated with an estrogen receptor gene restriction fragment length polymorphism. Cancer Res 1989;49(1):145–8.

[63] Parl FF, Cavener DR, Dupont WD. Genomic DNA analysis of the estrogen receptor gene in breast cancer. Breast Cancer Res Treat 1989;14(1):57–64.

[64] Yaich L, Dupont WD, Cavener DR, et al. Analysis of the PvuII restriction fragment-length polymorphism and exon structure of the estrogen receptor gene in breast cancer and peripheral blood. Cancer Res 1992;52:77–83.

[65] Andersen TI, Heimdal KR, Skrede M, et al. Oestrogen receptor (ESR) polymorphisms and breast cancer susceptibility. Hum Genet 1994;94(6):665–70.

[66] Roodi N, Bailey LR, Kao WY, et al. Estrogen receptor gene analysis in estrogen receptor-positive and receptor-negative primary breast cancer. J Natl Cancer Inst 1995;87(6): 446–51.

[67] Iwase H, Greenman JM, Barnes DM, et al. Sequence variants of the estrogen receptor (ER) gene found in breast cancer patients with ER negative and progesterone receptor positive tumors. Cancer Lett 1996;108(2):179–84.

[68] Southey MC, Batten L, Andersen CR, et al. CFTR deltaF508 carrier status, risk of breast cancer before the age of 40 and histological grading in a population-based case-control study. Int J Cancer 1998;79(5):487–9.

[69] Southey MC, Batten LE, McCredie MR, et al. Estrogen receptor polymorphism at codon 325 and risk of breast cancer in women before age forty. J Natl Cancer Inst 1998;90(7):532–6.

[70] Schubert EL, Lee MK, Newman B, et al. Single nucleotide polymorphisms (SNPs) in the estrogen receptor gene and breast cancer susceptibility. J Steroid Biochem Mol Biol 1999; 71(1–2):21–7.

[71] Curran JE, Lea RA, Rutherford S, et al. Association of estrogen receptor and glucocorticoid receptor gene polymorphisms with sporadic breast cancer. Int J Cancer 2001;95(4):271–5.

[72] Vasconcelos A, Medeiros R, Veiga I, et al. Analysis of estrogen receptor polymorphism in codon 325 by PCR-SSCP in breast cancer: association with lymph node metastasis. Breast J 2002;8(4):226–9.

[73] Kang HJ, Kim SW, Kim HJ, et al. Polymorphisms in the estrogen receptor-alpha gene and breast cancer risk. Cancer Lett 2002;178(2):175–80.

[74] Comings DE, Gade-Andavolu R, Cone LA, et al. A multigene test for the risk of sporadic breast carcinoma. Cancer 2003;97(9):2160–70.

[75] Shin A, Kang D, Nishio H, et al. Estrogen receptor alpha gene polymorphisms and breast cancer risk. Breast Cancer Res Treat 2003;80(1):127–31.

[76] Cai Q, Shu XO, Jin F, et al. Genetic polymorphisms in the estrogen receptor alpha gene and risk of breast cancer: results from the Shanghai Breast Cancer Study. Cancer Epidemiol Biomarkers Prev 2003;12(9):853–9.

[77] Han W, Kang D, Lee KM, et al. Full sequencing analysis of estrogen receptor-alpha gene polymorphism and its association with breast cancer risk. Anticancer Res 2003;23(6C): 4703–7.

[78] Cai Q, Gao YT, Wen W, et al. Association of breast cancer risk with a GT dinucleotide repeat polymorphism upstream of the estrogen receptor-alpha gene. Cancer Res 2003;63(18): 5727–30.

[79] Wedren S, Lovmar L, Humphreys K, et al. Oestrogen receptor alpha gene haplotype and postmenopausal breast cancer risk: a case control study. Breast Cancer Res 2004;6(4): R437–49.

[80] Boyapati SM, Shu XO, Ruan ZX, et al. Polymorphisms in ER-alpha gene interact with estrogen receptor status in breast cancer survival. Clin Cancer Res 2005;11(3):1093–8.

[81] Yu JC, Chen ST, Hsu GC, et al. Breast cancer risk associated with genotypic polymorphism of the genes involved in the estrogen-receptor-signaling pathway: a multigenic study on cancer susceptibility. J Biomed Sci 2006;13:419–32.

[82] Millikan RC, Player JS, Decotret AR, et al. Polymorphisms in DNA repair genes, medical exposure to ionizing radiation, and breast cancer risk. Cancer Epidemiol Biomarkers Prev 2005;14(10):2326–34.

ELSEVIER
SAUNDERS

Surg Clin N Am 87 (2007) 569–574

SURGICAL
CLINICS OF
NORTH AMERICA

Index

Note: Page numbers of article titles are in **boldface** type.

Moving?

Make sure your subscription moves with you!

To notify us of your new address, find your **Clinics Account Number** (located on your mailing label above your name), and contact customer service at:

E-mail: elspcs@elsevier.com

800-654-2452 (subscribers in the U.S. & Canada)
407-345-4000 (subscribers outside of the U.S. & Canada)

Fax number: 407-363-9661

Elsevier Periodicals Customer Service
6277 Sea Harbor Drive
Orlando, FL 32887-4800

*To ensure uninterrupted delivery of your subscription, please notify us at least 4 weeks in advance of move.

ELSEVIER